T0414435

CLINICAL NUTRITION

The Interface Between Metabolism,
Diet, and Disease

CLINICAL NUTRITION

The Interface Between Metabolism,
Diet, and Disease

Edited by
Leah Coles, PhD

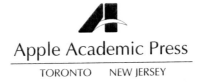

Apple Academic Press

TORONTO   NEW JERSEY

Apple Academic Press Inc. | Apple Academic Press Inc.
3333 Mistwell Crescent | 9 Spinnaker Way
Oakville, ON L6L 0A2 | Waretown, NJ 08758
Canada | USA

©2014 by Apple Academic Press, Inc.
Exclusive worldwide distribution by CRC Press, a member of Taylor & Francis Group

No claim to original U.S. Government works
Printed in the United States of America on acid-free paper

International Standard Book Number-13: 978-1-926895-97-0 (Hardcover)

Library of Congress Control Number: 2013950919

Library and Archives Canada Cataloguing in Publication

Clinical nutrition: the interface between metabolism, diet, and disease/ edited by Leah Coles, PhD.

Includes bibliographical references and index.
ISBN 978-1-926895-97-0
1. Diet therapy. I. Coles, Leah, editor of compilation

| RM258.C65 2013 | 615.8'54 | a | C2013-906624-1 |

Apple Academic Press also publishes its books in a variety of electronic formats. Some content that appears in print may not be available in electronic format. For information about Apple Academic Press products, visit our website at **www.appleacademicpress.com** and the CRC Press website at **www.crcpress.com**

ABOUT THE EDITOR

LEAH COLES, PhD

Leah Coles, PhD, completed her PhD in Human Nutrition at the Riddet Institute, Massey University, New Zealand. She is presently a Research Fellow in the Nutritional Interventions Lab at Baker IDI Heart and Diabetes Institute, Melbourne, Australia. Her current research involves clinical trials focused on functional foods and weight loss, particularly in relation to diabetes and cardiovascular disease. She has also published several peer-reviewed articles in the area of *in vitro* and *in vivo* (animal and human) digestibility studies and linked these with mathematical models to predict the available energy (ATP) content of foods.

CONTENTS

Acknowledgment and How to Cite .... *xi*

List of Contributors .... *xiii*

Introduction .... *xxi*

Part I: Micronutrient Supplementation

1. **A 12-Week Double-Blind Randomized Clinical Trial of Vitamin D3 Supplementation on Body Fat Mass in Healthy Overweight and Obese Women** 1

   Amin Salehpour, Farhad Hosseinpanah, Farzad Shidfar, Mohammadreza Vafa, Maryam Razaghi, Sahar Dehghani, Anahita Hoshiarrad, and Mahmoodreza Gohari

2. **Postprandial Effects of Calcium Phosphate Supplementation on Plasma Concentration-Double-Blind, Placebo-Controlled Cross-Over Human Study** 19

   Ulrike Trautvetter, Michael Kiehntopf, and Gerhard Jahreis

3. **Efficacy of Vitamin C as an Adjunct to Fluoxetine Therapy in Pediatric Major Depressive Disorder: A Randomized, Double-Blind, Placebo-Controlled Pilot Study** 33

   Mostafa Amr, Ahmed El-Mogy, Tarek Shams, Karen Vieira, and Shaheen E. Lakhan

Part II: Role of Clinical Nutrition in Preventing and Managing Organ Disease

4. **Nutrition Therapy for Liver Diseases Based on the Status of Nutritional Intake** 53

   Kenichiro Yasutake, Motoyuki Kohjima, Manabu Nakashima, Kazuhiro Kotoh, Makoto Nakamuta, and Munechika Enjoji

5. **Role of Nutrition in the Management of Hepatic Encephalopathy in End-Stage Liver Failure** 73

   Chantal Bémeur, Paul Desjardins, and Roger F. Butterworth

6. **Parenteral Nutrition Combined with Enteral Nutrition for Severe Acute Pancreatitis** 103

   Akanand Singh, Ming Chen, Tao Li, Xiao-Li Yang, Jin-Zheng Li, and Jian-Ping Gong

7. **Dietary Protein Intake and Renal Function** 121

William F. Martin, Lawrence E. Armstrong, and Nancy R. Rodriguez

8. **Phosphorus and Nutrition in Chronic Kidney Disease** 141

Emilio González-Parra, Carolina Gracia-Iguacel, Jesús Egido, and Alberto Ortiz

Part III: Dietary Treatments for Obesity and Type 2 Diabetes

9. **Ketogenic Enteral Nutrition as a Treatment for Obesity: Short Term and Long Term Results from 19,000 Patients** 157

Gianfranco Cappello, Antonella Franceschelli, Annalisa Cappello, and Paolo De Luca

10. **Nutrition Support to Patients Undergoing Gastrointestinal Surgery** 175

Nicola Ward

11. **Micronutrient Deficiency in Obese Subjects Undergoing Low Calorie Diet** 185

Antje Damms-Machado, Gesine Weser, and Stephan C. Bischoff

12. **Diabetes-Specific Nutrition Algorithm: A Transcultural Program to Optimize Diabetes and Prediabetes Care** 209

Jeffrey I. Mechanick, Albert E. Marchetti, Caroline Apovian,
Alexander Koglin Benchimol, Peter H. Bisschop, Alexis Bolio-Galvis,
Refaat A. Hegazi, David Jenkins, Enrique Mendoza, Miguel Leon Sanz,
Wayne Huey-Herng Sheu, Patrizio Tatti, Man-Wo Tsang, and Osama Hamdy

13. **Effect of Fruit Restriction on Glycemic Control in Patients with Type 2 Diabetes: A Randomized Trial** 241

Allan S. Christensen, Lone Viggers, Kjeld Hasselström, and Søren Gregersen

14. **Is There a Role for Carbohydrate Restriction in the Treatment and Prevention of Cancer?** 255

Rainer J. Klement and Ulrike Kämmerer

Part IV: Recent Developments and Future Trends in Clinical Nutrition

15. **Parenteral Nutrition Additive Shortages: The Short-Term, Long-Term and Potential Epigenetic Implications in Premature and Hospitalized Infants** 295

Corrine Hanson, Melissa Thoene, Julie Wagner, Dean Collier, Kassandra Lecci, and Ann Anderson-Berry

16. **An Observational Study Reveals that Neonatal Vitamin D Is Primarily Determined by Maternal Contributions: Implications of a New Assay on the Roles of Vitamin D Forms** 313

Spyridon N. Karras, Iltaf Shah, Andrea Petroczi, Dimitrios G. Goulis, Helen Bili, Fotini Papadopoulou, Vikentia Harizopoulou, Basil C. Tarlatzis, and Declan P. Naughton

17. **Weight Science: Evaluating the Evidence for a Paradigm Shift** 333

Linda Bacon and Lucy Aphramor

18. **Gauging Food and Nutritional Care Quality in Hospitals** 365

Rosa Wanda Diez-Garcia, Anete Araújo de Sousa, Rossana Pacheco da Costa Proença, Vania Aparecida Leandro-Merhi, and Edson Zangiacomi Martinez

Author Notes 391

Index 401

ACKNOWLEDGMENT AND HOW TO CITE

The chapters in this book were previously published in various places and in various formats. By bringing them together here in one place, we offer the reader a comprehensive perspective on recent investigations of clinical nutrition and diet and disease. Each chapter is added to and enriched by being placed within the context of the larger investigative landscape.

We wish to thank the authors who made their research available for this book, whether by granting their permission individually or by releasing their research as open source articles. When citing information contained within this book, please do the authors the courtesy of attributing them by name, referring back to their original articles, using the credits provided at the end of each chapter.

LIST OF CONTRIBUTORS

Mostafa Amr
Department of Psychiatry, Mansoura University, Mansoura, Egypt

Ann Anderson-Berry
College of Pediatrics, University of Nebraska Medical Center, Omaha, NE 981205, USA

Caroline Apovian
Nutrition and Weight Management Center, Boston University School of Medicine, Boston, MA USA

Lawrence E. Armstrong
Department of Kinesiology, University of Connecticut, Storrs, CT, USA

Lucy Aphramor
Coventry University, Applied Research Centre in Health and Lifestyle Interventions, Priory Street, Coventry, CV1 1FB, UK and University Hospitals Coventry and Warwickshire NHS Trust, Cardiac Rehab, Cardiology Suite, 1st Floor, East Wing, Walsgrave Hospital, Clifford Bridge Road, Coventry CV2 2DX, UK

Linda Bacon
University of California, Davis, and City College of San Francisco, Box S-80, City College of San Francisco, 50 Phelan Avenue, San Francisco, CA 94112, USA

Chantal Bémeur
Neuroscience Research Unit, CHUM, Saint-Luc Hospital, University of Montreal, 1058 St-Denis Street, Montreal, QC, Canada and Department of Nutrition, University of Montreal, Montreal, QC, Canada

Alexander Koglin Benchimol
Obesity and Eating Disorders Group, State Institute of Diabetes and Endocrinology of Rio de Janeiro, Rio de Janeiro, Brazil

Helen Bili
Unit of Reproductive Endocrinology, First Department of Obstetrics and Gynecology, Medical School, Aristotle University of Thessaloniki, Thessaloniki, Greece

Stephan C. Bischoff
Department of Nutritional Medicine, University of Hohenheim, Fruwirthstr. 12, ss70599, Stuttgart, Germany

Peter H. Bisschop
Division of Endocrinology and Metabolism, Academic Medical Center, University of Amsterdam, Amsterdam, The Netherlands

Alexis Bolio-Galvis
Department of General and Bariatric Surgery and Clinical Nutrition, Hospital Angeles Pedregal; Clinical Nutrition and General Surgery, Facultad Mexicana de Medicina, Universidad La Salle, México City, Mexico

Roger F. Butterworth
Neuroscience Research Unit, CHUM, Saint-Luc Hospital, University of Montreal, 1058 St-Denis Street, Montreal, QC, Canada

Annalisa Cappello
Clinical Nutrition Service of the Department of Surgery Paride Stefanini, University of Rome La Sapienza, Rome, Italy

Gianfranco Cappello
Clinical Nutrition Service of the Department of Surgery Paride Stefanini, University of Rome La Sapienza, Rome, Italy

Ming Chen
Department of General Surgery, People's Hospital of Tongliang County, Tongliang, Chongqing 402560, China

Allan S. Christensen
Department of Nutrition, Regional Hospital West Jutland, Jutland, Denmark

Dean Collier
College of Pharmacy, University of Nebraska Medical Center, Omaha, NE 986045, USA

Antje Damms-Machado
Department of Nutritional Medicine, University of Hohenheim, Stuttgart, Germany

Sahar Dehghani
Department of Nutrition, School of Public Health, Tehran University of Medical Sciences, Number 52, Alvand Street Arjantin Square, Tehran, Iran

Paolo De Luca
Clinical Nutrition Service of the Department of Surgery Paride Stefanini, University of Rome La Sapienza, Rome, Italy

Paul Desjardins
Neuroscience Research Unit, CHUM, Saint-Luc Hospital, University of Montreal, 1058 St-Denis Street, Montreal, QC, Canada

Anete Araújo de Sousa
Department of Nutrition, Federal University of Santa Catarina, Campus Universitário, Florianópolis, SC, 88040-900, Brazil

Rosa Wanda Diez-Garcia
Laboratory of Food Practices and Behavior – PrátiCA, Nutrition and Metabolism, Department of Internal Medicine, Faculty of Medicine of Ribeirão Preto, University of São Paulo, Av. Bandeirantes, 3900, Ribeirão Preto, SP 14049-900, Brazil

Jesús Egido
Division of Nephrology and Hipertensión, IIS-Fundación Jiménez Díaz, Autonoma University, 28040 Madrid, Spain

Ahmed El-Mogy
Department of Psychiatry, Mansoura University, Mansoura, Egypt

Munechika Enjoji
Clinical Research Center, Kyushu Medical Center, National Hospital Organization, Fukuoka 810-0065, Japan and Health Care Center and Faculty of Pharmaceutical Sciences, Fukuoka University, Fukuoka 814-0180, Japan

Antonella Franceschelli
Clinical Nutrition Service of the Department of Surgery Paride Stefanini, University of Rome La Sapienza, Rome, Italy

Mahmoodreza Gohari
Department of Biostatistics, Tehran University of Medical Sciences, Number 52, Alvand Street, Arjantin Square, Tehran, Iran

Jian-Ping Gong
Chongqing Key Laboratory of Hepatobiliary Surgery and Department of Hepatobiliary Surgery, The Second Affiliated Hospital of Chongqing Medical University, Chongqing 400010, China

Emilio González-Parra
Division of Nephrology and Hipertensión, IIS-Fundación Jiménez Díaz, Autonoma University, 28040 Madrid, Spain

Dimitrios G. Goulis
Unit of Reproductive Endocrinology, First Department of Obstetrics and Gynecology, Medical School, Aristotle University of Thessaloniki, Thessaloniki, Greece

Carolina Gracia-Iguacel
Division of Nephrology and Hipertensión, IIS-Fundación Jiménez Díaz, Autonoma University, 28040 Madrid, Spain

Søren Gregersen
Department of Endocrinology and Metabolism, Aarhus University Hospital, Aarhus, Denmark

Osama Hamdy
Division of Endocrinology, Diabetes and Metabolism, Joslin Diabetes Center, Harvard Medical School, Boston, MA USA

Corrine Hanson
School of Allied Health Professionals, University of Nebraska Medical Center, Omaha, NE 984045, USA

Vikentia Harizopoulou
Unit of Reproductive Endocrinology, First Department of Obstetrics and Gynecology, Medical School, Aristotle University of Thessaloniki, Thessaloniki, Greece

Kjeld Hasselström
Medical Department, Regional Hospital West Jutland, Jutland, Denmark

Refaat A. Hegazi
Research & Development, Abbott Nutrition, Columbus, OH USA

Anahita Hoshiarrad
National Nutrition and Food Technology Research Institute, Shahid Beheshti University of Medical Sciences, Number 42, Arghavan Street, Farahzadi Boulevard, Shahrak-e Gharb, Iran

Farhad Hosseinpanah
Obesity Research Center, Research Institute for Endocrine Sciences, Shahid Beheshti University of Medical Sciences, Floor 4th, Number 24, Parvaneh Street, Yemen Street, Chamran Exp, Tehran, Iran

Gerhard Jahreis
Department of Nutritional Physiology, Institute of Nutrition, Friedrich Schiller University of Jena, Dornburger Straße 24, Jena, D-07743, Germany

David Jenkins
Department of Nutritional Sciences, University of Toronto, Toronto, Ontario Canada

Ulrike Kämmerer
Department of Obstetrics and Gynaecology, University hospital of Würzburg, D-97080 Würzburg, Germany

Spyridon N. Karras
Unit of Reproductive Endocrinology, First Department of Obstetrics and Gynecology, Medical School, Aristotle University of Thessaloniki, Thessaloniki, Greece

Michael Kiehntopf
Institute of Clinical Chemistry and Laboratory Medicine, Jena University Hospital, Friedrich Schiller University Jena, Erlanger Allee 101, Jena, D-07747, Germany

Rainer J. Klement
Department of Radiation Oncology, University hospital of Würzburg, D-97080 Würzburg, Germany

Motoyuki Kohjima
Department of Gastroenterology, Kyushu Medical Center, National Hospital Organization, Fukuoka 810-0065, Japan

Kazuhiro Kotoh
Department of Medicine and Bioregulatory Science, Graduate School of Medical Sciences, Kyushu University, Fukuoka 812-8582, Japan

Shaheen E. Lakhan
Biosciences Department, Global Neuroscience Initiative Foundation, Los Angeles, California, USA and Neurological Institute, Cleveland Clinic, Cleveland, Ohio, USA

Vania Aparecida Leandro-Merh
Faculty of Nutrition, PUC Campinas, Av. John Boyd Dunlop, s/n., Campinas, SP, 13060-904, Brazil

Kassandra Lecci
Pharmacy and Nutrition Care Services, Nebraska Medical Center, Omaha, NE 984045, USA

Jin-Zheng Li
Chongqing Key Laboratory of Hepatobiliary Surgery and Department of Hepatobiliary Surgery, The Second Affiliated Hospital of Chongqing Medical University, Chongqing 400010, China

Tao Li
Department of General Surgery, People's Hospital of Tongliang County, Tongliang, Chongqing 402560, China

Albert E. Marchetti
Department of Preventive Medicine and Community Health, University of Medicine and Dentistry of New Jersey, Newark, NJ USA

William F. Martin
Department of Nutritional Sciences, University of Connecticut, Storrs, CT, USA

Edson Zangiacomi Martinez
Department of Social Medicine, Faculty of Medicine of Ribeirão Preto, University of São Paulo, Av. Bandeirantes, 3900, Ribeirão Preto, SP, 14049-900, Brazil

Jeffrey I. Mechanick
Division of Endocrinology, Diabetes, and Bone Disease, Mount Sinai School of Medicine, New York, NY USA

Enrique Mendoza
University of Panama School of Medicine, Panama City, Panama

Makoto Nakamuta
Clinical Research Center, Kyushu Medical Center, National Hospital Organization, Fukuoka 810-0065, Japan and Department of Gastroenterology, Kyushu Medical Center, National Hospital Organization, Fukuoka 810-0065, Japan

Manabu Nakashima
Health Care Center and Faculty of Pharmaceutical Sciences, Fukuoka University, Fukuoka 814-0180, Japan

Declan P. Naughton
School of Life Sciences, Kingston University London, London, UK

Alberto Ortiz
Division of Nephrology and Hipertensión, IIS-Fundación Jiménez Díaz, Autonoma University, 28040 Madrid, Spain

Fotini Papadopoulou
Department of Endocrinology, Diabetes and Metabolism, Panagia General Hospital, Thessaloniki, Greece

Andrea Petrocz
School of Life Sciences, Kingston University London, London, UK

Rossana Pacheco da Costa Proença
Department of Nutrition, Federal University of Santa Catarina, Campus Universitário, Florianópolis, SC, 88040-900, Brazil

Maryam Razaghi
Department of Nutrition, School of Public Health, Tehran University of Medical Sciences, Number 52, Alvand Street Arjantin Square, Tehran, Iran

Nancy R. Rodriguez
Department of Nutritional Sciences, University of Connecticut, Storrs, CT, USA

Amin Salehpour
Department of Nutrition, School of Public Health, Tehran University of Medical Sciences, Number 52, Alvand Street Arjantin Square, Tehran, Iran

Miguel Leon Sanz
Service of Endocrinology and Nutrition, University Hospital Doce de Octubre, Department of Medicine, Complutense University, Madrid, Spain

Iltaf Shah
School of Life Sciences, Kingston University London, London, UK

Tarek Shams
Department of Intensive Care, Mansoura University, Mansoura, Egypt

Wayne Huey-Herng Sheu
Division of Endocrinology and Metabolism, Taichung Veterans General Hospital, Taichung; College of Medicine, Chung-Shan Medical University, Taichung; School of Medicine, National Yang-Ming Medical University, Taipei, Taiwan

Farzad Shidfar
Department of Nutrition, School of Public Health, Tehran University of Medical Sciences, Number 52, Alvand Street Arjantin Square, Tehran, Iran

Akanand Singh
Chongqing Key Laboratory of Hepatobiliary Surgery and Department of Hepatobiliary Surgery, The Second Affiliated Hospital of Chongqing Medical University, Chongqing 400010, China

Basil C Tarlatzis
Unit of Reproductive Endocrinology, First Department of Obstetrics and Gynecology, Medical School, Aristotle University of Thessaloniki, Thessaloniki, Greece

Patrizio Tatti
Department of Endocrinology and Diabetology, ASL RMH, Rome, Italy

Melissa Thoene
Pharmacy and Nutrition Care Services, Nebraska Medical Center, Omaha, NE 984045, USA

Ulrike Trautvetter
Department of Nutritional Physiology, Institute of Nutrition, Friedrich Schiller University of Jena, Dornburger Straße 24, Jena, D-07743, Germany

Man-Wo Tsang
Division of Diabetes & Endocrinology, Department of Medicine & Geriatrics, United Christian Hospital, Hospital Authority, Hong Kong, China

Mohammadreza Vafa
Department of Nutrition, School of Public Health, Tehran University of Medical Sciences, Number 52, Alvand Street Arjantin Square, Tehran, Iran

Karen Vieira
Biosciences Department, Global Neuroscience Initiative Foundation, Los Angeles, California, USA

Lone Viggers
Department of Nutrition, Regional Hospital West Jutland, Jutland, Denmark

Julie Wagner
Alegent Health Bergan Mercy Medical Center, 7500 Mercy Road, Omaha, NE 68124, USA

Nicola Ward
Department of Pharmacy, Glenfield Hospital, University Hospitals of Leicester, NHS Trust, Leicester, UK

Gesine Weser
Department of Nutritional Medicine, University of Hohenheim, Stuttgart, Germany

Xiao-Li Yang
Chongqing Key Laboratory of Hepatobiliary Surgery and Department of Hepatobiliary Surgery, The Second Affiliated Hospital of Chongqing Medical University, Chongqing 400010, China

Kenichiro Yasutake
Department of Health and Nutrition Sciences, Faculty of Health and Social Welfare Sciences, Nishi-kyushu University, Kanzaki 842-8585, Japan and Clinical Research Center, Kyushu Medical Center, National Hospital Organization, Fukuoka 810-0065, Japan

INTRODUCTION

The field of clinical nutrition as a whole seeks to consider the nutrition of patients within the healthcare system, paying attention to the interactions between diet, nutrition, and disease. To that end, this book discusses nutrition as both a contributing and managing factor in relation to diseases such as obesity and diabetes. It also presents malnutrition as a contributing factor to such diseases and considers the efficacy of micronutrient supplementation. It ends by looking at some of the recent developments and future trends in the field of clinical nutrition.

The first chapter, by Salehpour and colleagues, examines the effect of Vitamin D on body fat mass. Vitamin D concentrations are linked to body composition indices, particularly body fat mass. Relationships between hypovitaminosis D and obesity, described by both BMI and waist circumference, have been mentioned. The authors investigated the effect of a 12-week vitamin D3 supplementation on anthropometric indices in healthy overweight and obese women. In a double-blind, randomized, placebo-controlled, parallel-group trial, 77 participants (age 38 ± 8.1 years, BMI 29.8 ± 4.1 kg/m^2) were randomly allocated into two groups: vitamin D ($25\,\mu g$ per day as cholecalciferol) and placebo ($25\,\mu g$ per day as lactose) for 12 weeks. Body weight, height, waist, hip, fat mass, 25(OH) D, iPTH, and dietary intakes were measured before and after the intervention. They found that Serum 25(OH)D significantly increased in the vitamin D group compared to the placebo group (38.2 ± 32.7 nmol/L vs. 4.6 ± 14.8 nmol/L; $P<0.001$) and serum iPTH concentrations were decreased by vitamin D3 supplementation (-0.26 ± 0.57 pmol/L vs. 0.27 ± 0.56 pmol/L; $P<0.001$). Supplementation with vitamin D3 caused a statistically significant decrease in body fat mass in the vitamin D group compared to the placebo group (-2.7 ± 2.1 kg vs. -0.47 ± 2.1 kg; $P<0.001$). However, body weight and waist circumference did not change significantly in both groups. A significant reverse correlation between changes in serum 25(OH) D concentrations and body fat mass was observed ($r=-0.319$, $P=0.005$). Among healthy overweight and obese women, increasing 25(OH) D concentrations by vitamin D3 supplementation led to body fat mass reduction.

Trautvetter and colleagues looked at the effects of calcium sulfate in chapter 2. The aim of their study was to examine the postprandial calcium and phosphate concentrations after supplementation with pentacalcium hydroxy-triphosphate (CaP). Ten men participated in this double-blind, placebo-controlled, cross-over study. The participants were divided into two groups. One group consumed bread enriched with CaP (plus 1 g calcium/d) and the other group a placebo product for three weeks. After a two week wash-out, the intervention was switched between the groups for another three weeks. Blood samples were drawn at the beginning (single administration) and at the end (repeated administration) of the intervention periods at 0, 30, 60, 120, 180 and 240 min. Between 0 and 30 min, a test meal, with or without CaP was consumed. The plasma concentrations of calcium and phosphate were examined. One participant dropped out due to personal reasons. CaP supplementation resulted in a significantly higher plasma calcium concentration after 240 min compared to placebo. After repeated CaP administration, the AUC for the increment in plasma calcium concentration was significantly higher compared to placebo. After single and repeated CaP supplementation, plasma phosphate concentration significantly decreased after 30, 60, 120 and 180 min compared to 0 min. The placebo administration resulted in significant decreases after 30, 60 and 120 min compared to 0 min. The results show that CaP contributes to an adequate calcium supply, but without increasing the plasma concentration of phosphate.

Chapter 3 examines the effects of Vitamin C when used in treating pediatric depression. Amr and colleagues argue that current antidepressants used to treat pediatric patients have the disadvantage of limited efficacy and potentially serious side effects. The purpose of this study was to assess the efficacy of vitamin C as an adjuvant agent in the treatment of pediatric major depressive disorder in a six-month, double-blind, placebo-controlled pilot trial. The study group (n=12) was given fluoxetine (10–20 mg/day) plus vitamin C (1000 mg/day) and control group (n=12) administered fluoxetine (10–20 mg/day) plus placebo. The data were analyzed by ANOVA and t-test for independent samples. Both groups demonstrated significantly improved scores on the Children's Depression Rating Scale (CDRS), the Children's Depression Inventory (CDI), and the Clinical Global Impression (CGI). ANOVA was significantly different on all clinical measurements (group effect, time effect, and interaction), with the exception of group effect and interaction for CGI. Patients treated for six months with fluoxetine and vitamin C showed a significant decrease in depressive symptoms in comparison to the fluoxetine plus placebo group as measured by the CDRS (t=11.36, P<0.0001) and CDI (t=12.27, P<0.0001), but not CGI (t=0.13, P=0.90). No serious adverse effects were observed. These preliminary results suggest that vitamin C may be an effective adjuvant agent in the treatment of MDD in pediatric patients.

Yusutake and colleagues look at the connections between nutrition and liver disease in chapter 4. The dietary intake of patients with nonalcoholic fatty liver disease (NAFLD) is generally characterized by high levels of carbohydrate, fat, and/or cholesterol, and these dietary patterns influence hepatic lipid metabolism in the patients. Therefore, careful investigation of dietary habits could lead to better nutrition therapy in NAFLD patients. The main treatment for chronic hepatitis C (CHC) is interferon-based antiviral therapy, which often causes a decrease in appetite and energy intake; hence, nutritional support is also required during therapy to prevent undernourishment, treatment interruption, and a reduction in quality of life. Moreover, addition of some nutrients that act to suppress viral proliferation is recommended. As a substitutive treatment, low-iron diet therapy, which is relatively safe and effective for preventing hepatocellular carcinoma, is also recommended for CHC patients. Some patients with liver cirrhosis (LC) have decreased dietary energy and protein intake, while the number of LC patients with overeating and obesity is increasing, indicating that the nutritional state of LC patients has a broad spectrum. Therefore, nutrition therapy for LC patients should be planned on an assessment of their complications, nutritional state, and dietary intake. Late evening snacks, branched-chain amino acids, zinc, and probiotics are considered for effective nutritional utilization.

Similarly, chapter 5 examines nutrition in patients with end-stage liver failure. Bémeur and colleagues show that malnutrition is common in patients with end-stage liver failure and hepatic encephalopathy, and is considered a significant prognostic factor affecting quality of life, outcome, and survival. The liver plays a crucial role in the regulation of nutrition by trafficking the metabolism of nutrients, their distribution and appropriate use by the body. Nutritional consequences with the potential to cause nervous system dysfunction occur in liver failure, and many factors contribute to malnutrition in hepatic failure. Among them are inadequate dietary intake, malabsorption, increased protein losses, hypermetabolism, insulin resistance, gastrointestinal bleeding, ascites, inflammation/infection, and hyponatremia. Patients at risk of malnutrition are relatively difficult to identify since liver disease may interfere with biomarkers of malnutrition. The supplementation of the diet with amino acids, antioxidants, vitamins as well as probiotics in addition to meeting energy and protein requirements may improve nutritional status, liver function, and hepatic encephalopathy in patients with end-stage liver failure.

Singh and colleagues argue in chapter 6 that nutritional support in severe acute pancreatitis (SAP) is controversial concerning the merits of enteral or parenteral nutrition in the management of patients with severe acute pancreatitis. Here, the authors assess the therapeutic efficacy of gradually combined treatment of parenteral nutrition (PN) with enteral nutrition (EN) for SAP. Methods. The clinical data of 130 cases of SAP were analyzed retrospectively. Of them, 59 cases were treated by general method of nutritional support (Group I) and the other 71 cases were treated by PN gradually combined with EN (Group II). The APACHE II score and the level of IL-6 in Group II were significantly lower than Group I . Complications, mortality, mean hospital stay, and the cost of hospitalization in Group II were 39.4 percent, 12.7 percent, 32 ± 9 days, and 30869.4 ± 12794.6 Chinese Yuan, respectively, which were significantly lower than those in Group I. The cure rate of Group II was 81.7 percent which is obviously higher than that of 59.3% in Group I. This study indicates that the combination of PN with EN not only can improve the natural history of pancreatitis but also can reduce the incidence of complication and mortality.

In chapter 7, Martin and colleagues examine the connections between protein intake and renal function. Recent trends in weight loss diets have led to a substantial increase in protein intake by individuals. As a result, the safety of habitually consuming dietary protein in excess of recommended intakes has been questioned. In particular, there is concern that high protein intake may promote renal damage by chronically increasing glomerular pressure and hyperfiltration. There is, however, a serious question as to whether there is significant evidence to support this relationship in healthy individuals. In fact, some studies suggest that hyperfiltration, the purported mechanism for renal damage, is a normal adaptive mechanism that occurs in response to several physiological conditions. This paper reviews the available evidence that increased dietary protein intake is a health concern in terms of the potential to initiate or promote renal disease. While protein restriction may be appropriate for treatment of existing kidney disease, we find no significant evidence for a detrimental effect of high protein intakes on kidney function in healthy persons after centuries of a high protein Western diet.

Chapter 8, in a similar vein, looks at the connections between renal function and phosphorus intake. Patients with renal impairment progressively lose the ability to excrete phosphorus. Decreased glomerular filtration of phosphorus is initially compensated by decreased tubular reabsorption, regulated by PTH and FGF23, maintaining normal serum phosphorus concentrations. González-Parra and colleagues show that there is a close relationship between protein and phosphorus intake. In chronic renal disease, a low dietary protein content slows the progression of kidney disease, especially in patients with proteinuria and decreases the supply of phosphorus, which has been directly related with progression of kidney disease and with patient survival. However, not all animal proteins and vegetables have the same proportion of phosphorus in their composition. Adequate labeling of food requires showing the phosphorus-to-protein ratio. The diet in patients with advanced-stage CKD has been controversial, because a diet with too low protein content can favor malnutrition and increase morbidity and mortality. Phosphorus binders lower serum phosphorus and also FGF23 levels, without decreasing diet protein content. But the interaction between intestinal dysbacteriosis in dialysis patients, phosphate binder efficacy, and patient tolerance to the binder could reduce their efficiency.

Cappello and colleagues examine the effects of nutrition on obesity in chapter 9. Only protein diet has been used successfully to prevent loss of lean body mass first in post-surgical and then in obese patients. The authors studied overweight and obese patients receiving short treatments of an exclusively protein-based nutritional solution as 24-hour enteral infusion. 19,036 patients (age 44.3 ± 13, M:F $= 2:5$) with an initial body mass index of 36.5 ± 7.1 underwent 10-day cycles of enteral nutrition through a fine nasogastric tube. The nutritional solution consisted solely of 50–65 g of proteins, plus vitamins and electrolytes. The 24-hour infusion was controlled with a small portable pump. Before and after each 10-day cycle body composition was checked with a Handy 3000 impedance analyzer. At the onset of treatment, average fat mass was 40.9 ± 12.8 kg while body cell mass was 42.7 ± 7.2 kg in males and 27.4 ± 4.6 kg in females. After an average of 2.5 cycles the patients lost 10.2 ± 7.0 kg of body weight, 5.8 ± 5.5 kg of fat mass and 2.2 ± 3.3 kg of body cell mass. No significant adverse effects were recorded except asthenia and constipation which were easily controlled with therapy. Long-term results were obtained from 15,444 patients and after an average of 362 ± 296 days we found a mean weight regain of 15.4%. The authors concluded that Ketogenic Enteral Nutrition treatment of over 19,000 patients induced a rapid 10% weight loss, 57% of which was Fat Mass. No significant adverse effects were found. The treatment is safe, fast, inexpensive and has good one-year results for weight maintenance.

In chapter 10, Ward looks at the effects of nutrition on patients undergoing gastrointestinal surgery. Nutritional depletion has been demonstrated to be a major determinant of the development of post-operative complications. Gastrointestinal surgery patients are at risk of nutritional depletion from inadequate nutritional intake, surgical stress and the subsequent increase in metabolic rate. Fears of postoperative ileus and the integrity of the newly constructed anastomosis have led to treatment typically entailing starvation with administration of intravenous fluids until the passage of flatus. However, it has since been shown that prompt postoperative enteral feeding is both effective and well tolerated. Enteral feeding is also associated with specific clinical benefits such as reduced incidence of postoperative infectious complications and an improved wound healing response. Further research is required to determine whether enteral nutrition is also associated with modulation of gut function. Studies have indicated that significant reductions in morbidity and mortality associated with perioperative Total Parenteral Nutrition (TPN) are limited to severely malnourished patients with gastrointestinal malignancy. Meta-analyses have shown that enteral nutrition is associated with fewer septic complications compared with parenteral feeding, reduced costs and a shorter hospital stay, so should be the preferred option whenever possible. Evidence to support pre-operative nutrition support is limited, but suggests that if malnourished individuals are adequately fed for at least 7–10 days preoperatively then surgical outcome can be improved. Ongoing research continues to explore the potential benefits of the action of glutamine on the gut and immune system for gastrointestinal surgery patients. To date it has been demonstrated that glutamine-enriched parenteral nutrition results in reduced length of stay and reduced costs in elective abdominal surgery patients. Further research is required to determine whether the routine supplementation of glutamine is warranted. A limitation for targeted nutritional support is the lack of a standardised, validated definition of nutritional depletion. This would enable nutrition support to be more readily targeted to those surgical patients most likely to derive significant clinical benefit in terms of improved post-operative outcome.

Damms-Machado and colleagues examine the prevalence of micronutrient deficiencies in obese individuals in chapter 11. These deficiencies are higher compared to normal-weight people, probably because of inadequate eating habits but also due to increased demands among overweight persons, which are underestimated by dietary reference intakes (DRI) intended for the general population. They therefore evaluated the dietary micronutrient intake in obese individuals compared to a reference population and DRI recommendations. Furthermore, the authors determined the micronutrient status in obese subjects undergoing a standardized DRI-covering low-calorie formula diet to analyze if the DRI meet the micronutrient requirements of obese individuals. In 104 subjects baseline micronutrient intake was determined by dietary record collection. A randomly assigned subgroup of subjects (n = 32) underwent a standardized DRI-covering low-calorie formula diet over a period of three months. Pre- and post-interventional intracellular micronutrient status in buccal mucosa cells (BMC) was analyzed, as well as additional micronutrient serum concentrations in 14 of the subjects. Prior to dietetic intervention, nutrition was calorie-rich and micronutrient-poor. Baseline deficiencies in serum concentrations were observed for 25-hydroxyvitamin-D, vitamin C, selenium, iron, as well as ß-carotene, vitamin C, and lycopene in BMC. After a three-month period of formula diet even more subjects had reduced micronutrient levels of vitamin

C (serum, BMC), zinc, and lycopene. There was a significant negative correlation between lipophilic serum vitamin concentrations and body fat, as well as between iron and C-reactive protein. The present pilot study shows that micronutrient deficiency occurring in obese individuals is not corrected by protein-rich formula diet containing vitamins and minerals according to DRI. In contrast, micronutrient levels remain low or become even lower, which might be explained by insufficient intake, increased demand and unbalanced dispersal of lipophilic compounds in the body.

In chapter 12, Mechanick and colleagues argue that type 2 diabetes (T2D) and prediabetes have a major global impact through high disease prevalence, significant downstream pathophysiologic effects, and enormous financial liabilities. To mitigate this disease burden, interventions of proven effectiveness must be used. Evidence shows that nutrition therapy improves glycemic control and reduces the risks of diabetes and its complications. Accordingly, diabetes-specific nutrition therapy should be incorporated into comprehensive patient management programs. Evidence-based recommendations for healthy lifestyles that include healthy eating can be found in clinical practice guidelines (CPGs) from professional medical organizations. To enable broad implementation of these guidelines, recommendations must be reconstructed to account for cultural differences in lifestyle, food availability, and genetic factors. To begin, published CPGs and relevant medical literature were reviewed and evidence ratings applied according to established protocols for guidelines. From this information, an algorithm for the nutritional management of people with T2D and prediabetes was created. Subsequently, algorithm nodes were populated with transcultural attributes to guide decisions. The resultant transcultural diabetes-specific nutrition algorithm (tDNA) was simplified and optimized for global implementation and validation according to current standards for CPG development and cultural adaptation. Thus, the tDNA is a tool to facilitate the delivery of nutrition therapy to patients with T2D and prediabetes in a variety of cultures and geographic locations. It is anticipated that this novel approach can reduce the burden of diabetes, improve quality of life, and save lives. The specific Southeast Asian and Asian Indian tDNA versions can be found in companion articles in this issue of Current Diabetes Reports.

Christensen and colleagues examine the effects of fruit restriction on patients with diabetes in chapter 13. Medical nutrition therapy is recognized as an important treatment option in type 2 diabetes. Most guidelines recommend eating a diet with a high intake of fiber-rich food including fruit. This is based on the many positive effects of fruit on human health. However some health professionals have concerns that fruit intake has a negative impact on glycemic control and therefore recommend restricting the fruit intake. The authors found no studies addressing this important clinical question. The objective was to investigate whether an advice to reduce the intake of fruit to patients with type 2 diabetes affects HbA1c, bodyweight, waist circumference and fruit intake. This was an open randomized controlled trial with two parallel groups. The primary outcome was a change in HbA1c during 12 weeks of intervention. Participants were randomized to one of two interventions; medical nutrition therapy + advice to consume at least two pieces of fruit a day (high-fruit) or medical nutrition therapy + advice to consume no more than two pieces of fruit a day (low-fruit). All participants had two consultations with a registered dietitian. Fruit intake was self-reported using 3-day fruit records and dietary recalls. All assessments were made by the "intention to treat" principle. The study population consisted of 63 men and women with newly diagnosed type 2 diabetes. All patients completed the trial. The high-fruit group increased fruit intake with 125 grams (CI 95%; 78 to 172) and the low-fruit group reduced intake with 51 grams (CI 95%; -18 to $^-$83). HbA1cdecreased in both groups with no difference between the groups (diff.: 0.19%, CI 95%; -0.23 to 0.62). Both groups reduced body weight and waist circumference, however there was no difference between the groups. A recommendation to reduce fruit intake as part of standard medical nutrition therapy in overweight patients with newly diagnosed type 2 diabetes resulted in eating less fruit. It had however no effect on HbA1c, weight loss or waist circumference. We recommend that the intake of fruit should not be restricted in patients with type 2 diabetes.

Chapter 14 looks at the effect of restricting carbohydrates on patients with cancer. Klement and Kämmerer argue that over the last years, evidence has accumulated suggesting that by systematically reducing the amount of dietary carbohydrates (CHOs) one could suppress, or at least delay, the emergence of cancer, and that proliferation of already existing tumor cells could be slowed down. This hypothesis is supported by the association between modern chronic diseases like the metabolic syndrome and the risk of developing or dying from cancer. CHOs or glucose, to which more complex carbohydrates are ultimately digested, can have direct and indirect effects on tumor cell proliferation: first, contrary to normal cells, most malignant cells depend on steady glucose availability in the blood for their energy and biomass generating demands and are not able to metabolize significant amounts of fatty acids or ketone bodies due to mitochondrial dysfunction. Second, high insulin and insulin-like growth factor (IGF)-1 levels resulting from chronic ingestion of CHO-rich Western diet meals, can directly promote tumor cell proliferation via the insulin/IGF1 signaling pathway. Third, ketone bodies that are elevated when insulin and blood glucose levels are low, have been found to negatively affect proliferation of different malignant cells in vitro or not to be usable by tumor cells for metabolic demands, and a multitude of mouse models have shown anti-tumorigenic properties of very low CHO ketogenic diets. In addition, many cancer patients exhibit an altered glucose metabolism characterized by insulin resistance and may profit from an increased protein and fat intake. In this review, the authors address the possible beneficial effects of low CHO diets on cancer prevention and treatment. Emphasis will be placed on the role of insulin and IGF1 signaling in tumorigenesis as well as altered dietary needs of cancer patients.

In chapter 15, Hanson and colleagues argue that nutrition support practitioners are currently dealing with shortages of parenteral nutrition micronutrients, including multivitamins (MVI), selenium and zinc. A recent survey from the American Society of Enteral and Parenteral Nutrition (ASPEN) indicates that this shortage is having a profound effect on clinical practice. A majority of respondents reported taking some aggressive measures to ration existing supplies. Most premature infants and many infants with congenital anomalies are dependent on parenteral nutrition for the first weeks of life to meet nutritional needs. Because of fragile health and poor reserves, they are uniquely susceptible to this problem. It should be understood that shortages and rationing have been associated with adverse outcomes, such as lactic acidosis and Wernicke encephalopathy from thiamine deficiency or pulmonary and skeletal development concerns related to inadequate stores of Vitamin A and D. In this review, the authors will discuss the current parenteral shortages and the possible impact on a population of very low birth weight infants. This review will also present a case study of a neonate who was impacted by these current shortages.

In chapter 16, by Karras and colleagues, vitamin D concentrations during pregnancy are measured to diagnose states of insufficiency or deficiency. The aim of this study is to apply accurate assays of vitamin D forms [single- hydroxylated [$25(OH)D_2$, $25(OH)D_3$], double-hydroxylated [$1\alpha,25(OH)_2D_2$, $1\alpha,25(OH)_2D_3$], epimers [3-epi-$25(OH)D_2$, 3-epi-$25(OH)$ D_3] in mothers (serum) and neonates (umbilical cord) to i) explore maternal and neonatal vitamin D biodynamics and ii) to identify maternal predictors of neonatal vitamin D concentrations. All vitamin D forms were quantified in 60 mother- neonate paired samples by a novel liquid chromatography -mass spectrometry (LC-MS/MS) assay. Maternal characteristics [age, ultraviolet B exposure, dietary vitamin D intake, calcium, phosphorus and parathyroid hormone] were recorded. Hierarchical linear regression was used to predict neonatal $25(OH)D$ concentrations. Mothers had similar concentrations of $25(OH)D_2$ and $25(OH)D_3$ forms compared to neonates (17.9 ± 13.2 vs. 15.9 ± 13.6 ng/mL, p=0.289) with a ratio of 1:3. The epimer concentrations, which contribute approximately 25% to the total vitamin D levels, were similar in mothers and neonates (4.8 ± 7.8 vs. 4.5 ± 4.7 ng/mL, p=0.556). No correlation was observed in mothers between the levels of the circulating form ($25OHD_3$) and its active form. Neonatal $25(OH)D_2$ was best predicted by maternal characteristics, whereas $25(OH)D_3$ was strongly associated to maternal vitamin D forms ($R^2=0.253$ vs. 0.076 and $R^2=0.109$ vs. 0.478, respectively). Maternal characteristics explained 12.2% of the neonatal $25(OH)D$, maternal $25(OH)D$ concentrations explained 32.1%, while epimers contributed an additional 11.9%. By applying a novel highly specific vitamin D assay, the present study is the first to quantify 3-epi-$25(OH)D$ concentrations in mother - newborn pairs. This accurate assay highlights a considerable proportion of vitamin D exists as epimers and a lack of correlation between the circulating and active forms. These results highlight the need for accurate measurements to appraise vitamin D status. Maternal characteristics and circulating forms of vitamin D, along with their epimers explain 56% of neonate vitamin D concentrations. The roles of active and epimer forms in the maternal - neonatal vitamin D relationship warrant further investigation.

Bacon and Aphramor discuss current trends in weight management science in chapter 17. Current guidelines recommend that "overweight" and "obese" individuals lose weight through engaging in lifestyle modification involving diet, exercise and other behavior change. This approach reliably induces short term weight loss, but the majority of individuals are unable to maintain weight loss over the long term and do not achieve the putative benefits of improved morbidity and mortality. Concern has arisen that this weight focus is not only ineffective at producing thinner, healthier bodies, but may also have unintended consequences, contributing to food and body preoccupation, repeated cycles of weight loss and regain, distraction from other personal health goals and wider health determinants, reduced self-esteem, eating disorders, other health decrement, and weight stigmatization and discrimination. This concern has drawn increased attention to the ethical implications of recommending treatment that may be ineffective or damaging. A growing trans-disciplinary movement called Health at Every Size (HAES) challenges the value of promoting weight loss and dieting behavior and argues for a shift in focus to weight-neutral outcomes. Randomized controlled clinical trials indicate that a HAES approach is associated with statistically and clinically relevant improvements in physiological measures (e.g., blood pressure, blood lipids), health behaviors (e.g., eating and activity habits, dietary quality), and psychosocial outcomes (such as self-esteem and body image), and that HAES achieves these health outcomes more successfully than weight loss treatment and without the contraindications associated with a weight focus. This paper evaluates the evidence and rationale that justifies shifting the health care paradigm from a conventional weight focus to HAES.

In the final chapter, chapter 18, Diez-Garcia and colleagues explore nutritional care in hospitals. Food and nutritional care quality must be assessed and scored, so as to improve health institution efficacy. This study aimed to detect and compare actions related to food and nutritional care quality in public and private hospitals. Investigation of the Hospital Food and Nutrition Service (HFNS) of 37 hospitals by means of structured interviews assessing two quality control corpora, namely nutritional care quality (NCQ) and hospital food service quality (FSQ). HFNS was also evaluated with respect to human resources per hospital bed and per produced meal. Comparison between public and private institutions revealed that there was a statistically significant difference between the number of hospital beds per HFNS staff member ($p = 0.02$) and per dietitian ($p < 0.01$). The mean compliance with NCQ criteria in public and private institutions was 51.8% and 41.6%, respectively. The percentage of public and private health institutions in conformity with FSQ criteria was 42.4% and 49.1%, respectively. Most of the actions comprising each corpus, NCQ and FSQ, varied considerably between the two types of institution. NCQ was positively influenced by hospital type (general) and presence of a clinical dietitian. FSQ was affected by institution size: large and medium-sized hospitals were significantly better than small ones. Food and nutritional care in hospital is still incipient, and actions concerning both nutritional care and food service take place on an irregular basis. It is clear that the design of food and nutritional care in hospital indicators is mandatory, and that guidelines for the development of actions as well as qualification and assessment of nutritional care are urgent.

— **Leah Coles, PhD**

PART I

MICRONUTRIENT SUPPLEMENTATION

A 12-WEEK DOUBLE-BLIND RANDOMIZED CLINICAL TRIAL OF VITAMIN D3 SUPPLEMENTATION ON BODY FAT MASS IN HEALTHY OVERWEIGHT AND OBESE WOMEN

AMIN SALEHPOUR, FARHAD HOSSEINPANAH,
FARZAD SHIDFAR, MOHAMMADREZA VAFA,
MARYAM RAZAGHI, SAHAR DEHGHANI,
ANAHITA HOSHIARRAD, and MAHMOODREZA GOHARI

1.1 BACKGROUND

Obesity is a chronic condition of nutrients accumulation [1,2] in which excess energy aggregates in the form of fat mass [3]. Based on the thrifty genotype hypothesis [4], since metabolic efficiency is raised in negative energy states, important interactions between gene and obesogenic environment (including food abundance and low physical activity [5]) result in improper metabolic programming and epigenic change in utero; hence in this condition obesity is an inevitable outcome [6]. Fat mass distribution specifically visceral distribution, produces toxic milieu by initiating metabolic and inflammatory cascade, which is followed by endocrine, cardiovascular and malignant events. The risk of mortality rises synergistically with increase in BMI over than $30 \, kg/m^2$ [1].

Serum 25-hydroxyvitamin D concentrations are low in obese adults [7,8] and linked to components of body composition, particularly body fat mass [9,10]. Alterations in the vitamin D endocrine system have been reported in obesity [11,12]. Lumb et al believed that vitamin D is stored in adipose and muscle tissues after absorption, and is slowly released into the blood stream [13,14]. It was thought that vitamin D deficiency caused obesity, and is proposed that hypothalamus diagnoses low calcidiol concentrations in circulation and induces higher body set point by increase in appetite and decrease in energy consumption via stimulating Agouti Related Protein/Neuropeptide Y (AgRP/NPY) and suppressing pro-Opiomelanocortin/Cocaine- Amphetamine- Regulated Transcription (POMC/CART) pathway [15,16]. Wortsman et al confirmed insufficiency of vitamin D in the obese people indicating that they need to higher doses of vitamin D [17].

Evidence implies that dairy product consumption, and high calcium and/or vitamin D intakes can repress fatty acid synthase enzyme (FAS) by decreasing intracellular Ca^{+2} in adiposities [18-21]. Recent literature reveals that vitamin D receptor (VDR) gene polymorphisms are associated with adiposity phenotypes [22]. It has been postulated that both 1,25(OH)2D and VDR have imperative roles in adipocyte differentiation [23,24]. The differentiation of pre-adipocytes to mature adipocytes in vitro is halted by 1,25(OH)2D3 [24]. Contrarily, high serum 1,25(OH)2 D concentrations may increase lipogenesis by stimulating of FAS [25].

Alterations in the vitamin D endocrine system are causally associated with augmented adiposity or result from augmented fat mass storage of vitamin D [17]. Accumulating evidence for involvement of vitamin D in fat mass metabolism [25] was the impetus for this clinical trial in which we tested the effect of vitamin D3 supplementation on body composition in overweight and obese women.

1.2 METHODS

1.2.1 SUBJECTS

We conducted the study between November 2009 and April 2010 in the Heart and Vascular Laboratory in Pharmacology Department of Tehran

University of Medical Sciences, Tehran, Iran. Recruitment began in August 2009 by advertisements on university and ended in November 2009. The criteria for eligibility were age between 18-50 years old, a BMI $\geq 25 \, kg/m^2$, an apparently healthy status based on self-reports from the subjects, free from metabolic bone disease, gastrointestinal disease, diabetes mellitus, cardiovascular disease, renal disease, no medications, no vitamin supplements, none pregnant or lactating. We excluded individuals with changes in body weight more than 3 kg within last three months, following weight-loss programs, taking weight loss drugs, smoking and drinking alcohol. Of a total of 140 subjects initially selected, eighty five subjects who met the above inclusion criteria were recruited.

The present study was approved by the Ethics Committee of the Tehran University of Medical Sciences and Iranian Registry of Clinical Trial (registration no. IRCT138809092709N2) and written informed consent and subject assent were obtained.

1.2.2 DESIGN

Individuals were randomly allocated in a double-blind parallel manner from randomized number in an 85-person list; 42 women were assigned to the vitamin D group and 43 women to the placebo group. The vitamin D group had to take vitamin D3 supplement tablet of 25 µg/d as cholecalciferol; Merck Pharma GmbH, Germany, while the placebo group took tablet of 25 µg/d as lactose; Merck Pharma GmbH, Germany. The intervention was conducted for 90 days. To ensure and assess compliance, vitamin D supplements were issued at baseline, exchanged for a new package at both 4 wk and 8 wk, and returned to the research staff at post testing, and pills were counted later for compliance, which was 87.1% in the vitamin D and 87.4% in the placebo groups. To remain blinded, one research assistant who was not involved in data collection coordinated the supplement assignment schedule.

In a per-protocol analysis, eight subjects were excluded during the intervention (Figure 1); in the placebo group, four subjects were unwilling to continue the 12-week intervention for personal reasons and another subject used oral contraceptive pills. In the vitamin D group, one subject followed a weight reduction program, one got pregnant and one

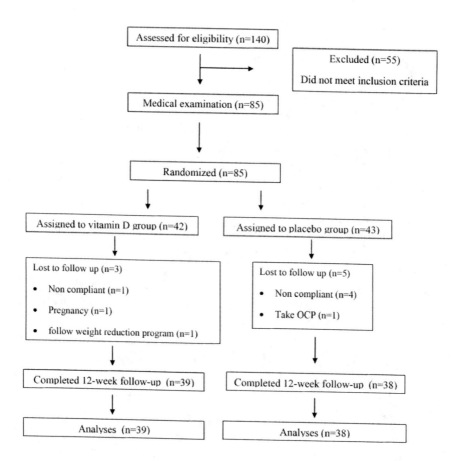

FIGURE 1: Follow of participants throughout the intervention.

was unwilling to continue the 12-week intervention for personal reasons. Eventually 77 subjects completed the study, 39 in the vitamin D group and 38 in the placebo group.

After a 12-h overnight fast, blood specimens were collected from the antecubital vein into the tubes. After centrifugation for 20 min (3000 g), the serum samples were frozen consecutively and stored at -80°C.

We assessed energy and nutrient intakes by 24 h food recall and validated food frequency questionnaires [26]. A nutritionist completed questionnaires during monthly face to face interviews. Because the Iranian food composition table (FCT) is incomplete (limited to only raw materials and few nutrients) [27], each food and beverage was analyzed for nutrient intake using Nutritionist IV software (Version 4.1, First Databank Division, The Hearst Corporation, San Bruno, CA) to assess macronutrient and micronutrient contents of foods. The Iranian FCT was used as an alternative for traditional Iranian food items, such as kashk, which are not included in the Food Composition Tables for USA (USDA FCT) [28]. The average of MET-minutes/week was calculated by multiplying the time of exercise by the respective metabolic equivalent task (MET) using the International Physical Activity Questionnaires (IPAQ) [29].

We measured body weight to the nearest 0.1 kg and height in light indoor clothes using a digital scale (model 763; Seca GmbH & Co, KG, Hamburg, Germany). Waist and hip circumference were measured on a horizontal plane at the level of the iliac crest by an Ergonomic Circumference Measuring Tape (model 201; Seca GmbH & Co, KG, Hamburg, Germany). Body mass index was calculated as weight in kilograms divided by the square of the height in meters. We assessed body fat mass and fat free mass by Bioelectrical Impedance Analysis (model 4000; Body Stat Quad Scan, Douglas Isle of Man, British Isles) after five minutes resting, with standard errors of estimate (accuracy) of 4.1%. All anthropometric indices were obtained using the WHO standard procedures [30].

1.2.3 BIOCHEMICAL MEASUREMENTS

Intact PTH was measured by immunoenzymo-metric assay (IEMA) (Immunodiagnostic Systems Ltd, Boldon, UK). Intra- and interassay CVs for intact PTH were 5.5%, and 8.3%, respectively. Serum 25(OH) D was measured by enzyme immunoassay (EIA) (Immunodiagnostic Systems Ltd, Boldon, UK). Intra- and interassay CVs for 25(OH) D were 6.9%, and 8.1%, respectively. Calcium was measured by colorimetric enzymatic (Pars Azmoon, Tehran, Iran), the kit expected range was 2.15-2.57 mmol/L. The assay sensitivity was 0.05 mmol/L, and intra- and interassay coefficients of variation were 2.4% and 3%, respectively. Phosphorus was measured by enzymatic photometric UV test (Pars Azmoon Co., Tehran, Iran); the kit expected range was 0.83-1.45 mmol/L. The assay sensitivity was 0.22 mmol/L, and intra- and interassay coefficients of variation were 3.2% and 4.1%, respectively.

1.2.4 STATISTICAL ANALYSIS

Descriptive statistics are presented as mean ± SD. We examined the normality of data by Kolmogorov-Smirnov and Shapiro-Wilk tests. All data had been normally distributed. For the primary analysis, we used an analysis of covariance (ANCOVA) to adjust mean differences on biochemical variables. Simple Pearson correlations were computed between changes in 25(OH) D and iPTH concentrations and body fat mass. All statistical analyses were performed using SPSS (version 16; SPSS Inc, Chicago, IL). All tests were two-sided and P values <0.05 were considered statistically significant.

1.3 RESULTS

Participant characteristics are given in Table 1. Baseline characteristics were similar in the vitamin D and placebo groups (Table 1). Serum 25(OH) D concentrations increased to (75±22 nmol/L vs. 51.5±31 nmol/L; P<0.001), respectively in the vitamin D group, in comparison to the placebo group after 12 weeks (Table 2). Although serum iPTH concentrations decreased in the vitamin D group, these concentrations increased in the placebo group (-0.26±0.5 pmol/L vs. 0.27±0.5 pmol/L; P<0.001), respectively. In the vitamin D group, weight loss was (-0.3±1.5 kg) whereas in the placebo group, it was (-0.1 ± 1.7 kg), differences were not statistically significant between the two groups. Waist circumference decreased in the vitamin D group, but increased in the placebo group (-0.3 ± 4.3 cm vs. 0.4 ± 4.1 cm), respectively. Hip circumference decreased (-0.39 ± 2.4 cm in the vitamin D group and -0.9 ± 2.4 cm in the placebo group), differences were not statistically significant between the two groups. Body fat mass decreased in the vitamin D and placebo groups (-2.7 ± 2 kg and -0.4 ± 2 kg; $P < 0.001$). There were significant inverse correlations between changes in serum 25(OH) D concentrations and body fat mass ($r = -0.319$, $P = 0.005$) (Figure 2), and iPTH concentrations ($r = -0.318$, $P = 0.005$). A significant positive and correlation was observed between changes in serum iPTH concentrations and body fat mass ($r = 0.32$, $P = 0.004$) (Figure 3), while there were no significant correlations between serum 25(OH)D concentrations and body fat mass or iPTH concentrations.

1.4 DISCUSSION

The present study shows that a 12 week supplementation with 25 µg vitamin D3 in overweight and obese women with mean serum 25(OH)D concentrations of 41.8 ± 31.4 nmol/L decreases body fat mass, but does not affect body weight and waist circumference.

There is a large body of growing evidence showing that dairy products, and calcium and vitamin D intake play a role in the regulation of body fat mass [31-33]. Data also indicates that vitamin D may increase lean body mass [34] and inhibit the development of adipocytes. These effects of vitamin D may be mediated by 1,25(OH)2D3 or via suppression of PTH [35].

However, there are few clinical trials of vitamin D supplementation on body composition and most of them have assessed effects of combined calcium and vitamin D supplementation. Moreover, these studies are heterogeneous with regard to doses and types of vitamin D, lengths of follow up, outcome ascertainment methods, prevalence of vitamin D deficiency and other characteristics in studied subjects, which have led to inconsistent results. Our study is one of the few clinical trials which have investigated the effect of vitamin D3 supplementation in overweight or obese women with low 25(OH)D concentrations on body compositions.

The 12 week vitamin D3 supplementation did not significantly affect body weight, waist or hip circumference. However, a modest fat mass reduction of 7% was associated with a significant increase of 25OHD levels by 103% and a significant decrease of PTH levels by 14%. The initial serum 25(OH)D concentrations were low in both groups.

TABLE 1: Baseline characteristics of subject groups who received vitamin D3 supplements (25 µ/d) or placebo before the intervention

Characteristics	Vitamin D group	Placebo group	P-value
Age (y)	38±72	37±8	0.29
Body weight (kg)	73.9±10.2	75.1±11.9	0.61
Height (cm)	156.5±5.8	159.3±5.6	0.035
Waist circumference (cm)	89.9±8.7	91.2±12.1	0.59
Hip circumference (cm)	108±8.5	108.2±8.1	0.91
BMI (kg/m^2)	30.1±3.9	29.5±4.4	0.54
Fat mass (kg)	30.2±6.9	29±8.7	0.53
Fat free mass (kg)	43.7±5.1	45.9±4.7	0.05
Physical activity (MET-minutes/week)	902±1245	702±996	0.43
Energy intake (kcal/d)	1866±927	2060±834	0.33
Carbohydrate intake (g/d)	280±134	329±140	0.12
Fiber intake (g/d)	16±9	18±10	0.23
Protein intake (g/d)	64±29	76±35	0.10
Fat intake (g/d)	55±44	49±24	0.43
Dietary calcium intake (mg/d)	873±586	677±386	0.08
Dietary vitamin D intake (µg/d)	0.53±0.6	0.39±0.37	0.22
25(OH) D (nmol/L)^2	36.8±30	46.9±32	0.15
iPTH (pmol/L)^2	1.4±0.7	1.4±0.7	0.84
Calcium (mmol/L)	2.2±0.09	2.3±0.1	0.004
Phosphorus (mmol/L)	1.1±0.1	1.1±0.1	0.6

[a]*Mean ± SD (all such values).*
[b]*25(OH) D, 25-hydroxyvitamin D; PTH, parathyroid hormone. To convert 25(OH) D values to ng/mL, divide by 2.5. To convert PTH values to pg/mL, divide by 0.11.*

Recently, in a double-blind, placebo-controlled trial in overweight and obese participants, Rosenblum et al [32] reported that after a 16 week calcium and vitamin D supplementation with either regular or reduced energy (lite) orange juice (three 240 mL glasses of orange juice fortified with 350 mg Ca and 100 IU vitamin D per serving), the average weight loss did not differ significantly between groups, but in the regular orange juice trial, the reduction of visceral adipose tissue (VAT) was significantly greater in the CaD group than in controls (-12.7 ± 25.0 cm^2 vs. -1.3 ± 13.6 cm^2; P=0.024, respectively) and in the lite orange juice trial, the reduction of VAT was significantly greater in the CaD group than in controls (-13.1 ± 18.4 cm^2 vs. -6.4 ± 17.5 cm^2; P=0.039, respectively) after control for baseline VAT. They suggested that calcium and vitamin D supplementation contributes to a beneficial reduction of VAT. Dong et al [36] in a 16 week randomized, blinded, controlled clinical trial of 2000 IU vitamin D3 supplementation in forty nine black youth, evaluated the relation between 25(OH)D concentrations and total body fat mass by dual-energy x-ray absorptiometry. The experimental group compared with the controls reached significantly higher 25(OH)D concentrations at 16 wk (85.7±30.1 nmol/liter vs. 59.8±18.2 nmol/liter, P<0.001, respectively) and partial correlation analyses indicated that total body fat mass at baseline was significantly and inversely associated with 25(OH)D concentrations in response to the 2000 IU supplement (R=-0.46; P=0.03). Zhou et al [37] in a large-scale, placebo controlled, double-blind, 4-year longitudinal clinical trial, investigated the effect of calcium and vitamin D supplementation on obesity in postmenopausal women, randomly assigned into one of three groups: 1) supplemental calcium (1400 mg/d or 1500 mg/d) plus vitamin D placebo (Ca-only group); 2) supplemental calcium (1400 mg/d or 1500 mg/d) plus supplemental vitamin D3 (1100 IU/d) (Ca+D group); or, 3) two placebos. No significant difference was observed for body mass index between groups, but changes in trunk fat (for Ca-only and Ca+D groups compared to the placebo group preserved lower trunk fat 2.4%, 1.4% vs. 5.4%, P=0.015 at year 3) and trunk lean (for Ca-only and Ca+D groups preserved more trunk lean compared to the placebo group, -0.6%, -1.0% vs. -2.1%, P=0.004 at year 4), were significantly different between groups. Major et al [38] conducted a randomized, double-blind, placebo-controlled study to compare the effects of a 15 week weight-reducing program (-700 kcal/d) coupled with a calcium plus vitamin D supplementation (600 mg elemental calcium and 5 mg vitamin D, twice a day or placebo), on the body fat of sixty-three overweight or obese women.

The calcium+D supplementation did not induce statistically significant increase in fat mass loss. However, when analyses were limited to very low-calcium consumers only (initial calcium intake ≤600 mg/d), significant time × treatment interaction were observed in body weight (P<0·009), BMI (P<0·008) and fat mass (P<0.02). Waist circumference decreased in both groups and there were significant treatment effects (P=0.03). Zittermann et al [39] investigated the effect of vitamin D (83 μg/d) on weight loss in overweight subjects with a mean 25(OH)D concentration of 30 nmol/L in a double-blind manner for 12 months while participating in a weight-reduction program. Their results showed that although weight loss was not affected significantly by vitamin D supplementation, waist circumference however decreased in both groups and there were significant treatment effects (P=0.022). Body fat mass did not alter after the intervention.

It has been suggested that high levels of calcitrophic hormones such as 1α,25,dihydroxyvitamin D and iPTH can modulate intracellular Ca^{+2} concentrations, so increasing Ca^{+2} flux to adiposities, which stimulate fatty acid synthase enzyme, may increase lipogenesis and inhibit lipolysis [25]. According to this hypothesis, 1α, 25dihydroxyvitamin D is known as a key factor that provokes triglyceride accumulation in adiposities [18] a finding not confirmed by others [39]. Vitamin D insufficiency and secondary hyperparathyroidism lead to PTH related phospholipase C activation in adiposities, a process, which is followed by increase in intracellular calcium [40,41]. Chronic increase in $[Ca^{+2}]$ may attenuate the ability of catecholamines in activating of lipolysis by increasing the activity of Ca^{+2} related cAMP phosphodiesterase [42]. Meanwhile, with increasing of $[Ca^{+2}]$, induction of fatty acid synthase is strengthened, which facilitates de novo lipogenesis [43]. Thus hyperparathyroidism can affect weight gain [44,45].

The primary limitation of our study is that we could not assess body composition by Dual X-Ray Absorptiometry (DXA) as a gold standard method. However, Bioelectrical Impedance Analysis is a validated and reliable method to assess body composition. A second limitation is that Resting Metabolic Rate (RMR) was not determined in subjects. Although our main goal was to examine the effect of vitamin D3 supplementation on body composition. A third potential limitation is not evaluating sun exposure, a confounding factor, which can not be completely ruled out. However, the subjects were requested not to use sunscreen during the intervention.

TABLE 2. Anthropometric, dietary and serum variables in the subject groups after vitamin D3 supplementation and changes in variables between measurement periods

Characteristics	Vitamin D group		Placebo group		P-valuea
	Week 12	Changeb	Week 12	Change	
Body weight (kg)	73.5±10.43	-0.3±1.5	75±12.3	-0.1±1.7	0.71
Waist circumference (cm)	89.5±8.8	-0.3±4.3	91.6±13	0.4±4.1	0.38
Hip circumference (cm)	107.6±7.9	-0.39±2.4	107.3±7.2	-0.9±2.4	0.36
BMI (kg/m²)	30±4	-0.13±0.6	29.5±4.6	-0.04±0.6	0.50
Fat mass(kg)	28.2±7.5	-2.7±2.1	28.6±8.9	-0.47±2.1	<0.001
Fat free mass (kg)	45.5±4.9	1.8±2.1	46.2±5	0.4±2.1	<0.001
Physical activity (MET-minutes/week)	892±1488	-10±1627	1081±1372	379±1137	0.23
Energy intake (kcal/d)	2010±1289	143.7±1358.4	1852±992	-208±920.9	0.32
Carbohydrate intake (g/d)	312±186	31.8±194.6	294±164	-34.3±143	0.23
Fiber intake (g/d)	16±12	1±11.7	14±7	-4.3±11.3	0.10
Protein intake (g/d)	72±53	7.8±54.3	66±32	-9.3±35.6	0.29
Fat intake (g/d)	53±43	-2.3±52.2	45±36	-4.2±39.3	0.48
Dietary calcium intake (mg/d)	829±533	-43.9±674.4	625±454	-51.8±509.5	0.18
Dietary vitamin D intake (μg/d)	0.4±0.47	-0.09±0.77	0.37±0.35	-0.04±0.52	0.70
25(OH) D (nmol/L)	75±22	38.2±32	51.5±31	4.6±14	<0.001
PTH (pmol/L)	1.2±0.5	-0.2±0.5	1.7±0.8	0.2±0.5	<0.001
Calcium (mmol/L)	2.2±0.1	-0.02±0.1	2.3±0.09	-0.02±0.1	0.81
Phosphorus (mmol/L)	0.9±0.09	-0.12±0.1	1±0.09	-0.09±0.1	0.21

aAn analysis of covariance (ANCOVA) was used to adjust mean differences on all dependent variables.
bAfter 12 weeks.
Mean ± SD (all such values).

1.5 CONCLUSIONS

To summarize, based on result of the 12 week vitamin D3 supplementation, we concluded body fat mass decreased in healthy overweight and obese women via increase in serum 25(OH) D and decrease in iPTH

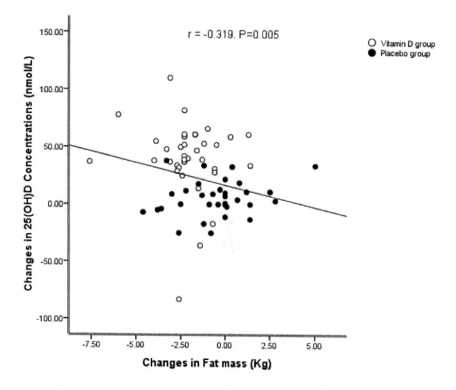

FIGURE 2: Relation between alterations of serum 25(OH) D concentrations and body fat mass.

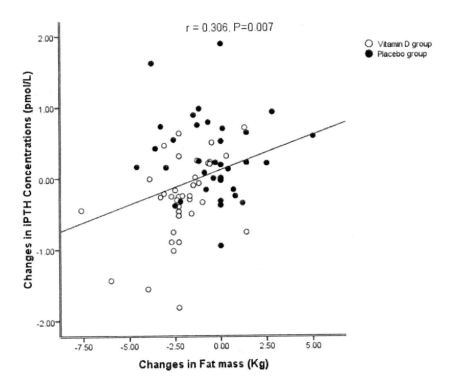

FIGURE 3: Relation between alterations of serum iPTH concentrations and body fat mass.

concentrations. Further investigation into whether vitamin D may play a role in regulation of body composition is warranted.

REFERENCES

1. Welborn TA, Dhaliwal SS, Bennett SA: Waist-hip ratio is the dominant risk factor predicting cardiovascular death in australia. Med J Aust 2003, 179:580-585.

2. Welborn TA, Dhaliwal SS: Preferred clinical measures of central obesity for predicting mortality. Eur J Clin Nutr 2007, 61:1373-1379.

3. Marieke B, Snijder MB, van Dam RM, Visser M, Deeg DJH, Dekker JM, Bouter LM, Seidell JC, Lips P: Adiposity in relation to vitamin D status and parathyroid hormone levels: a population-based study in older men and women. J Clin Endocrinol Metab 2005, 90:4119-4123.

4. Neel JV: Diabetes mellitus: a "thrifty" genotype rendered detrimental by "progress"? Am J Hum Genet 1962, 14:353-362.

5. Wareham N: Physical activity and obesity prevention. Obes Rev 2007, 8(Suppl):109-114.

6. Buffington C, Walker B, Cowan GS, Scruggs D: Vitamin D deficiency in morbidly obese. Obes Surg 1993, 3:421-424.

7. Zamboni G, Soffiati M, Giavarina D, Tato L: Mineral metabolism in obese children. Acta Paediatr Scand 1988, 77:741-746.

8. Yanoff LB, Parikh SJ, Spitalnik A, Denkinger B, Sebring NG, Slaughter P, McHugh T, Remaley AT, Yanovski JA: The prevalence of hypovitaminosis d and secondary hyperparathyroidism in obese black americans. Clin Endocrinol 2006, 64:s23-s29.

9. Liel Y, Ulmer E, Shary J, Hollis BW, Bell NH: Low circulating vitamin d in obesity. Calcif Tissue Int 1988, 43:199-201.

10. Danescu LG, Levy S, Levy J: Vitamin d and diabetes mellitus. Endocrine 2009, 35:11-7.

11. Bell NH, Epstein S, Greene A, Shary J, Oexmann MJ, Shaw S: Evidence for alteration of the vitamin d endocrine system in obese subjects. J Clin Invest 1985, 76:370-373.

12. Sutherland ER, Goleva E, Jackson LP, Stevens AD, Leung DY: Vitamin d levels, lung function, and steroid response in adult asthma. Am J Respir Crit Care Med 2010, 181:699-704.

13. Cowley MA, Pronchuk N, Fan W, Dinulescu DM, Colmers WF, Cone RD: Integration of npy, agrp, and melanocortin signals in the hypothalamic paraventricular nucleus: evidence of a cellular basis for the adipostat. Neuron 1999, 24(Suppl 1):155-163.

14. Bays HE, Gonzalez-Campoy JM, Bray GA, Kitabchi AE, Bergman DA, Schorr AB, Rodbard HW, Henry RR: Pathogenic potential of adipose tissue and metabolic consequences of adipocyte hypertrophy and increased visceral adiposity. Expert Rev Cardio Ther 2008, 6:343-368.

15. Schwartz MW, Niswender KD: Adiposity signaling and biological defense against weight gain: absence of protection or central hormone resistance? J Clin Endocrinol Metab 2004, 89(Suppl 12):5889-5897.

16. Posey KA, Clegg DJ, Printz RL, Byun J, Morton GJ, Vivekanandan-Giri A, Pennathur S, Baskin DG, Heinecke JW, Woods SC, Schwartz MW, Niswender KD: Hypothalamic proinflammatory lipid accumulation, inflammation, and insulin resistance in rats fed a high-fat diet. Am J Physiol Endocrinol Metab 2009, 296:E1003-E1012.

17. Wortsman J, Matsuoka LY, Chen TC, Lu Z, Holick MF: Decreased bioavailability of vitamin d in obesity. Am J Clin Nutr 2000, 72:690-693.

18. Zemel MB, Shi H, Greer B, Dirienzo D, Zemel PC: Regulation of adiposity by dietary calcium. FASEB J 2000, 14:1132-1138.

19. Teegarden D: Calcium intake and reduction of fat mass. J Nutr 2003, 133:249S-251S.

20. Zemel MB: Proposed role of calcium and dairy food components in weight management and metabolic health. Physician Sport Med 2009, 37:29-39.

21. Spence LA, Cifelli CJ, Miller GD: The role of dairy products in healthy weight and body composition in children and adolescents. Curr Nutr Food Sci 2011, 7(Suppl 1):40-49(10).

22. Ochs-Balcom HM, Chennamaneni R, Millen AE, Shields PG, Marian C, Trevisan M, Freudenheim JL: Vitamin d receptor gene polymorphisms are associated with adiposity phenotypes. Am J Clin Nutr 2011, 93:5-10.

23. Wood RJ: Vitamin d and adipogenesis: new molecular insights. Nutr Rev 2008, 66:40-46.

24. Kong J, Li YC: Molecular mechanism of 1,25-dihydroxyvitamin d3 inhibition of adipogenesis in 3T3-L1 cells. Am J Physiol Endocrinol Metab 2006, 290:E916-E924.

25. Zemel MB: Regulation of adiposity and obesity risk by dietary calcium: mechanisms and implications. J Am Coll Nutr 2002, 21:146S-151S.

26. Hosseini Esfahani F, Asghari G, Mirmiran P, Azizi F: Reproducibility and relative validity of food group intake in a food frequency questionnaire developed for the tehran lipid and glucose study. J Epidemiol 2010, 20:150-158.

27. Azar M, Sarkisian E: Food Composition Table of Iran. National Nutrition and Food Research Institute, Shaheed Beheshti University, Tehran; 1980.

28. Ars.usda.gov. http://www.nal.usda.gov/fnic/foodcomp/ webciteArs.usda.gov. http://www.nal.usda.gov/fnic/foodcomp/

29. Craig CL, Marshall AL, Sjostrom M, Bauman AE, Booth ML, Ainsworth BE: International physical activity questionnaire: 12-country reliability and validity. Med Sci Sports Exercise 2003, 35:1381-1395.

30. World Health Organization Physical Status: The Use 478 and Interpretation of Anthropometry. Technical Report 479 Series no. 854. WHO, Geneva; 1995.

31. Siddiqui SM, Chang E, Li J, Burlage C, Zou M, Buhman KK, Koser S, Donkin SS, Teegarden D: Dietary intervention with vitamin d, calcium, and whey protein reduced fat mass and increased lean mass in rats. Nutr Res 2008, 28:783-790.

32. Rosenblum JL, Castro VM, Moore CE, Kaplan LM: Calcium and vitamin d supplementation is associated with decreased abdominal visceral adipose tissue in overweight and obese adults. Am J Clin Nutr 2012, 95(Suppl 1):101-108.

33. Adams JS, Hewison M: Update in vitamin d. J Clin Endocrinol Metab 2010, 95:471-478.

34. Reid IR: Relationships between fat and bone. Osteoporos Int 2008, 19:595-606.

35. Ward KA, Das G, Berry JL, Roberts SA, Rawer R, Adams JE, Mughal Z: Vitamin d status and muscle function in post-menarchal adolescent girls. J Clin Endocrinol Metab 2009, 9:559-563.

36. Dong Y, Stallmann-Jorgensen IS, Pollock NK, Harris RA, Keeton D, Huang Y, Li K, Bassali R, Guo D, Thomas J, Pierce GL, White J, Holick MF, Zhu H: A 16-week randomized clinical trial of 2000 international units daily vitamin d3 supplementation in black youth: 25-hydroxyvitamin d, adiposity, and arterial stiffness. J Clin Endocrinol Metab 2010, 95:4584-4591.

37. Zhou J, Zhao LJ, Watson P, Zhang Q, Lappe JM: The effect of calcium and vitamin d supplementation on obesity in postmenopausal women: secondary analysis for a large-scale, placebo controlled, double-blind, 4-year longitudinal clinical trial. Nutr Metab 2010, 7:62-70.

38. Major GC, Alarie FP, Dore J, Tremblay A: Calcium plus vitamin d supplementation and fat mass loss in female very low-calcium consumers: potential link with a calcium-specific appetite control. Brit J Nutr 2009, 101:659-663.

39. Zittermann A, Frisch S, Berthold HK, Götting C, Kuhn J, Kleesiek K, Stehle P, Koertke H, Koerfer R: Vitamin d supplementation enhances the beneficial effects of weight loss on cardiovascular disease risk markers. Am J Clin Nutr 2009, 89:1321-1327.

40. Begum N, Sussman KE, Draznin B: Calcium-induced inhibition of phosphoserine phosphatase in insulin target cells is mediated by the phosphorylation and activation of inhibitor 1. J Biol Chem 1992, 267:5959-5963.

41. Ni Z, Smogorzewski M, Massry SG: Effects of parathyroid hormone on cytosolic calcium of rat adipocytes. Endocrinology 1994, 135:1837-1844.

42. Xue B, Greenberg AG, Kraemer FB, Zemel MB: Mechanism of intracellular calcium ([ca2+]i) inhibition of lipolysis in human adipocytes. FASEB J 2001, 15:2527-2529.

43. Kim JH, Mynatt RL, Moore JW, Woychik RP, Moustaid N, Zemel MB: The effects of calcium channel blockade on agouti-induced obesity. FASEB J 1996, 10:1646-1652.

44. Shrago E, Spennetta T: The carbon pathway for lipogenesis in isolated adipocytes from rat, guinea pig, and human adipose tissue. Am J Clin Nutr 1976, 29:540-545.

45. Guo ZK, Cella LK, Baum C, Ravussin E, Schoeller DA: De novo lipogenesis in adipose tissue of lean and obese women: application of deuterated water and isotope ratio mass spectrometry. Int J Obes Relat Metab Disord 2000, 24:932-937.

This chapter was originally published under the Creative Commons Attribution License. Salehpour, A., Hosseinpanah, F., Shidfar, F., Vafa, M., Razaghi, M., Dehghani, S., Hoshiarrad, A., and Gohari, M. 12-Week Double-Blind Randomized Clinical Trial of Vitamin D3 Supplementation on Body Fat Mass in Healthy Overweight and Obese Women. Nutrition Journal. 2012; 11(78). doi:10.1186/1475-2891-11-78.

CHAPTER 2

POSTPRANDIAL EFFECTS OF CALCIUM PHOSPHATE SUPPLEMENTATION ON PLASMA CONCENTRATION-DOUBLE-BLIND, PLACEBO-CONTROLLED CROSS-OVER HUMAN STUDY

ULRIKE TRAUTVETTER, MICHAEL KIEHNTOPF, and GERHARD JAHREIS

2.1 BACKGROUND

Hyperphosphatemia is recognized as a risk factor for mortality in chronic kidney disease [1]. In addition, serum phosphate concentration within the upper limits of normal is associated with a greater prevalence of vascular and valvular calcification in patients with moderate chronic kidney disease [2]. In the last years, our research group performed human studies involving calcium phosphate supplementation [3-5]. Most studies with calcium phosphate focus on the beneficial effects relating to intestinal metabolism, e.g. bile acid metabolism, fatty acid excretion, and modulation of the microbiota [5-8]. This is because amorphous calcium phosphate is formed in the human gut and, moreover, is able to precipitate intestinal substances, such as bile or fatty acids [6,7,9]. However, calcium phosphate is poorly absorbed in the gut. Evidence comes from studies showing unchanged fasting plasma concentrations of calcium and phosphate after calcium phosphate supplementation [4]. Nevertheless, measuring fasting concentrations is not a convincing method to examine the influence of calcium phosphate supplementation on calcium and phosphate status. Furthermore, Heaney et al. showed that solubility of a calcium supplement has very little influence on its absorbability and that absorption of calcium from food sources is determined mainly by other food components [10]. In addition, it is necessary to test every calcium product for absorbability [11]. Therefore, in this human study, we examined the postprandial calcium and phosphate concentrations after calcium phosphate supplementation of both a single dose and after three weeks.

2.2 METHODS

2.2.1 SUPPLEMENT

For purposes of supplementation, we used pentacalcium hydroxy-triphosphate ($Ca_5(PO_4)_3OH$; cfb; Budenheim Germany; CaP) in this study. CaP was incorporated in whole wheat bread to achieve an additional calcium intake of 1 g/d (0.5 g phosphorus/d). Participants consumed approximately 135 g of this bread daily. Placebo bread was prepared in exactly the same way, but without the CaP supplement.

2.2.2 SUBJECTS

The study was conducted between July and September 2010 in the Institute of Nutrition, Department of Nutritional Physiology at the Friedrich Schiller University Jena. Ten omnivorous men participated in this double-blind, placebo-controlled, cross-over study. Eligibility criteria for participants included age between 20 and 35 years and good physical health. A further criterion was that participants remain at the blood withdrawal centre for at least 5 hours between 7.30 am till 12.30 pm. Volunteers were provided with detailed information regarding purpose, course, and possible risks involved in the study. All participants gave their written informed

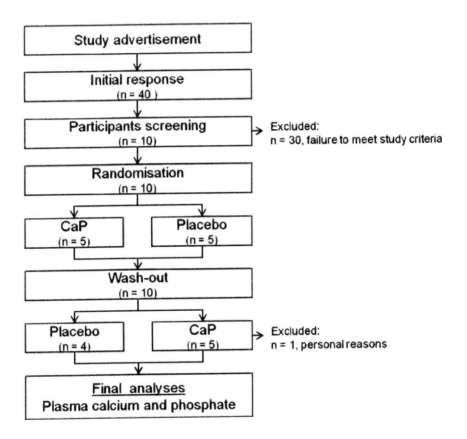

FIGURE 1: Study flowchart. CaP: pentacalcium hydroxy-triphosphate.

consent. The study protocol was approved by the Ethical Committee of the Friedrich Schiller University, Jena (No.:2833-05/10). Of the initial ten volunteers, one participant dropped out due to personal reasons. The main study outcomes comprised blood concentrations of calcium and phosphate (Figure 1).

2.2.3 STUDY DESIGN

Participants were divided into two groups. For a period of three weeks, one group consumed bread containing CaP whereas the other group consumed the placebo product. This was followed by a two-week wash-out phase. Thereafter, the intervention changed between the two groups for a further three weeks. Thus, the study design allowed that every participant was his own control. The intervention periods are divided in two parts. At the beginning the participants ate the test bread with or without CaP onetime and then blood was taken (single administration). Afterwards the participants consumed the test bread three weeks daily and then blood was taken again (repeated administration). Consequently, the study involved four types of administrations: single CaP administration, single placebo administration, repeated CaP administration and repeated placebo administration. In addition, participants consumed a defined diet for three days before each blood sample was taken (Figure 2).

The defined diet containing the complete food supply for three days was prepared and pre-weighed in the study centre. The subjects were instructed to consume no other foods than provided. Any food residues were weighed and food intake was calculated.

On the day of blood withdrawal, participants came fasting to the Institute of Transfusion Medicine of the Jena University Hospital. Blood samples were drawn after 0, 30, 60, 120, 180 and 240 minutes, immediately cooled, and transported to the study centre.

Between time point 0 and 30 minutes, the participants consumed a test meal. The test meal consisted of bread with or without CaP (according to the intervention), 20 g butter, 25 g ham, 15 g sweet hazelnut spread and a banana. During the 240 min the participants were allowed to drink water ad libitum.

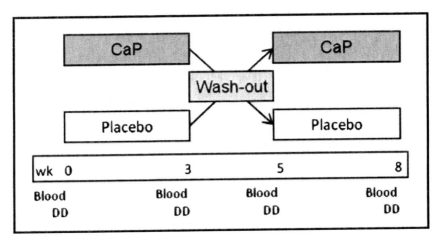

FIGURE 2: Design of the double-blind, placebo-controlled cross-over study. wk: week; CaP: pentacalcium hydroxy-triphosphate; blood: blood sampling at time points 0, 30, 60, 120, 180 and 240 minutes; between 0 and 30 minutes, the participants consumed a test meal with or without CaP; DD: defined diet for three days before blood sampling.

2.2.4 SAMPLE PREPARATION

Samples of each food component of the defined diet were frozen and stored at −20°C until analysis. Blood was collected in lithium heparin tubes. Plasma was obtained by centrifugation at 2500 x g for 15 minutes at 20°C. Aliquots were frozen at −80°C until analysis.

2.2.5 FOOD ANALYSIS

The intake of energy, fat, proteins, and carbohydrates was verified using the Prodi® 5.4 software (Nutri-Science GmbH, Freiburg, Germany). For intake of minerals, the respective contents in the provided foods were analysed instead of using the calculation software. Mineral contents of all food samples were determined employing the iCAP 6000 ICP Spectrometer

(Thermo Scientific, Waltham, USA). Before analysis, the samples were ashed at 525°C. The ash was dissolved in HCl (25%) and diluted with distilled water.

2.2.6 ANALYSIS OF CALCIUM AND PHOSPHATE

Calcium and phosphate in plasma were quantified using the autoanalyser ARCHITECT C16000 (Abbott, Illinois, USA) according to the manufacturer's recommendations.

2.2.7 CALCULATIONS AND STATISTICAL METHODS

Samples from each participant were coded to protect volunteer identity and to mask treatment groups during the analysis. The areas under the curves (AUC) from 0 to 240 min were calculated using the trapezoidal method. The calculation based on the increment in plasma calcium and phosphate concentrations.

All values in the text and tables were expressed as mean±standard deviation. For reasons of clarity and comprehensibility, values in figures were expressed only as means. Data analysis was performed using the statistical software package PASW Statistics 18 (SPSS Inc., Chicago, USA). Differences were considered significant at $p \leq 0.05$. The effect of time was tested only to baseline using paired Student's t-test. The effect of supplementation was tested with paired Student's t-test. The sample size for calcium and phosphate was $n=9$.

2.3 RESULTS

Nine subjects completed the four blood samples and test meals. The baseline characteristics and the nutrient intake of the test meal and defined diet are presented in Tables 1 and 2.

TABLE 1: Baseline characteristics of participants who completed the study

	Subject (n= 9)
Age [y]	27±4
Height [cm]	178±5
Weight [kg]	73.2±7.5
BMI [kg/m²]	23.1±2.3

TABLE 2: Mean nutrient composition of the test meal and the defined diet

	Test meal (per meal)		Defined (per day)	
Energy [MJ]	2,6±0,1		10,4±1,4	
Carbohydrates [g]	82,1±3,4		292,9±41,2	
Fat [g]	23,5±0,1		101,6±19,1	
Protein [g]	16,7±0,3		85,3±6,3	
	CaP	Placebo	CaP	Placebo
Ca [mg]	1160±1	55±1	2019±75,2	926±57
from CaP [mg]	1104	0	1104	0
P [mg]	868±4	346±5	2050±127	1542±104
from CaP [mg]	519	0	519	0

N = 9; data are expressed as mean ± standard deviation; CaP pentacalcium hydroxytriphosphate, Ca calcium, P phosphorus.

The calcium and phosphorous concentrations of the CaP bread was 1129 mg/135 g bread and 749 mg/135 g bread, respectively. The placebo bread contained 26 mg calcium/135 g bread and 229 mg phosphorus/135 g bread, respectively.

Following single administration with CaP, calcium concentration increased significantly after 120 ($p = 0.043$) and 240 min ($p \leq 0.001$) compared to 0 min. The three week administration of CaP led to an increase of calcium concentration after 60 ($p = 0.026$), 180 ($p = 0.011$) and 240 ($p = 0.001$) min compared to 0 min (Figure 3). Both the single and the repeated administration of CaP resulted in a significantly higher calcium concentration after 240 min (p=0.005, p=0.006) compared to placebo. After repeated administration, the AUC for the increment in calcium concentration was significantly higher after CaP administration compared to placebo (p=0.007).

After single and repeated CaP supplementation, the phosphate concentration significantly decreased after 30 (single: p≤0.001, repeated: p=0.002), 60 (single: p≤0.001; repeated: p≤0.001), 120 (single: p=0.006, repeated: p=0.006) and 180 (single: p=0.043, repeated: p=0.041) min compared to 0 min. The placebo administration resulted in similar significant decreases after 30 (single: p≤0.001; repeated: p=0.001), 60 (single: p≤0.001; repeated: p≤0.001) and 120 (single: p=0.007; repeated: p=0.011) min compared to 0 min.

Following single CaP and placebo administration, the calcium-phosphorus product significantly decreased compared to 0 (CaP: 2.5 mmol2/l2; placebo: 2.6 mmol2/l2) after 30 (CaP: 2.3 mmol2/l2, p≤0.001; placebo: 2.3 mmol2/l2, p=0.003), 60 (CaP: 2.1 mmol2/l2, p≤0.001; placebo: 2.1 mmol2/l2, p≤0.001), 120 (CaP: 2.1 mmol2/l2, p=0.006; placebo: 2.2 mmol2/l2, p=0.008) and 180 (CaP: 2.3 mmol2/l2, p=0.049; placebo: 2.3 mmol2/l2, p=0.031) min, respectively. After repeated CaP and placebo administration, the calcium-phosphorus product significantly decreased after 30 (CaP: 2.4 mmol2/l2, p=0.001; placebo: 2.4 mmol2/l2, p=0.001), 60 (CaP: 2.1 mmol2/l2, p=0.001; placebo: 2.2 mmol2/l2, p≤0.001) and 120 (CaP: 2.1 mmol2/l2, p=0.011; placebo: 2.2 mmol2/l2, p=0.012) min compared to 0 min (CaP: 2.6 mmol2/l2, placebo: 2.6 mmol2/l2). At 0 min, the calcium-phosphorus product was significantly higher after CaP administration compared to placebo administration (p=0.031).

2.4 DISCUSSION

Calcium has a tightly regulated homeostasis rendering it unsuitable for comparing fasting calcium concentrations for the purpose of determining the effect of supplementation on calcium status. Although, there are some studies in the literature in which the calcium concentration was determined following a short time interval after calcium intake [12-16]. For

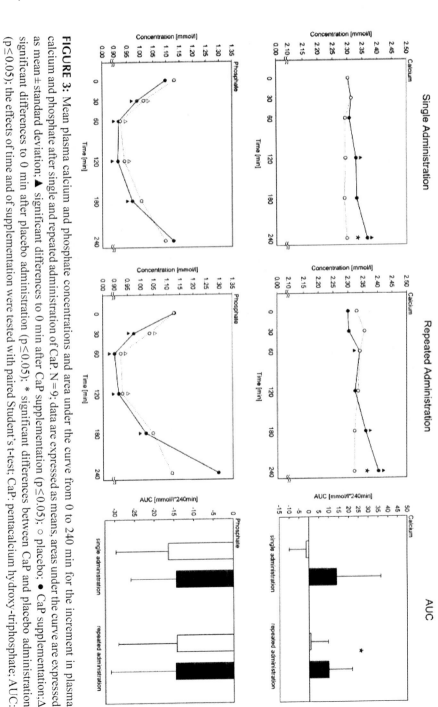

FIGURE 3: Mean plasma calcium and phosphate concentrations and area under the curve from 0 to 240 min for the increment in plasma calcium and phosphate after single and repeated administration of CaP. N=9; data are expressed as means, areas under the curve are expressed as mean±standard deviation; ▲ significant differences to 0 min after CaP supplementation (p≤0.05); ○ placebo; ● CaP supplementation;△ significant differences to 0 min after placebo administration (p≤0.05); * significant differences between CaP and placebo administration (p≤0.05); the effects of time and of supplementation were tested with paired Student's t-test; CaP: pentacalcium hydroxy-triphosphate; AUC: area under the curve.

instance, Heaney et al. compared the bioavailability of calcium from two fortification systems. A combination of tricalcium phosphate and calcium lactate (500 mg calcium, orange juice) led to an increase in serum calcium of almost 0.35 mg/dl (0.09 mmol/l) after two hours [14]. In the study of Green et al., the change in the calcium concentration after tricalcium phosphate (1200 mg calcium, powder mixed in water) was 0.1 mmol/l [12]. In present study, plasma calcium concentration rose by approximately 0.06 mmol/l in four hours after single administration and by about 0.1 mmol/l after repeated administration. The significantly higher calcium concentration at 240 min after single and repeated CaP administration and the significantly higher AUC for the increment in calcium concentration after repeated CaP administration compared to placebo suggest that part of the calcium from the CaP supplement was absorbed. Supplementation with CaP led to an increase in blood calcium concentration, which is comparable to other studies.

Because hyperphosphatemia is linked with vascular calcification, cardiovascular mortality, and progression of chronic kidney disease, phosphate intake is an aspect that is controversially discussed [17-19]. In the present study, there was no difference in the plasma phosphate concentration between CaP and placebo after 240 min. In another study by Reginster et al. comprising 10 male subjects, the serum phosphorus concentration did not change after supplementation with tricalcium phosphate (1000 mg Ca) within a time frame of 360 min [20]. In contrast, both Yang et al. and Shires et al. showed an increase in phosphorus concentration after an intake of 1200 mg calcium [21,22].

Interestingly, after all administrations (single CaP and placebo administration, repeated CaP and placebo administrations), phosphate concentration significantly decreased at first, followed by a rise to basal concentration (Figure 2). Karp et al. showed similar results for plasma phosphate concentration after supplementation with different calcium supplements and potassium citrate [23]. Because of a decrease in bone resorption, the authors assumed a decrease in the release of phosphate from bone for potassium citrate only [23]. Moreover, hypophosphatemia can be a result of phosphate shifts from the blood into the cells, such as after ingestion of glucose, fructose, and feeding following starvation (phosphorylation processes) [24]. A glucose load can induce a transient reduction in serum phosphate levels [24], probably due to secretion of gastrointestinal hormones and subsequent stimulation of calcitonin [25]. Calcitonin induces an inhibition of osteoclasts and a reduction in the release of phosphorus from bone into blood. However, the association between gastrointestinal hormones and calcitonin has only been shown in rodents and not in humans [26].

Alternatively, the decreasing concentration of phosphate in the present study can also be explained by a dilution effect as participants were allowed to drink water ad libitum after the test meal. Between time points 60–120 min, the phosphate concentration increased again to baseline levels indicating that intestinal phosphate absorption took place within this time frame. Indeed, in the study by Karp et al., the participants were also allowed to drink water ad libitum[23]. In contrast, studies in which liquid intake were restricted showed either an immediate increase or a constant phosphate concentration [20-22].

Hence, the present results indicate that the increased phosphate intake due to the CaP supplementation, did probably not lead to an increased phosphate absorption in the gut. This conclusion is supported by comparably postprandial phosphate concentrations and the similar AUC for the increment in phosphate concentration after CaP and placebo administrations. In order to confirm these results, isotopic tracer studies are indicated. However, the results show that phosphate from this CaP supplement did not lead to an increase in plasma phosphate concentration.

2.5 CONCLUSION

In conclusion, our results show that CaP contributes to an adequate calcium supply, but without increasing the plasma concentration of phosphate. Indeed, the major part of the phosphate from the CaP supplement is precipitated as amorphous calcium phosphate in the human gut, an aspect that has been shown in several human studies [3,5,27,28].

REFERENCES

1. Eddington H, Hoefield R, Sinha S, Chrysochou C, Lane B, Foley RN, Hegarty J, New J, O'Donoghue DJ, Middleton RJ, Kalra PA: Serum phosphate and mortality in patients with chronic kidney disease. Clin J Am Soc Nephrol 2010, 5:2251-2257.
2. Adeney KL, Siscovick DS, Ix JH, Seliger SL, Shlipak MG, Jenny NS, Kestenbaum BR: Association of serum phosphate with vascular and valvular calcification in moderate CKD. J Am Soc Nephrol 2009, 20:381-387.
3. Ditscheid B, Keller S, Jahreis G: Cholesterol metabolism is affected by calcium phosphate supplementation in humans. J Nutr 2005, 135:1678-1682. Grimm M, Muller A, Hein G, Funfstuck R, Jahreis G: High phosphorus intake only slightly affects serum minerals, urinary pyridinium crosslinks and renal function in young women. Eur J Clin Nutr 2001, 55:153-161.
4. Trautvetter U, Ditscheid B, Kiehntopf M, Jahreis G: A combination of calcium phosphate and probiotics beneficially influences intestinal lactobacilli and cholesterol metabolism in humans. Clin Nutr 2012, 31:230-237.
5. Govers MJ, Van der Meer R: Effects of dietary calcium and phosphate on the intestinal interactions between calcium, phosphate, fatty acids, and bile acids. Gut 1993, 34:365-370.
6. Van der Meer R, Lapre JA, Govers M, Kleibeuker JH: Mechanisms of the intestinal effects of dietary fats and milk products on colon carcinogenesis. Cancer Lett 1997, 114:75-83.
7. Bovee-Oudenhoven I, Van der Meer R: Protective effects of dietary lactulose and calcium phosphate against Salmonella infection. Scand J Gastroenterol Suppl 1997, 222:112-114.
8. Ditscheid B, Keller S, Jahreis G: Faecal steroid excretion in humans is affected by calcium supplementation and shows gender-specific differences. Eur J Nutr 2009, 48:22-30.
9. Heaney RP, Recker RR, Weaver CM: Absorbability of calcium sources: the limited role of solubility. Calcif Tissue Int 1990, 46:300-304.
10. Rafferty K, Walters G, Heaney RP: Calcium fortificants: Overview and strategies for improving calcium nutriture of the US population. J Food Sci 2007, 72:R152-R158.
11. Green JH, Booth C, Bunning R: Acute effect of high-calcium milk with or without additional magnesium, or calcium phosphate on parathyroid hormone and biochemical markers of bone resorption. Eur J Clin Nutr 2003, 57:61-68.
12. Hanzlik RP, Fowler SC, Fisher DH: Relative bioavailability of calcium from calcium formate, calcium citrate, and calcium carbonate. J Pharmacol Exp Ther 2005, 313:1217-1222.
13. Heaney RP, Rafferty K, Dowell MS, Bierman J: Calcium fortification systems differ in bioavailability. J Am Diet Assoc 2005, 105:807-809.

14. Heller HJ, Greer LG, Haynes SD, Poindexter JR, Pak CY: Pharmacokinetic and pharmacodynamic comparison of two calcium supplements in postmenopausal women. J Clin Pharmacol 2000, 40:1237-1244.
15. Heller HJ, Stewart A, Haynes S, Pak CY: Pharmacokinetics of calcium absorption from two commercial calcium supplements. J Clin Pharmacol 1999, 39:1151-1154.
16. Ellam TJ, Chico TJ: Phosphate: the new cholesterol? The role of the phosphate axis in non-uremic vascular disease. Atherosclerosis 2012, 220:310-318.
17. Gonzalez-Parra E, Tunon J, Egido J, Ortiz A: Phosphate: a stealthier killer than previously thought? Cardiovasc Pathol 2012, 21:372-381.
18. Uribarri J: Phosphorus homeostasis in normal health and in chronic kidney disease patients with special emphasis on dietary phosphorus intake. Semin Dial 2007, 20:295-301.
19. Reginster JY, Denis D, Bartsch V, Deroisy R, Zegels B, Franchimont P: Acute biochemical variations induced by four different calcium salts in healthy male volunteers. Osteoporos Int 1993, 3:271-275.
20. Shires R, Kessler GM: The absorption of tricalcium phosphate and its acute metabolic effects. Calcif Tissue Int 1990, 47:142-144.
21. Yang RS, Liu TK, Tsai KS: The acute metabolic effects of oral tricalcium phosphate and calcium carbonate. Calcif Tissue Int 1994, 55:335-341.
22. Karp HJ, Ketola ME, Lamberg-Allardt CJ: Acute effects of calcium carbonate, calcium citrate and potassium citrate on markers of calcium and bone metabolism in young women. Br J Nutr 2009, 102:1341-1347.
23. Berner YN, Shike M: Consequences of phosphate imbalance. Annu Rev Nutr 1988, 8:121-148.
24. Yamada C, Yamada Y, Tsukiyama K, Yamada K, Udagawa N, Takahashi N, Tanaka K, Drucker DJ, Seino Y, Inagaki N: The murine glucagon-like peptide-1 receptor is essential for control of bone resorption. Endocrinology 2008, 149:574-579.
25. Bjerre Knudsen L, Madsen LW, Andersen S, Almholt K, de Boer AS, Drucker DJ, Gotfredsen C, Egerod FL, Hegelund AC, Jacobsen H: Glucagon-like Peptide-1 receptor agonists activate rodent thyroid C-cells causing calcitonin release and C-cell proliferation. Endocrinology 2010, 151:1473-1486.
26. Lapre JA, De Vries HT, Van der Meer R: Dietary calcium phosphate inhibits cytotoxicity of fecal water. Am J Physiol Gastrointest Liver Physiol 1991, 261:G907-912.
27. Van der Meer R, Termont DS, De Vries HT: Differential effects of calcium ions and calcium phosphate on cytotoxicity of bile acids. Am J Physiol 1991, 260:G142-147.

This chapter was originally published under the Creative Commons Attribution License. Trautvetter, U., Kiehntopf, M., and Jahreis, G . Postprandial Effects of Calcium Phosphate Supplementation on Plasma Concentration-Double-Blind, Placebo-Controlled Cross-Over Human Study. Nutrition Journal. 2013; 12(30). doi:10.1186/14752891-12-30.

EFFICACY OF VITAMIN C AS AN ADJUNCT TO FLUOXETINE THERAPY IN PEDIATRIC MAJOR DEPRESSIVE DISORDER: A RANDOMIZED, DOUBLE-BLIND, PLACEBO-CONTROLLED PILOT STUDY

MOSTAFA AMR, AHMED EL-MOGY, TAREK SHAMS, KAREN VIEIRA, and SHAHEEN E. LAKHAN

3.1 INTRODUCTION

The prevalence of depression in community settings has been estimated to be between 0.4% and 2.5% in children and 0.4% and 8.3% in adolescents [1]. However, in a more recent community study of children without depression who were initially assessed between the ages of 9 and 13 years, more than 7% of boys and almost 12% of girls developed a depressive disorder by the age of 16 [2].

While the diagnosis of major depressive disorder (MDD) in younger patients generally follows the criteria set forth in the Diagnostic and Statistical Manual of Mental Disorders, 4th edition, text revision (DSM-IV-TR) [3], the treatment of pediatric depression presents many challenges. Not only do children with MDD have multiple co-morbid disorders [4,5], psychosocial and academic problems, and are at increased risk for suicide attempts, self-harm, and substance abuse [1,6-10], treatment options are often limited and ineffective, poorly tolerated, and generally present long delays in delivering a therapeutic benefit [11-14].

One of the few antidepressants approved for use in children is the selective serotonin reuptake inhibitor (SSRI) fluoxetine [15]. The first study that demonstrated the positive effects of using fluoxetine to treat depression in child and adolescent patients was published in 1997 [16], following a small trial in which no difference was observed between fluoxetine treatment and placebo [17]. Overall, five clinical trials have been conducted which show the positive effects of using fluoxetine to treat pediatric depression [16,18-21]. In addition, the improvement response rate on the Clinical Global Impressions (CGI) for antidepressant use was found to be between 52% and 61% for fluoxetine patients versus 33% to 37% for patients treated with placebo [22]. The CGI measures whether or not depressive symptoms have improved after treatment.

Despite being one of the most popular treatments for pediatric patients, in 2004 the use of prescription medication such as fluoxetine as well as other antidepressant medications declined by approximately 20% in the United States [23]. This shift in prescription patterns is likely due to warnings issued by regulatory agencies, initially in the United Kingdom [24] and later in the United States [25], against the use of SSRIs to treat depression in pediatric populations due to the possible link between antidepressant usage and an increased incidence of suicidal ideations or attempts. Subsequently, there is a compelling need for better understanding of the pathophysiology of MDD as well as the development of novel treatment methods that can be used to improve the current clinical management of pediatric depression.

Nutrients like vitamin C (ascorbic acid) have become of interest in adjuvant therapy settings for the management of depressive symptoms due to the fact that psychological abnormalities are among the characteristics of vitamin C deficiency [26-29]. A recent population-based survey revealed that 60% of the patients in the acute medical wards of a Montreal teaching hospital were vitamin C deficient, while this deficiency was only detected in 16% of people attending the hospital's outpatient center [30]. There is also preliminary evidence that the administration of vitamin C may be able to reduce the severity of MDD in both children [31] and adults [32], as well as improve mood in healthy individuals [33-35]. In addition, a recent study reported a 35% reduction in average mood disturbance in hospitalized patients following treatment with vitamin C (1000 mg/day) [36]. In one particular study that investigated mood, patients who were acutely hospitalized were either treated with vitamin C or vitamin D as a deficiency in both of these vitamins has been associated with psychological abnormalities [32]. The results showed that only vitamin C led to an improved mood. More specifically, treating the vitamin C deficiency led to a decrease in mood disturbance while vitamin D supplementation had no effect on mood. Similar findings were observed in non-critically ill hospitalized patients who were treated with vitamin C for hypovitaminosis C [36]. Moreover, an animal study showed that the co-administration of vitamin C was found to potentiate the action of subeffective doses of fluoxetine (1 mg/kg) [37]. This synergistic antidepressant effect of vitamin C and fluoxetine suggests that this vitamin could be helpful in improving conventional pharmacotherapy for pediatric MDD and potentially reduce side effects.

This study would be the first to examine the efficacy of vitamin C as an adjunct to SSRIs in the treatment of pediatric depression. In addition, the low potential toxicity, inexpensiveness, and over-the-counter availability, we sought to investigate whether oral supplementation of vitamin C would improve clinical depressive symptoms. Therefore, the present study was designed to measure the effect of vitamin C on the Children's Depression Rating Scale (CDRS), the Children's Depression Inventory (CDI), and the CGI scores in pediatric patients with depression taking fluoxetine.

3.2 METHODS

3.2.1 TRIAL DESIGN

The study was a prospective, double-blind, placebo-controlled, six-month clinical trial. Two parallel groups of outpatient pediatric patients with depression in Mansoura University Hospital, Egypt participated in the study from October 2009 to September 2011. The study was approved by the institution's review board.

3.2.2 PARTICIPANTS

The authors screened pediatric patients (less than 18 years of age) who were referred to the outpatient psychiatry clinic for MDD based on a semi-structured interview and DSM-IV-TR criteria [3]. Exclusion criteria included clinically significant organic or neurological disorder, psychotic disorder or depression with psychotic features, a history of substance abuse or dependence, or prior use of psychotropic medication. Young patients with bipolar disorder may experience adverse psychological effects such as mania and hypomania due to antidepressants and were therefore, excluded from the study. It has been shown that patients who are young in age at the onset of bipolar disorder demonstrate an illness progression that is characterized by high rates of switching into mania or hypomania in response to antidepressant treatment [38]. Among the 32 patients screened during this period, five were excluded (two had depression with psychotic features, two had a history of hypomania, and one had a substance abuse disorder). The remaining 27 patients agreed to participate in this study after informed consent from at least one parent was obtained. The patients did not receive any other treatment such as cognitive behavioral therapy during the trial period. This trial was performed in accordance with the Declaration of Helsinki and subsequent revisions [39]. Written consent was obtained from each patient's parent or guardian before entering the study.

3.2.3 INTERVENTION

Vitamin C and placebo were formulated into capsules by the Mansoura University Hospital. The patients were randomly allocated to either the treatment or control group using a computer-generated list of random numbers. Fourteen patients were assigned to the treatment group and were given fluoxetine (10–20 mg/day) plus vitamin C (1000 mg/day; 500 mg BID). Thirteen patients were assigned to the control group and were given fluoxetine (10–20 mg/day) plus placebo. Patients less than eight years of age received fluoxetine (10 mg/day), whereas patients eight years of age or older were given 10 mg/day of fluoxetine for one week and 20 mg/day all subsequent weeks as per the prescribing information [40]. There are several published studies which support the administration of 20 mg/day of fluoxetine for children at least eight years of age [16,18,20,21], and it is within FDA indication. The use of fluoxetine for children under the age of eight is off-label. A dose of 1000 mg/day of vitamin C (500 mg BID) was chosen based on human studies suggest that psychiatric patients generally require higher levels of vitamin C to improve symptoms than the doses that are recommended for healthy individuals [32,41]. The recommended dose of vitamin C for healthy individuals is 70 mg/day, while a dose of 1000 mg/day needs to be consumed before symptoms begin to improve in psychiatric patients [41].

Patients in the placebo group received two identical capsules (morning and evening). No other psychotropic medications were prescribed. Three subjects were removed from the trial due to noncompliance (two patients from the vitamin C group and one from the placebo group). Patients were assessed using CDRS, an Arabic version of CDI, and CGI at the baseline as well as 3 and 6 months after the start of treatment. The scores for the CDRS were based on parent ratings, CDI on children ratings, and CGI on clinician ratings. Examinations of patients during the treatment period were performed by a psychiatrist trained in the use of these instruments.

3.2.4 INSTRUMENTS

The Children's Depression Rating Scale (CDRS) is a 16-item measure used to determine the severity of depression in children and adolescents aged 6 to 12 [42]. The CDRS is derived from the Hamilton Rating Scale for Depression (HAM-D) [43] and is based on parent, child, and school-teacher interviews. CDRS scores show good concordance with research diagnostic criteria for depression [44] and correlate highly with other in-terview and self-report measures of depression severity [45].

The Children's Depression Inventory (CDI) is a 27-item, self-rated, symptom-oriented scale suitable for children and adolescents aged 7 to 17 [46]. The CDI is sensitive to changes in depressive symptoms over time, making it a useful index for the severity of MDD. The CDI is reported to have high internal consistency and test-retest reliability [47]. The CDI assessment utilized in this study was based on the previously developed instrument [46] and was translated and normalized for Arab children by Gharib (1988) [48]. Reliability and validity data for the Arabic version are comparable to those provided for the original instrument.

The Clinical Global Impressions Scale (CGI) is a 3-item, observer-rated scale that measures illness severity, global improvement or change, and therapeutic response [49]. The CGI is rated on a 7-point scale with each component being rated separately; the instrument does not yield a global score. Over the past 30 years, the CGI has been shown to correlate well with standard, well-known research drug efficacy scales, including the Hamilton Rating Scale for Depression, the Brief Psychiatric Rating Scale, and the Scale for the Assessment of Negative Symptoms across a wide range of psychiatric indications [50].

3.2.5 STATISTICAL ANALYSIS

Student's t-tests and chi-squared tests were used to evaluate possible differences in baseline demographics. Two-way repeated measures analysis of variance (ANOVA) were used to assess the effects of treatment (treatment versus placebo), time (months of visit), and an interaction between the treatment and time. Significant differences in the mean scores for each visit were assessed through unpaired Student's t-tests. Quantitative variables were tested for normal distributions by the Kolmogorov-Smirnov test. The variables were presented as means ± standard deviations (SD). Statistical significance was set at the 5% level. SPSS for Windows version 13 was used for the statistical analysis of the data obtained from the study.

3.3 RESULTS

3.3.1 DEMOGRAPHIC CHARACTERISTICS AND ATTRITION

Thirty-two patients were initially examined, but five patients did not satisfy the inclusion criteria. Therefore 27 patients enrolled in the study; 14

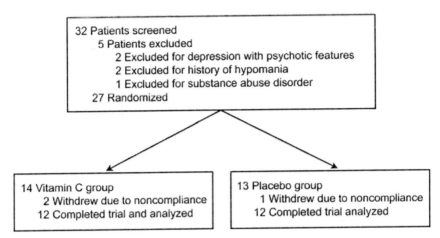

FIGURE 1: Diagram demonstrating the disposition of all patients screened for the study.

assigned to the vitamin C group and 13 to the placebo group. Twenty-four patients aged between 7 and 14 completed the six-month trial. Two patients from the vitamin C group and one patient from the placebo group were removed from the trial due to noncompliance (Figure 1).

The characteristics of the two study groups are summarized in Table 1. The two groups were well matched, and there were no statistically significant differences between the groups with regard to demographic factors or duration of illness.

3.3.2 EFFECT ON CDRS, CDI AND CGI SCORES

The clinical severity of the depression was comparable at baseline and not significantly different across all three clinical instruments. As shown in Figure 2, mean scores for CDRS, CDI, and CGI gradually improved in both study groups during the trial. ANOVA was significantly different on all clinical measurements (group effect, time effect, and interaction), with the exception of group effect and interaction for CGI. The results of ANOVA are presented in Table 2.

TABLE 1: Demographic data of the participants in fluoxetine + vitamin C and fluoxetine + placebo groups

Characteristic	Vitamin C group	Placebo group	P
Age (years)	10.3 ±2.2	9.9 ±2.1	0.653
Sex (M/F)	7/5	8/4	0.673
Duration of illness (months)	4.3 ±1.1	4.5 ±0.1	0.5370

Statistical significance defined as P<0.05.

Table 2: Repeated-measures analysis of variance assessments at baseline and after 3 and 6 months in fluoxetine + vitamin C and fluoxetine + placebo groups

	Group effect			Time effect			Interaction		
Variable	F	Df	P	F	Df	P	F	Df	P
CDRS	155.90	1, 11	<0.0001	294.59	1.6, 17	<0.0001	25.14	1.4, 18.4	<0.0001
CDI	89.69	1, 11	<0.0001	512.77	1.8, 19.4	<0.0001	57.21	1.8, 19.8	<0.0001
CGI	0.000	1, 11	1.000	447.95	1.6, 17.2	<0.0001	0.68	1.1, 12.1	0.438

Statistical significance defined as P<0.05. CDI: Children's Depression Inventory; CDRS: Children's Depression Rating Scale; CGI: Clinical Global Impression.

The most striking effects were observed for the interaction between treatment and time: CDRS (F=25.16, df=1.4, 18.4, P<0.0001) and CDI (F=57.21, df=1.8, 19.8, P<0.0001). There was no significant interaction effect in CGI scores (F=0.68, df=1.1, 12.1, P=0.438).

The clinical changes demonstrated with vitamin C intake compared to placebo were noted by the third month of the study (Table 3). At three months, a significant difference was observed on CDRS (t=9.85, P<0.0001) and CDI (t=10.77, P<0.0001), but not CGI (t=0.15, P=0.88). By the end of trial (six months), the vitamin C group showed a significantly larger decrease in depressive symptoms compared to the placebo group as measured by CDRS (t=11.36, P<0.0001) and CDI (t=12.27, P<0.0001). However, the effect on CGI was not significantly different (t=0.13, P=0.90) at six months.

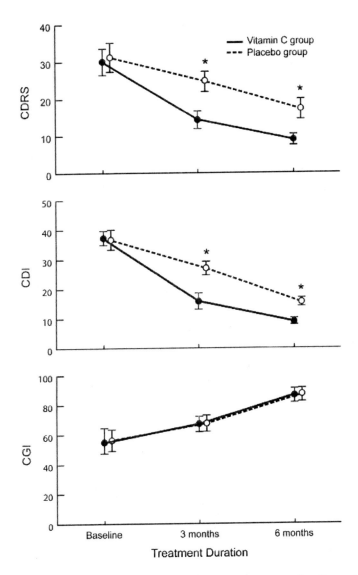

FIGURE 2: Mean and SD changes in CDRS, CDI, and CGI scores at baseline and after 3 and 6 months in fluoxetine + vitamin C and fluoxetine + placebo groups. Asterisk indicates statistical significance defined as P<0.05. CDI: Children's Depression Inventory; CDRS: Children's Depression Rating Scale; CGI: Clinical Global Impression; SD: standard deviation.

TABLE 3: CDRS, CDI, and CGI scores at baseline and after 3 and 6 months in fluoxetine + vitamin C and fluoxetine + placebo groups

Variable	Treatment duration	Vitamin C group	Placebo group	t	P
CDRS	Baseline	30.1 ±3.56	31.3 ±3.89	0.77	0.45
	3 months	14.4 ±2.39	24.7 ±2.73	9.85	<0.0001
	6 months	9.0 ±1.50	17.3 ±2.73	11.36	<0.0001
CDI	Baseline	37.3 ±2.38	36.7 ±3.33	−0.42	0.68
	3 months	15.8 ±2.75	27.0 ±2.30	10.77	<0.0001
	6 months	9.0 ±1.12	15.5 ±1.45	12.27	<0.0001
CGI	Baseline	54.7 ±7.19	56.3 ±7.23	0.57	0.58
	3 months	67.1 ±5.04	67.4 ±5.55	0.15	0.88
	6 months	86.5 ±4.91	86.7 ±4.41	0.13	0.90

Values given are mean ± standard deviation. The statistics listed were measured with t-test. Statistical significance defined as $P<0.05$. CDI: Children's Depression Inventory; CDRS: Children's Depression Rating Scale; CGI: Clinical Global Impression.

3.3.3 CLINICAL COMPLICATIONS AND ADVERSE EFFECTS

No major adverse effects were observed.

3.4 DISCUSSION

These results show that orally administered vitamin C as an adjunct to fluoxetine treatment leads to significantly greater decreases in depressive symptoms in comparison to fluoxetine treatment alone. This was demonstrated by the decrease in depressive symptoms, which was observed in the improved CDRS and CDI scores. A significant effect was not observed for the CGI, but this may be related to the response items for this instrument. For instance, symptoms were scored according to whether "much improvement" or "very much improvement" was observed [49]. Although there may have been a slight increase in CGI scores, response items such as these may have made it difficult to detect a significant improvement of symptoms. The differences between the scores may have also been related to the individuals who supplied the ratings for each instrument. More specifically, the scores for the CDRS were based on parent ratings, the scores for the CDI were based on children ratings, and the scores for the CGI were based on clinician ratings. The scores from the CGI were computed based on clinical criteria such as that which is listed in the DSM-IV-TR as well as semi-structured interviews. Therefore, the clinician's rating and score interpretations adhered to strict guidelines and training, whereas the ratings from parents and children may have been more subjective leading to significantly different scores. Nonetheless, these preliminary findings, including the results of ANOVA suggest that vitamin C may be an effective adjuvant agent for the treatment of depression in pediatric patients. Furthermore, the results support the notion that vitamin C has antidepressant-like properties and are in accordance with previous animal research that demonstrated vitamin C's ability to potentiate the action of conventional antidepressants [37].

Despite the lack of research investigating the effects of vitamin C in pediatric patients with MDD, previous studies have suggested that vitamin C improves clinical symptoms in other psychiatric disorders [51-53], and that vitamin C supplementation can be used to positively modulate mood [33-35]. Furthermore, Khanzode et al., (2003) showed that plasma levels of vitamin C were decreased in depressive patients [54]. In a more recent study, Chang et al., (2007) described a case in which a patient with depression developed scurvy, suggesting that reduced plasma levels of vitamin C due to inadequate vitamin C intake could be associated with the pathophysiology of depression [29]. Other studies have also shown that depressive symptoms are associated with scurvy [55-57].

While the exact role of vitamin C in the etiology of MDD is not well understood, a growing body of evidence suggests that oxidative stress, characterized by an accumulation of free radicals due to an organism's inhibited antioxidant capacity, may play a primary or secondary role in the pathogenesis of neurological and psychiatric diseases like MDD [58,59]. The brain is much more vulnerable to oxidative free radicals than other tissues since it utilizes 20% of the oxygen consumed by the body, contains large amounts of polyunsaturated fatty acids and iron, and typically has low concentrations of antioxidant enzymes [60]. Previous studies have shown that MDD may be accompanied by disturbances in the balance between pro- and anti-oxidative processes, demonstrated by decreased blood plasma levels of the antioxidants enzymes superoxide dismutase, catalase, and glutathione peroxidase and an increased level of lipid peroxidation by-products in patients with depression versus healthy controls [54,61,62].

While antidepressant drugs may affect the oxidative or antioxidative systems [54], partly due to their effects on the immune [63] and P450 systems [64], adjunctive therapy with vitamin C may provide additional protection as it is the brain's most abundant antioxidant and plays an important role in preventing free radical-induced damage [65,66]. In addition to its neuroprotective properties, vitamin C has also been identified as a neuromodulator in the brain, modulating both dopamine- and glutamate-mediated neurotransmission [67-69]. As there is a considerable amount of pharmacological evidence demonstrating the efficacy of antidepressants with dopaminergic effects in the treatment of depression [70], vitamin C's complex interaction with the dopaminergic system may be another potential mechanism of action. However this effect appears to be dose-dependent. Wambebe and Sokomba (1986) showed that administering 50–200 mg/kg of vitamin C to rats enhanced dopamine-mediated behavioral effects [71], while higher dosages have been shown to antagonize such effects [68].

There are a number of other potential biological substrates that underlie vitamin C's effects on depression and mood. For example, Binfaré et al. [37] identified the involvement of 5-HT1A receptors in the antidepressant-like effect of vitamin C. Additionally, adjuvant administration of vitamin C may also prove useful in decreasing the risk of suicidal thoughts and behaviors linked to antidepressant therapy in pediatric patients [72]. Meta-analyses of placebo-controlled studies have indicated that antidepressants may cause a significant, although small and short-term, risk of self-harm or suicide-related events in children and adolescents with MDD, no completed suicides were reported in any trial included in the analysis [73,74]. Li et al. [75] reported that a history of attempted suicide was shown to be associated with a low level of antioxidant vitamins and carotenoids. Therefore, increasing plasma vitamin C levels in children and adolescents who are being treated with antidepressants may help mitigate some of this risk. However, as suicidal thoughts and behaviors were not measured in the present study, future clinical research is needed to test this hypothesis.

3.4.1 LIMITATIONS

The present study has several limitations, one being its small sample size. While pilot clinical trials can play an important role in the early assessment of novel treatment methods when they are well designed and evaluated [76], further studies with larger sample sizes are needed to substantiate the results of this study. Secondly, drawing conclusions from a combined sample of children and adolescents with regard to the response to medication should be done with precaution as there is reason to believe that children respond differently than adolescents to antidepressants [77]. Also, due to the low potential for adverse drug reactions related to vitamin C in this study, the effect of doses higher than 1000 mg/day should be considered in future studies.

Measuring plasma vitamin C levels pre- and post-treatment may also be of interest, but although these levels were not measured, previous studies have demonstrated the association between hypovitaminosis C (vitamin C deficiency) and psychological abnormalities and this deficiency is highly prevalent in acutely hospitalized patients [32,36]. Furthermore, the increase in plasma and mononuclear leukocyte vitamin C from subnormal to normal concentrations after the administration of vitamin C administration implicate that the metabolic properties of hypovitaminosis C are consistent with deficiency as opposed to different mechanisms such as tissue redistribution [36]. These findings also indicate that patients with depression, such as those who participated in this study, may experience vitamin C deficiency and that the decrease in depressive symptoms that was observed may be directly attributed to the synergistic antidepressant effect of vitamin C and fluoxetine. Future studies that involve measuring plasma vitamin C levels may further support these findings. Finally, in the current study, participants were only treated and assessed for a short period of time (six months). The most striking effects were observed for the interaction between treatment and time and this finding suggests that longer trials are needed to better assess the efficacy of vitamin C as an adjunct to fluoxetine therapy.

3.5 CONCLUSION

Treatment with 1000 mg/day of vitamin C potentiated the efficacy of fluoxetine in pediatric patients being treated for MDD. Furthermore, vitamin C was shown to be a particularly attractive therapeutic adjuvant due to the absence of substantial side effects and its inexpensive cost. The observed improvements in CDRS and CDI scores also imply that this type of treatment effectively increases blood plasma levels of vitamin C as it has been shown that ascorbic acid deficiency is associated with psychological abnormalities [26-29]. Future, large-scale clinical trials are warranted to evaluate the therapeutic efficacy of vitamin C for the treatment of depression in pediatric patients as well as its effectiveness as an adjuvant treatment to antidepressants.

REFERENCES

1. Birmaher B, Ryan N, Williamson D, Brent D, Kaufman J, Dahl R, Perel J, Nelson B: Childhood and adolescent depression: a review of the past 10 years. Part I. J Am Acad Child Adolesc Psychiatry 1996, 35:1427-1439.
2. Costello E, Mustillo S, Erkanli A, Keeler G, Angold A: Prevalence and development of psychiatric disorders in childhood and adolescence. Arch Gen Psychiatry 2003, 60:837-844.
3. American Psychiatric Association: Diagnostic and statistical manual of mental disorders. 4th edition. Washington, DC: American Psychiatric Association; 2000.
4. Goodyer I, Herbert J, Secher S, Pearson J: Short-term outcome of major depression: I. Comorbidity and severity at presentation as predictors of persistent disorder. J Am Acad Child Adolesc Psychiatry 1997, 36:179-187.
5. Hughes C, Preskorn S, Weller E, Weller R, Hassanein R, Tucker S: The effect of concomitant disorders in childhood depression on predicting treatment response. Psychopharmacol Bull 1990, 26:235-238.
6. Birmaher B, Arbelaez C, Brent D: Course and outcome of child and adolescent major depressive disorder. Child Adolesc Psychiatr Clin N Am 2002, 11:619-637.
7. Lewinsohn P, Allen N, Seeley J, Gotlib I: First onset versus recurrence of depression: differential processes of psychosocial risk. J Abnorm Psychol 1999, 108:483-489.
8. Pine D, Cohen P, Gurley D, Brook J, Ma Y: The risk for early-adulthood anxiety and depressive disorders in adolescents with anxiety and depressive disorders. Arch Gen Psychiatry 1998, 55:56-64.
9. Weissman M, Wolk S, Goldstein R, Moreau D, Adams P, Greenwald S, Klier C, Ryan N, Dahl R, Wickramaratne P: Depressed adolescents grownup. JAMA 1999, 281:1707-1713.

10. Weissman M, Wolk S, Wickramaratne P, Goldstein R, Adams P, Greenwald S, Ryan N, Dahl R, Steinberg D: Children with prepubertal-onset major depressive disorder and anxiety grown up. Arch Gen Psychiatry 1999, 56:794-801.

11. Berton O, Nestler E: New approaches to antidepressant drug discovery: beyond monoamines. Nat Rev Neurosci 2006, 7:137-151.

12. Holtzheimer P, Nemeroff C: Advances in the treatment of depression. NeuroRx Journal 2006, 3:42-56.

13. Nemeroff C, Owens M: Treatment of mood disorders. Nat Neurosci 2002, 5:1068-1070.

14. Calles JJ: Depression in children and adolescents. Primary Care: Clinics in Office Practice 2007, 34:243-258.

15. Boylan K, Romero S, Birmaher B: Psychopharmacologic treatment of pediatric major depressive disorder. Psychopharmacology 2007, 191:27-38.

16. Emslie G, Rush A, Weinberg W, Kowatch R, Hughes C, Carmody T, Rintelmann J: A double-blind, randomized, placebo-controlled trial of fluoxetine in children and adolescents with depression. Arch Gen Psychiatry 1997, 54:1031-1037.

17. Simeon J, Dinicola V, Ferguson H, Copping W: Adolescent depression: a placebo-controlled fluoxetine treatment study and follow-up. Progress in Neuropsychopharmacology Biological Psychiatry 1990, 14:791-795.

18. Emslie G, Heiligenstein J, Wagner K, Hoog S, Ernest D, Brown E, Nilsson M, Jacobson J: Fluoxetine for acute treatment of depression in children and adolescents: a placebocontrolled, randomized clinical trial. J Am Acad Child Adolesc Psychiatry 2002, 41:1205-1215.

19. March J, Silva S, Petrycki S, Curry J, Wells K, Fairbank J: Fluoxetine, cognitive-behavioral therapy, and their combination for adolescents with depression: Treatment for Adolescents With Depression Study (TADS) randomized controlled trial. JAMA 2004, 292:807-820.

20. Bridge J, Jyengar S, Salary C, Barbe R, Birmaher B, Pincus H: Clinical response and risk for suicidal ideation and suicide attempts in pediatric antidepressant treatment. Journal of the Amercian Medical Association 2007, 297:1683-1696.

21. Emslie G, Kennard B, Mayes T, Nightingale-Teresi J, Carmody T, Hughes C: Fluoxetine versus placebo in preventing relapse of major depression in children and adolescents. Am J Psychiatry 2008, 165:459-467.

22. Bridge J, Salary C, Birmaher B, Asare A, Brent D: The risks and benefits of antidepressant treatment for youth depression. Ann Med 2005, 37:404-412.

23. Rosack J: New data show declines in antidepressant prescribing. Psychiatr News 2005, 40:1.

24. Selective serotonin reuptake inhibitors: use in children and adolescents with major depressive disorder. [http:// www.mhra.gov.uk/ home/ groups/ pl-p/ documents/ drugsafetymessage/ con019492.pdf]

25. Labeling change request letter. http://www.fda.gov/cder/drug/antidepressants/SSRI-labelChange.htm

26. Kinsman R, Hood J: Some behavioral effects of ascorbic acid deficiency. Am J Clin Nutr 1971, 24:455-464.

27. Levine M, Conry-Cantilena C, Wang Y, Welch R, Washko P, Dhariwal K, Park J, Lazarev A, Graumlich J, King J, Cantilena L: Vitamin C pharmacokinetics in

healthy volunteers: evidence for a recommended dietary allowance. Proc Natl Acad Sci 1996, 93:3704-3709.

28. Milner C: Ascorbic acid in chronic psychiatric patients: A controlled trial. Br J Psychiatry 1963, 109:294.

29. Chang C, Chen M, Wang T, Chang W, Lin C, Liu C: Scurvy in a patient with depression. Dig Dis Sci 2007, 52:1259-1261.

30. Gan R, Eintracht S, Hoffer L: Vitamin C deficiency in a university teaching hospital. J Am Coll Nutr 2008, 27:428-433.

31. Cocchi P, Silenzi M, Calabri G, Salvi G: Antidepressant effect of vitamin C. Pediatrics 1980, 65:862-863.

32. Zhang M, Robitaille L, Eintracht S, Hoffer L: Vitamin C provision improves mood in acutely hospitalized patients. Nutrition 2011, 27:530-533.

33. Brody S: High-dose ascorbic acid increases intercourse frequency and improves mood: A randomized controlled clinical trial. Biol Psychiatry 2002, 52:371-374.

34. Kennedy D, Veasey R, Watson A, Dodd F, Jones E, Maggini S, Haskell C: Effects of high-dose B vitamin complex with vitamin C and minerals on subjective mood and performance in healthy males. Psychopharmacology 2010, 211:55-68.

35. Gosney M, Hammond H, Shenkin A, Allsup S: Effect of micronutrient supplementation on mood in nursing home residents. Gerontology 2008, 54:292-299.

36. Evans-Olders R, Eintracht S, Hoffer L: Metabolic origin of hypovitaminosis C in acutely hospitalized patients. Nutrition 2010, 26:1070-1074.

37. Binfaré R, Rosa A, Lobato K, Santos A, Rodrigues A: Ascorbic acid administration produces an antidepressant-like effect: evidence for the involvement of monoaminergic neurotransmission. Progress in Neuropsychopharmacology & Biological Psychiatry 2009, 33:530-540.

38. Valentí M, Pacchiarotti I, Bonnín C, Rosa A, Popovic D, Nivoli A, Goikolea J, Murru A, Undurraga J, Colom F, Vieta E: Risk factors for antidepressant-related switch to mania. J Clin Psychiatry 2012, 73:e271-e276.

39. World Medical Association: World medical association declaration of helsinki: ethical principles for medical research involving human subjects. J Postgrad Med 2002, 48:206.

40. Highlights of Prescribing Information. http://pi.lilly.com/us/zyprexa-pi.pdf webcite

41. Subotičanec K, Folnegović-Šmalc V, Korbar M, Meštrović B, Buzina R: Vitamin C status in chronic schizophrenia. Biol Psychiatry 1990, 28:959-966.

42. Poznanski E, Cook S, Carroll B: A depression rating scale for children. Pediatrics 1979, 64:442-450.

43. Hamilton M: A rating scale for depression. J Neurol Neurosurg Psychiatry 1960, 12:56-62.

44. Poznanski E, Grossman J, Buchsbaum Y, Banegas M, Freeman L, Gibbons R: Preliminary studies of the reliability and validity of the Children's Depression Rating Scale. J Am Acad Child Psychiatry 1984, 23:191-197.

45. Shain B, Naylor M, Alessi N: Comparison of self-rated and clinician-rated measure of depression in adolescents. Am J Psychiatry 1990, 147:793-795.

46. Kovacs M: Rating scales to assess depression in school-age children. Acta Paedopsychiatr 1981, 46:305-315.

47. Saylor C, Finch A, Spirito A, Bennett B: The Children's Depression Inventory: A systematic evaluation of psychometric properties. J Consult Clin Psychol 1984, 52:955-967.

48. Gharib A: Children's depression inventory. Cairo: Dar Al-Nahda; 1988.
49. Guy W: ECDEU Assessment Manual for Psychopharmacology —Revised (DHEW Publ No ADM 76–338). Rockville, MD: U.S. Department of Health, Education, and Welfare, Public Health Service, Alcohol, Drug Abuse, and Mental Health Administration, NIMH Psychopharmacology Research Branch, Division of Extramural Research Programs; 1976.
50. Brusner J, Targum S: The clinical global impressions scale: Applying a research tool in clinical practice. Psychiatry (Edgmont) 2007, 4:28-37.
51. Dakhale GNKS, Khanzode SS, Saoji A: Supplementation of vitamin C with atypical antipsychotics reduces oxidative stress and improves the outcome of schizophrenia. Psychopharmacology 2005, 182:494-498.
52. Hoffer A, Osmond H: Scurvy and schizophrenia. Diseases Of The Nervous System 1967, 24:273.
53. VanderKamp H: A biochemical abnormality in schizophrenia involving ascorbic acid. Int J Neuropsychiatry 1966, 2:204.
54. Khanzode S, Dakhale G, Khanzode S, Saoji A, Palasodkar R: Oxidative damage and major depression: the potential antioxidant action of selective serotonin reuptake inhibitors. Redox Rep 2003, 8:365-370.
55. DeSantis J: Scurvy and psychiatric symptoms. Perspect Psychiatr Care 1993, 29:18-22.
56. Nguyen R, Cowley D, Muir J: Scurvy: a cutaneous clinical diagnosis. Aust J Dermatol 2003, 44:48-51.
57. Stöger H, Wilders-Truschnig M, Schmid M, Petek W, Samonigg H: Scurvy after a suicide attempt by starvation. Deutsche Medizinische Wochenschrift 1994, 119:589-592.
58. Ng F, Berk M, Dean O, Bush A: Oxidative stress in psychiatric disorders: evidence base and therapeutic implications. Int J Neuropsychopharmacol 2008, 11:851-876.
59. Maes M, De Vos N, Pioli R, Demedts P, Wauters A, Neels H, Christophe A: Lower serum vitamin E concentrations in major depression: Another marker of lowered antioxidant defenses in that illness. J Affect Disord 2000, 58:241-246.
60. Sarandol A, Sarandol E, Eker S, Erdinc S, Vatansever E, Kirli S: Major depressive disorder is accompanied with oxidative stress: short-term antidepressant treatment does not alter oxidative–antioxidative systems. Hum Psychopharmacol Clin Exp 2007, 22:67-73.
61. Bilici M, Efe H, Koroglu M, Uydu H, Bekaroglu M, Deger O: Antioxidative enzyme activities and lipid peroxidation in major depression: alterations by antidepressant treatments. J Affect Disord 2001, 64:43-51.
62. Ozcan M, Gulec M, Ozerol E, Polat R, Akyol O: Antioxidant enzyme activities and oxidative stress in affective disorders. Int Clin Psychopharmacol 2004, 19:89-95.
63. Ravindran V, Ravindran G, Sivakanesan R, Rajaguru S: Biochemical and nutritional assessment of tubers from 16 cultivars of sweet potato (Ipomoea batatas L.). J Agric Food Chem 1995, 43:2646-2651.
64. Stahl S: Classical antidepressants, serotonin selective reuptake inhibitors, and noradrenergic reuptake inhibitors. In Essential Psychopharnacology. Edited by SM S. Cambridge: Cambridge University Press; 2000::199-245.
65. Seregi A, Schaefer A, Komlos M: Protective role of brain ascorbic acid content against lipid peroxidation. Experientia 1978, 34:1056-1057.

66. Oke A, May L, Adams R: Ascorbic acid distribution pattern in human brain. In Third conference on Vit C. Edited by Bums J, Reverse J, Machlin L. New York: Annals of New York Academy of Sciences; 1987::1-12.
67. Grunewald R: Ascorbic acid in the brain. Brain Res Rev 1993, 18:123-133.
68. Rebec G, Pierce R: A vitamin as neuromodulator: Ascorbate release into the extracellular fluid of the brain regulates dopaminergic and glutamatergic transmission. Prog Neurobiol 1994, 43:537-565.
69. Rice M: Ascorbate regulation and its neuroprotective role in the brain. Trends Neurosci 2000, 3:209-216.
70. Papakostas G: Dopaminergic-based pharmacotherapies for depression. Eur Neuropsychopharmacol 2006, 16:391-402.
71. Wambebe C, Sokomba E: Some behavioral and EEG effects of ascorbic acid in rats. Psychopharmacology 1986, 89:167-170.
72. Wohlfarth T, van Zwieten B, Lekkerkerker F, Gispen-de Wied C, Ruis J, Elferink A, Storosum J: Antidepressants use in children and adolescents and the risk of suicide. Eur Neuropsychopharmacol 2006, 16:79-83.
73. Dubicka B, Hadley S, Roberts C: Suicidal behaviour in youths with depression treated with new-generation antidepressants: meta-analysis. Br J Psychiatry 2006, 189:393-398.
74. Hammad TALT, Racoosin J: Suicidality in pediatric patients treated with antidepressant drugs. Arch Gen Psychiatry 2006, 63:332-339.
75. Li Y, Zhang J: Serum concentrations of antioxidant vitamins and carotenoid are low in individuals with a history of attempted suicide. Nutr Neurosci 2007, 10:51-58.
76. Matthews J: Small clinical trials: are they all bad? Stat Med 1995, 14:115-126.
77. Moreno C, Roche A, Greenhill L: Pharmacotherapy of child and adolescent depression. Child Adolesc Psychiatr Clin N Am 2006, 15:977-998.

This chapter was originally published under the Creative Commons Attribution License. Amr, M., El-Mogy, A., Shams, T., Vieira, K., and Lakhan, S. E. Efficacy of Vitamin C as an Adjunct to Fluoxetine Therapy in Pediatric Major Depressive Disorder: A Randomized, Double-Blind, Placebo-Controlled Pilot Study. Nutrition Journal. 2013; 12(31). doi:10.1186/1475-2891-12-31.

PART II

ROLE OF CLINICAL NUTRITION IN PREVENTING AND MANAGING ORGAN DISEASE

CHAPTER 4

NUTRITION THERAPY FOR LIVER DISEASES BASED ON THE STATUS OF NUTRITIONAL INTAKE

KENICHIRO YASUTAKE, MOTOYUKI KOHJIMA, MANABU NAKASHIMA, KAZUHIRO KOTOH, MAKOTO NAKAMUTA, and MUNECHIKA ENJOJI

4.1 INTRODUCTION

The liver is one of the main organs of nutritional metabolism, including protein synthesis, glycogen storage, and detoxification. These functions become damaged to a greater or lesser extent in patients with liver diseases, resulting in various metabolic disorders, and their disturbed nutritional condition is associated with disease progression. Therefore, dietary counseling and nutritional intervention can support other medical treatments in some liver diseases.

Nonalcoholic fatty liver disease (NAFLD) is a disease caused by excessive dietary intake, which leads to hepatocytic triglyceride accumulation, obesity, and insulin resistance; hence, nutrition therapy is a basic treatment for NAFLD. NAFLD has a wide spectrum of pathologic conditions from simple steatosis to steatosis with necroinflammation and fibrosis, the condition termed nonalcoholic steatohepatitis (NASH). Nutritional intake in NAFLD patients is characterized as energy overload by a high-carbohydrate and high-fat diet, or excessive cholesterol intake. In patients with chronic hepatitis C (CHC), nutritional support is expected to promote the effect of antiviral treatment, for example, n-3 polyunsaturated fatty acids (PUFAs) inhibit HCV replication, and a low-iron diet is effective in reducing hepatic injury. Various nutritional problems as well as clinical symptoms lie in liver cirrhosis (LC), the end stage of chronic hepatitis, complications of influence and prognosis. Therefore, nutrition therapy is important in preventing these problems. In this paper, nutritional aspects and beneficial nutrition therapies are outlined in patients with NAFLD/NASH, CHC, and LC.

4.2 PROFILE OF NUTRITIONAL INTAKE IN NAFLD PATIENTS

4.2.1 HIGH-CARBOHYDRATE DIET INCLUDING EXCESSIVE INTAKE OF SOFT DRINKS

Studies of NAFLD patients found that they had an increased daily consumption of sugar or sugar-containing beverages by twice or more when compared with their matched controls [1–3]. Imaging indicated that fatty liver disease worsened with an increase in the number of bottles of soft drinks consumed, suggesting that consumption of sugar-containing beverages is a significant predictor of NAFLD [3]. Moreover, in NASH patients, the percentage of simple sugars or carbohydrates contributing to total energy intake was considerably higher compared with that in simple steatosis patients [4]. These findings are explained by the following mechanism; excessive carbohydrates/sugar intake activates sterol regulatory element-binding protein-1c (SREBP-1c), which acts as a transcription factor to activate de novo fatty acid synthesis in hepatocytes [5].

4.2.2 HIGH-FAT DIET

It has been recognized that energy overload by excessive fat intake causes NAFLD [6]. When dietary habits were compared between NASH patients and healthy individuals, the intake of saturated fatty acids was found to be significantly higher in NASH patients [7]. In model animals with an equivalent daily calorie intake, increasing the fat/energy ratio with a high-fat diet resulted in an increase in body weight, upregulation of blood glucose levels, progression of steatosis, and marked inflammation of the liver [8], indicating a close association between excessive fat intake and NASH. In this regard, it is proposed that peroxisome proliferator-activated receptor- (PPAR-) activation may play an important role [5].

4.2.3 EXCESSIVE CHOLESTEROL INTAKE

In an investigation of nutritional intake, dietary cholesterol levels were significantly higher in NASH patients compared with healthy individuals [7]. Also in our study, dietary cholesterol levels were significantly higher in the order of nonobese NAFLD patients, obese NAFLD patients, and healthy controls [9]. In animal models, in which dietary energy intake was within normal limits, a high-cholesterol diet induced NAFLD without obesity [10–12]. Excessive cholesterol intake leads to an increase in its metabolites, oxysterols, which are agonistic ligands for liver X receptor (LXR), resulting in activation of the LXR-SREBP-1c pathway and de novo fatty acid synthesis in hepatocytes [13, 14]. Furthermore, in the NAFLD liver, hepatocytic cholesterol is excessive but de novo cholesterol synthesis is further activated hence, lipid metabolism is dysregulated [13, 14].

4.3 NUTRITION THERAPY FOR NAFLD PATIENTS

4.3.1 TREATMENT FOR OBESE PATIENTS (ORDINARY TYPE OF NAFLD)

When nutrition therapy is considered for NAFLD patients, the actual nutritional intake and content should first be examined in detail to determine which nutrient is the main cause of NAFLD, that is, carbohydrates, fat, or cholesterol. Because the state of nutritional intake and hepatic expression patterns of lipid metabolism-associated factors are different between obese and nonobese NAFLD patients, the target of nutrition therapy is also different in the two groups.

It is common knowledge that the main cause of NAFLD is excessive dietary energy intake in obese patients. In practice, a reduction in nutritional intake by metabolic surgery or dietary counseling improves the condition of NAFLD in obese patients [15, 16]. Usually, the profile of nutritional intake in obese NAFLD patients shows excessive intake of carbohydrates and fat. Therefore, normalizing their intake of these nutrients, which leads to weight reduction, can correct a vicious cycle of abnormal hepatic lipid metabolism. However, it is often hard for patients to maintain weight reduction. Additional therapies for weight reduction, including inhibitors against gastric and pancreatic lipases, such as orlistat, and new antagonists against endocannabinoid receptors, are now being developed although these have not proved to be effective or without side effects.

As additional nutritional means, PUFAs and vitamin E with antioxidant effects may be effective in NAFLD. In a clinical trial of NAFLD patients, treatment with ethyl icosapentate, a type of n-3 PUFA, for 12 months improved liver function to some extent in a biochemical evaluation [17]. n-3 PUFAs exhibit their effect by suppressing the activity of SREBP-1c and de novo fatty acid synthesis. It means that n-3 PUFAs may be effective for patients in whom the main cause of NAFLD is excessive intake of carbohydrates or a shortage of PUFAs, but less effective in NAFLD caused by excessive fat intake. Vitamin E exhibits a greater effect in patients with NASH compared with patients with simple steatosis because of its strong antioxidant activity [18].

4.3.2 TREATMENT FOR NONOBESE PATIENTS

A substantial proportion of NAFLD patients are nonobese and/or are without insulin-resistance in Japan [19, 20]. In our study of nutritional intake, mean intake levels of proteins, fat, carbohydrates, and total energy were not excessive in nonobese patients [9]. However, dietary cholesterol intake was markedly excessive, while intake of PUFAs was insufficient in nonobese patients compared with obese patients and healthy individuals [9]. These characteristic findings may be closely associated with the pathogenesis of NAFLD. In our study, expression levels of lipogenic transcription factor LXR, of which agonistic ligands are oxysterols, were significantly higher in nonobese patients compared with obese patients [13, 14]. Thus, in nonobese NAFLD patients, an excess of cholesterol and its metabolites (oxysterols), leading to activation of de novo fatty acid synthesis via the LXR-SREBP-1c pathway, should be considered as a main cause of steatosis. As a nutritional treatment for these patients, intake of food containing a high level of cholesterol should be restricted. Accordingly, a Niemann-Pick C1-like 1 (NPC1L1) inhibitor (ezetimibe), which decreases cholesterol absorption in the intestine, is a reasonable treatment relevant to nutrition therapy. In practice, ezetimibe treatment in nonobese NAFLD patients improves liver injury and steatosis [21]. Also in animal models, inactivation of NPC1L1, a critical mediator of cholesterol absorption, shows protective effects against diet-induced hypercholesterolemia and fatty liver, and ezetimibe treatment improves liver steatosis and insulin resistance in obese rat models [22, 23].

n-3 PUFAs can improve insulin resistance and NAFLD by lowering the hepatic tumor necrosis factor level. n-3 PUFAs also suppress fatty acid synthesis by controlling SREBP-1c expression negatively and promote fatty acid -oxidation by activating PPAR expression [24, 25]. These facts suggest the possibility that a shortage of PUFA intake leads to NAFLD independent of dietary energy intake. Because a shortage of PUFA intake is found in nonobese NAFLD patients, n-3 PUFA-rich fish and supplements of n-3 PUFAs, such as EPA and docosahexaenoic acid, are recommended as nutrition therapy. Some herbal compounds, such as curcuma, have antioxidant effects and they are expected to show therapeutic effects on NAFLD.

4.4 PROFILE OF NUTRITIONAL INTAKE IN CHC PATIENTS

Presently, the main strategy for CHC is interferon (IFN)-based antiviral therapy and liver protective treatments. In Japan, a high energy, high protein, and high vitamin diet was previously recommended for CHC patients. This principle had spread and become established by broadening the meaning of nutrition therapy reported by Patek and Post, which was adequate for improving the prognosis of alcoholic hepatitis in heavy drinkers [26]. Generally, the nutritional intake of CHC patients is almost similar to that of healthy individuals [27]. However, during IFN-based antiviral treatment, weight loss is apparent in 11–29% of patients because of decreased appetite and malnutrition [28–32]. Although reducing iron by phlebotomy and a low iron diet are also effective for liver injury in CHC patients [33–35], some patients still take iron-rich food and supplements because they believe the incorrect information that glycogen- and iron-rich corbiculae, curcuma, and bovine liver, which are traditional food used to treat acute hepatitis in folk remedies, show therapeutic effects for chronic hepatitis.

4.5 NUTRITION THERAPY FOR CHC PATIENTS

4.5.1 NUTRITION THERAPY DURING IFN-BASED ANTIVIRAL THERAPY

In CHC patients, HCV infection causes a disturbance of glucose and lipid metabolism, and liver steatosis [36–38], which reduces the effect by IFN-based antiviral therapy and affects liver fibrosis [39–42]. However, some patients have a glucose and lipid metabolism disorder, and obesity due to lifestyle-related disease independent of HCV infection.

A recent meta-analysis indicated that insulin resistance reduces the antiviral effect of IFN-based therapy, regardless of HCV genotype [43, 44]. Therefore, before starting antiviral therapy, it is better to improve some metabolic disorders including obesity and insulin resistance by diet therapy and exercise therapy. After starting IFN-based therapy, body weight decreases due to decreased appetite and some digestive symptoms in many patients [28, 29]. A recent study showed that resting energy expenditure did not increase during IFN-based antiviral therapy, and weight loss during the therapy was ascribed to a decrease in energy intake [29]. Although there are no guidelines on how nutrition therapy should be conducted, a decrease in quality of life or malnutrition must be prevented for avoiding an interruption in antiviral therapy.

Various nutrients have lately been identified to be associated with suppression or promotion of HCV proliferation and attract considerable notice [45]. It is known that -carotene, vitamin D, linoleic acid, arachidonic acid, eicosapentaenoic acid, docosahexaenoic acid, iron, and zinc have suppressive effects, while retinol, vitamin E, vitamin K, vitamin C, cholesterol, and selenium have promoting effects on HCV proliferation. For example, when the serum concentration of vitamin D was maintained at 32 ng/mL or more by daily administration of 2,000 IU vitamin D3, the antiviral effect of IFN-based treatment in CHC patients was markedly improved [46]. There is a fair possibility that a shortage of PUFA intake worsens the antiviral effect of IFN-based treatment in CHC patients [47]. Also, in an in vitro study, HCV proliferation was markedly suppressed by treatment with PUFAs, such as arachidonic acid, eicosapentaenoic acid, and docosahexaenoic acid [48, 49]. Additionally, it has been reported that -carotene-containing food and herbal food show an adjuvant effect for IFN-based antiviral therapy [50, 51]. Accordingly, these nutrients are expected to be used as adjuvants in antiviral therapy for patients with HCV infection.

4.5.2 NUTRITION THERAPY FOR PATIENTS WITH IRON ACCUMULATION

In CHC patients, hepatic iron uptake is accelerated and excessive iron accumulation is often apparent in hepatocytes [52–59]. When excessive iron changes to Fe^{3+} from Fe^{2+}, free radicals are produced and the oxidative stress causes injury of cell-membrane and DNA, leading to hepatitis progression. To prevent the iron-mediated injury, phlebotomy and low iron diet therapy is effective [33–35]. Long-term phlebotomy with low-iron diet therapy lowers the risk of development of hepatocellular carcinoma (HCC) from CHC [60]. In Japan, the desired daily iron intake is <6 g in low-iron diet therapy. There are two forms of dietary iron: heme iron, which is present in fish and meat, and nonheme iron, which is present in vegetables. The absorption rate of iron is 10–40% in fish and meat, and

0.3–5% in vegetables; therefore, dietary intake of heme iron must be especially considered in dietary counseling. It is known that a considerable quantity of iron is contained in lean meat, red flesh, internal organs, and the dark flesh of a fish; thus, the specific foods to eat should be specified. However, in low-iron diet therapy, too great a limitation of dietary intake or food selection can result in total nutritional imbalance. Therefore, regular dietary monitoring is required for low-iron diet therapy.

4.6 PROFILE OF NUTRITIONAL INTAKE IN LC PATIENTS

LC is a consequence of all forms of chronic hepatic injury characterized by destruction of hepatic architecture and vascular structures with deposition of fibrotic tissue, which leads to functional decompensation. In some LC patients, intake of various nutrients decreases, which accelerates hepatic dysfunction including a metabolic disorder, resulting in protein energy malnutrition (PEM) [61–65]. Some investigations have shown that LC patients have a trend to take more energy via carbohydrates, which may reflect their insufficient glycogen storage, and fasting accelerates the oxidation of fat [66–68].

A recent increase in the obese population is a difficult worldwide problem, and the increase is also marked in LC patients [69]. This phenomenon indicates that a previous trend of malnutrition has changed into excessive energy intake in LC patients. Recently, there has been an increase in NASH causing LC. As described above, nutrition therapy for NASH patients is to correct their excessive dietary energy intake. Also, at present, in LC caused by alcohol and HCV infection, nutritional intake leans toward being either sufficient or excessive [68, 70]. In our study of compensated LC patients with HCV infection, dietary energy intake and/or protein intake were excessive in 70% of patients and their intake of energy, proteins, and fat was significantly higher than that of healthy individuals [70]. Mean body mass index (BMI) of patients with NASH causing LC was 27.6 kg/m², while more than 30% of patients with viral hepatitis causing LC were also obese (kg/m²) [69]. Although the nutritional state of LC patients cannot be estimated by BMI alone, a recent trend of increased nutritional intake is apparent in LC patients. The nutritional state of LC patients has become diversified by recent changes in dietary habits and by the progression of nutrition therapy, including treatment with branched-chain amino acids (BCAAs).

4.7 NUTRITION THERAPY FOR LC PATIENTS

4.7.1 Nutrition Therapy for LC with PEM As a guideline for energy intake and protein intake, the European Society for Clinical Nutrition and Metabolism (ESPEN) advocated the consensus nutrition standard for LC patients: 35–40 kcal/kg/day in energy and 1.2–1.5 kcal/kg/day in proteins [71]. However, the standard is not always pertinent and should be altered depending on conditions, such as race, intensity of daily activity, PEM, glucose intolerance, protein intolerance, and obesity. Therefore, flexible handling of the guideline is needed. For nutritional assessment of patients with LC, calorimetry may be the best way.

Regarding pathophysiology of PEM in LC patients, appetite stimulation signals from the hypothalamus are suppressed via downregulation of cholecystokinin clearance or cytokine secretion from internal organs, and additionally, ascitic fluid/intestinal edema induces appetite loss [61–63]. Moreover, in a metabolic disorder in LC, resting energy expenditure is upregulated and accompanied by an increased combustion rate of fat, resulting in downregulation of the nonprotein respiratory quotient. These changes are explained by a reduction in hepatic functional reserve, glycogen storage, and insulin sensitivity. In protein metabolism, serum BCAA values decrease markedly because of increased BCAA consumption in skeletal muscle as a substrate for efficient energy production and a substrate for compensatory metabolization of ammonia [72, 73]. When energy nutrition and protein nutrition in viral LC patients were assessed by indirect calorimetry and serum albumin level, respectively, 62% of patients had energy malnutrition, 75% of patients had protein malnutrition, and 50% of patients had energy and protein malnutrition [65]. As a measure for energy malnutrition, a late evening snack (LES) is recommended. When the number of meals is divided into 4–6 per day, nitrogen balance improves [74]. Also glucide intake at night shows a similar effect

[75]. The disruption of muscle protein is suppressed by BCAA intake at night and glucose tolerability is improved by BCAA with glucide intake at night [76, 77]. Because a simple LES addition induces energy overload promoting obesity and glucose intolerance, it is important that <200 kcal are allocated to the LES from the standard daily total energy intake. Concrete examples of LES are a snack mainly consisting of carbohydrates, general enteral nutrients, BCAA-rich enteral nutrition, and so on [76, 78–82]. It has been reported in LC patients with LES that energy metabolism (respiration quotient), serum-free fatty acid levels, and urine 3-methylhystidine levels improve in a week, and serum albumin levels, nitrogen balance, and QOL improve within 3 months [76, 78, 79].

The incidence of protein metabolism disorder is high in LC, and the disorder becomes more marked with the progression of cirrhosis. BCAA-rich enteral nutrition or oral BCAA granules are used for protein metabolism disorder in order to improve nitrogen balance and undernutrition. BCAA-rich enteral nutrition is adequate for patients with chronic hepatic failure, protein intolerance, and a history of hepatic encephalopathy, and BCAA granules are suitable for patients with adequate dietary intake but with hypoalbuminemia resulting from the protein metabolism disorder. In studies in decompensated LC patients, there was a high evidence level that BCAA-rich enteral nutrition and BCAA granules improved hypoalbuminemia, edema, ascitic fluid, event-free survival rates, and QOL [69, 78, 83–85]. However, the clinical response to BCAA was better at an early stage of hepatic failure [86].

PEM is based on the metabolic disorder and, at present, LES and oral BCAA supplementation are strongly recommended after assessment of the metabolic disorder and severity of malnutrition. However, more evidence is being accumulated on an ordinary diet therapy for LC patients with PEM, and new standard may be presented hereafter.

4.7.2 NUTRITION THERAPY FOR LC WITH GLUCOSE INTOLERANCE

Insulin resistance/hyperinsulinemia and glucose intolerance are often shown in LC patients and are associated with a reduction in glucose uptake in the liver and peripheral tissues [87]. It is nutritionally important that improving hyperinsulinemia brings about normalization of insulin-dependent glucose uptake and glycogen synthesis [88]. Nutrition therapy for LC patients with glucose intolerance requires a lower standard of energy intake to prevent hyperinsulinemia and hyperglycemia. In Japan, the standard of 25–30 kcal/kg ideal body weight/day is an advisable range. Dietary fiber-rich meals with a low glycemic index, a lower content of simple carbohydrates, and more exercise, as well as -glucosidase inhibitor (-GI) or insulin with -GI treatment, improve hyperinsulinemia and hyperglycemia in LC patients [89–92]. Zinc supplementation is also effective for improving hyperglycemia [93].

4.7.3 NUTRITION THERAPY FOR LC WITH A HISTORY OF HEPATIC ENCEPHALOPATHY

Hepatic encephalopathy is caused by highly impaired hepatic function and portosystemic shunt formation. Hepatic disruption of ammonia processing and urea synthesis is ascribed to hyperammonemia and a decrease in Fischer's ratio and BCAA/Tyr ratio. Nutritional induction factors of hepatic encephalopathy are excessive intake of dietary proteins and constipation. A protein-restricted diet of <40 g/day and BCAA supplementation has been generally recommended for patients with episodic hepatic encephalopathy or decompensated cirrhosis [94]. Because long-term protein restriction promotes catabolism of body proteins and PEM, it must be combined with BCAA supplementation. Increasing the intake of insoluble dietary fiber-rich vegetables serves to improve and prevent constipation. However, it is difficult to control serum ammonia levels by diet therapies alone, and synthetic disaccharides, such as lactulose, and nonabsorbable antibiotics are utilized for treatment. Recently, lactulose and/or probiotic therapy have been shown to decrease serum ammonia levels [95]. Additionally, zinc supplementation is also effective in improving ammonia metabolism [96, 97].

4.7.4 NUTRITION THERAPY FOR LC WITH OBESITY

Obesity is a risk factor for various cancers and is closely associated with the incidence of HCC [69, 98]. In a large-scale Japanese study of LC patients, the percentage of PEM patients (BMI < $18.5 \, kg/m^2$) was 5.5%, while the percentage of obese patients (BMI > $25 \, kg/m^2$) was 28.3% [69]. A high BMI level as well as a high -fetoprotein level, a low albumin level, and complications of diabetes were associated with a significantly high hazard ratio for HCC in LC patients. Obese LC patients, even under diet therapy, were more likely to develop HCC than nonobese LC patients, but addition of oral BCAA granules to diet therapy reduced the incidence of HCC [69]. It has been shown that oral BCAA granules increase serum albumin levels independent of dietary intake [83]. The mechanism may be that BCAA improve insulin sensitivity in muscle, increase albumin in reduced form, and reduce oxidative stress [99–101]. Thus, in obese LC patients, oral BCAA treatment is recommended in addition to correcting nutritional intake. Excessive nutrients should be assessed in each patient, and the time course of nutritional parameters, such as serum albumin and lean body mass, should be determined for appropriate nutritional therapy. However, the level to which body weight should be reduced has not been examined sufficiently in obese LC patients.

4.8 CONCLUSIONS

In NAFLD/NASH patients, elucidation of excessive nutrients by careful investigation of their dietary intake leads to better nutrition therapy. To obtain better results for antiviral therapy in CHC patients, nutritional care/ support is a significant strategy. In CHC patients, low-iron diet therapy is effective for diminishing liver injury and preventing HCC. The nutritional state of LC patients has a wide spectrum. Therefore, nutrition therapy for

LC patients should be planned after an assessment of their complications, nutritional state, and dietary intake.

REFERENCES

1. N. Assy, G. Nasser, I. Kamayse et al., "Soft drink consumption linked with fatty liver in the absence of traditional risk factors," Canadian Journal of Gastroenterology, vol. 22, no. 10, pp. 811–816, 2008.

2. X. Ouyang, P. Cirillo, Y. Sautin et al., "Fructose consumption as a risk factor for non-alcoholic fatty liver disease," Journal of Hepatology, vol. 48, no. 6, pp. 993–999, 2008.

3. A. Abid, O. Taha, W. Nseir, R. Farah, M. Grosovski, and N. Assy, "Soft drink consumption is associated with fatty liver disease independent of metabolic syndrome," Journal of Hepatology, vol. 51, no. 5, pp. 918–924, 2009.

4. K. Toshimitsu, B. Matsuura, I. Ohkubo et al., "Dietary habits and nutrient intake in non-alcoholic steatohepatitis," Nutrition, vol. 23, no. 1, pp. 46–52, 2007.

5. T. Yamazaki, A. Nakamori, E. Sasaki, S. Wada, and O. Ezaki, "Fish oil prevents sucrose-induced fatty liver but exacerbates high-safflower oil-induced fatty liver in ddY mice," Hepatology, vol. 46, no. 6, pp. 1779–1790, 2007.

6. S. Solga, A. R. Alkhuraishe, J. M. Clark et al., "Dietary composition and nonalcoholic fatty liver disease," Digestive Diseases and Sciences, vol. 49, no. 10, pp. 1578–1583, 2004.

7. G. Musso, R. Gambino, F. De Michieli et al., "Dietary habits and their relations to insulin resistance and postprandial lipemia in nonalcoholic steatohepatitis," Hepatology, vol. 37, no. 4, pp. 909–916, 2003.

8. S. K. Ha and C. Chae, "Inducible nitric oxide distribution in the fatty liver of a mouse with high fat diet-induced obesity," Experimental Animals, vol. 59, no. 5, pp. 595–604, 2010.

9. K. Yasutake, M. Nakamuta, Y. Shima et al., "Nutritional investigation of non-obese patients with non-alcoholic fatty liver disease: the significance of dietary cholesterol," Scandinavian Journal of Gastroenterology, vol. 44, no. 4, pp. 471–477, 2009.

10. M. Kainuma, M. Fujimoto, N. Sekiya et al., "Cholesterol-fed rabbit as a unique model of nonalcoholic, nonobese, non-insulin-resistant fatty liver disease with characteristic fibrosis," Journal of Gastroenterology, vol. 41, no. 10, pp. 971–980, 2006.

11. N. Matsuzawa, T. Takamura, S. Kurita et al., "Lipid-induced oxidative stress causes steatohepatitis in mice fed an atherogenic diet," Hepatology, vol. 46, no. 5, pp. 1392–1403, 2007.

12. K. Wouters, P. J. van Gorp, V. Bieghs et al., "Dietary cholesterol, rather than liver steatosis, leads to hepatic inflammation in hyperlipidemic mouse models of nonalcoholic steatohepatitis," Hepatology, vol. 48, no. 2, pp. 474–486, 2008.

13. N. Higuchi, M. Kato, Y. Shundo et al., "Liver X receptor in cooperation with SREBP-1c is a major lipid synthesis regulator in nonalcoholic fatty liver disease," Hepatology Research, vol. 38, no. 11, pp. 1122–1129, 2008.

14. M. Nakamuta, T. Fujino, R. Yada et al., "Impact of cholesterol metabolism and the LXRα-SREBP-1c pathway on nonalcoholic fatty liver disease," International Journal of Molecular Medicine, vol. 23, no. 5, pp. 603–608, 2009.

15. J. B. Dixon, P. S. Bhathal, N. R. Hughes, and P. E. O'Brien, "Nonalcoholic fatty liver disease: improvement in liver histological analysis with weight loss," Hepatology, vol. 39, no. 6, pp. 1647–1654, 2004.

16. M. C. Elias, E. R. Parise, L. D. Carvalho, D. Szejnfeld, and J. P. Netto, "Effect of 6-month nutritional intervention on non-alcoholic fatty liver disease," Nutrition, vol. 26, no. 11-12, pp. 1094–1099, 2010.

17. M. Capanni, F. Calella, M. R. Biagini et al., "Prolonged n-3 polyunsaturated fatty acid supplementation ameliorates hepatic steatosis in patients with non-alcoholic fatty liver disease: a pilot study," Alimentary Pharmacology and Therapeutics, vol. 23, no. 8, pp. 1143–1151, 2006.

18. T. Hasegawa, M. Yoneda, K. Nakamura, I. Makino, and A. Terano, "Plasma transforming growth factor-β1 level and efficacy of α-tocopherol in patients with non-alcoholic steatohepatitis: a pilot study," Alimentary Pharmacology and Therapeutics, vol. 15, no. 10, pp. 1667–1672, 2001.

19. S. I. Kojima, N. Watanabe, M. Numata, T. Ogawa, and S. Matsuzaki, "Increase in the prevalence of fatty liver in Japan over the past 12 years: analysis of clinical background," Journal of Gastroenterology, vol. 38, no. 10, pp. 954–961, 2003.

20. A. Nonomura, Y. Enomoto, M. Takeda et al., "Clinical and pathological features of non-alcoholic steatohepatitis," Hepatology Research, vol. 33, no. 2, pp. 116–121, 2005.

21. M. Enjoji, K. Machida, M. Kohjima et al., "NPC1L1 inhibitor ezetimibe is a reliable therapeutic agent for non-obese patients with nonalcoholic fatty liver disease," Lipids in Health and Disease, vol. 9, p. 29, 2010.

22. J. P. Davies, C. Scott, K. Oishi, A. Liapis, and Y. A. Ioannou, "Inactivation of NPC1L1 causes multiple lipid transport defects and protects against diet-induced hypercholesterolemia," Journal of Biological Chemistry, vol. 280, no. 13, pp. 12710–12720, 2005.

23. M. Deushi, M. Nomura, A. Kawakami et al., "Ezetimibe improves liver steatosis and insulin resistance in obese rat model of metabolic syndrome," FEBS Letters, vol. 581, no. 29, pp. 5664–5670, 2007.

24. Ghafoorunissa, A. Ibrahim, L. Rajkumar, and V. Acharya, "Dietary (n-3) long chain polyunsaturated fatty acids prevent sucrose-induced insulin resistance in rats," Journal of Nutrition, vol. 135, no. 11, pp. 2634–2638, 2005.

25. M. Teran-Garcia, A. W. Adamson, G. Yu et al., "Polyunsaturated fatty acid suppression of fatty acid synthase (FASN): evidence for dietary modulation of NF-Y binding to the Fasn promoter by SREBP-1c," Biochemical Journal, vol. 402, no. 3, pp. 591–600, 2007.

26. A. J. Patek and J. Post, "Treatment of cirrhosis of the liver by a nutritious diet and supplements rich in vitamin B complex," Journal of Clinical Investigation, vol. 20, no. 5, pp. 481–505, 1941.

27. M. Iwasa, K. Iwata, M. Kaito et al., "Efficacy of long-term dietary restriction of total calories, fat, iron, and protein in patients with chronic hepatitis C virus," Nutrition, vol. 20, no. 4, pp. 368–371, 2004.

28. C. Hamer, "The impact of combination therapy with peginterferon alfa-2a and riba-virin on the energy intake and body weight of adult hepatitis C patients," Journal of Human Nutrition and Dietetics, vol. 21, no. 5, pp. 486–493, 2008.

29. M. Fioravante, S. M. Alegre, D. M. Marin, et al., "Weight loss and resting energy ex-penditure in patients with chronic hepatitis C before and during standard treatment," Nutrition, vol. 28, no. 6, pp. 630–634, 2012.

30. M. W. Fried, "Side effects of therapy of hepatitis C and their management," Hepatol-ogy, vol. 36, no. 5, supplement 1, pp. S237–S244, 2002.

31. M. P. Manns, J. G. McHutchison, S. C. Gordon et al., "Peginterferon alfa-2b plus ribavirin compared with interferonalfa-2b plus ribavirin for initial treatment of chronic hepatitis C: a randomised trial," Lancet, vol. 358, no. 9286, pp. 958–965, 2001.

32. M. W. Fried, M. L. Shiffman, K. R. Reddy et al., "Peginterferon alfa-2a plus ribavi-rin for chronic hepatitis C virus infection," The New England Journal of Medicine, vol. 347, no. 13, pp. 975–982, 2002.

33. H. Hayashi, T. Takikawa, N. Nishimura, M. Yano, T. Isomura, and N. Sakamoto, "Improvement of serum aminotransferase levels after phlebotomy in patients with chronic active hepatitis C and excess hepatic iron," American Journal of Gastroen-terology, vol. 89, no. 7, pp. 986–988, 1994.

34. M. Iwasa, M. Kaito, J. Ikoma et al., "Dietary iron restriction improves aminotrans-ferase levels in chronic hepatitis C patients," Hepato-Gastroenterology, vol. 49, no. 44, pp. 529–531, 2002.

35. M. Yano, H. Hayashi, S. Wakusawa et al., "Long term effects of phlebotomy on biochemical and histological parameters of chronic hepatitis C," American Journal of Gastroenterology, vol. 97, no. 1, pp. 133–137, 2002.

36. Y. Shintani, H. Fujie, H. Miyoshi et al., "Hepatitis C virus infection and diabetes: direct involvement of the virus in the development of insulin resistance," Gastroen-terology, vol. 126, no. 3, pp. 840–848, 2004.

37. N. Bach, S. N. Thung, and F. Schaffner, "The histological features of chronic hepa-titis C and autoimmune chronic hepatitis: a comparative analysis," Hepatology, vol. 15, no. 4, pp. 572–577, 1992.

38. J. H. Lefkowitch, E. R. Schiff, G. L. Davis et al., "Pathological diagnosis of chronic hepatitis C: a multicenter comparative study with chronic hepatitis B," Gastroenter-ology, vol. 104, no. 2, pp. 595–603, 1993.

39. M. Romero-Gómez, M. Del Mar Viloria, R. J. Andrade et al., "Insulin resistance impairs sustained response rate to peginterferon plus ribavirin in chronic hepatitis C patients," Gastroenterology, vol. 128, no. 3, pp. 636–641, 2005.

40. T. Poynard, V. Ratziu, J. McHutchison et al., "Effect of treatment with peginterferon or interferon alfa-2b and ribavirin on steatosis in patients infected with hepatitis C," Hepatology, vol. 38, no. 1, pp. 75–85, 2003.

41. J. M. Hui, A. Sud, G. C. Farrell et al., "Insulin resistance is associated with chronic hepatitis C and virus infection fibrosis progression," Gastroenterology, vol. 125, no. 6, pp. 1695–1704, 2003.

42. L. F. Hourigan, G. A. Macdonald, D. Purdie et al., "Fibrosis in chronic hepatitis C correlates significantly with body mass index and steatosis," Hepatology, vol. 29, no. 4, pp. 1215–1219, 1999.

43. M. Eslam, R. Aparcero, T. Kawaguchi et al., "Meta-analysis: Insulin resistance and sustained virological response in hepatitis C," Alimentary Pharmacology and Therapeutics, vol. 34, no. 3, pp. 297–305, 2011.

44. P. Deltenre, A. Louvet, M. Lemoine, et al., "Impact of insulin resistance on sustained response in HCV patients treated with pegylated interferon and ribavirin: a meta-analysis," Journal of Hepatology, vol. 55, no. 6, pp. 1187–1194, 2011.

45. M. Yano, M. Ikeda, K. I. Abe et al., "Comprehensive analysis of the effects of ordinary nutrients on hepatitis C virus RNA replication in cell culture," Antimicrobial Agents and Chemotherapy, vol. 51, no. 6, pp. 2016–2027, 2007.

46. S. Abu-Mouch, Z. Fireman, J. Jarchovsky, A. R. Zeina, and N. Assy, "Vitamin D supplementation improves sustained virologic response in chronic hepatitis C, (genotype 1)-naive patients," World Journal of Gastroenterology, vol. 17, no. 47, pp. 5184–5190, 2011.

47. K. Yasutake, M. Ichinose, M. Bekki, et al., "Significance of dietary intake during combined peg-interferon plus ribavirin therapy for chronic hepatitis C: relationship between polyunsaturated fatty acid and early virologic response," Journal of the Japan Dietetic Association, vol. 55, no. 1, pp. 32–39, 2012 (Japanese).

48. G. Z. Leu, T. Y. Lin, and J. T. A. Hsu, "Anti-HCV activities of selective polyunsaturated fatty acids," Biochemical and Biophysical Research Communications, vol. 318, no. 1, pp. 275–280, 2004.

49. S. B. Kapadia and F. V. Chisari, "Hepatitis C virus RNA replication is regulated by host geranylgeranylation and fatty acids," Proceedings of the National Academy of Sciences of the United States of America, vol. 102, no. 7, pp. 2561–2566, 2005.

50. P. Vitaglione, V. Fogliano, S. Stingo, L. Scalfi, N. Capraso, and F. Morisco, "Development of a tomato-based food for special medical purposes as therapy adjuvant for patients with," European Journal of Clinical Nutrition, vol. 61, no. 7, pp. 906–915, 2007.

51. L. B. Seeff, T. M. Curto, G. Szabo et al., "Herbal product use by persons enrolled in the hepatitis C antiviral long-term treatment against cirrhosis (HALT-C) trial," Hepatology, vol. 47, no. 2, pp. 605–612, 2008.

52. H. L. Bonkovsky, B. F. Banner, and A. L. Rothman, "Iron and chronic viral hepatitis," Hepatology, vol. 25, no. 3, pp. 759–768, 1997.

53. A. M. Di Bisceglie, C. A. Axiotis, J. H. Hoofnagle, and B. R. Bacon, "Measurements of iron status in patients with chronic hepatitis," Gastroenterology, vol. 102, no. 6, pp. 2108–2113, 1992.

54. A. Piperno, R. D'Alba, S. Fargion et al., "Liver iron concentration in chronic viral hepatitis: a study of 98 patients," European Journal of Gastroenterology and Hepatology, vol. 7, no. 12, pp. 1203–1208, 1995.

55. S. Haque, B. Chandra, M. A. Gerber, and A. S. F. Lok, "Iron overload in patients with chronic hepatitis C: a clinicopathologic study," Human Pathology, vol. 27, no. 12, pp. 1277–1281, 1996.

56. A. M. Di Bisceglie, H. L. Bonkovsky, S. Chopra et al., "Iron reduction as an adjuvant to interferon therapy in patients with chronic hepatitis C who have previously not responded to interferon: a multicenter, prospective, randomized, controlled trial," Hepatology, vol. 32, no. 1, pp. 135–138, 2000.

57. A. Erhardt, A. Maschner-Olberg, C. Mellenthin et al., "HFE mutations and chronic hepatitis C: H63D and C282Y heterozygosity are independent risk factors for liver fibrosis and cirrhosis," Journal of Hepatology, vol. 38, no. 3, pp. 335–342, 2003.

58. H. L. Bonkovsky, N. Troy, K. McNeal et al., "Iron and HFE or TfR1 mutations as comorbid factors for development and progression of chronic hepatitis C," Journal of Hepatology, vol. 37, no. 6, pp. 848–854, 2002.

59. R. J. Fontana, J. Israel, P. LeClair et al., "Iron reduction before and during interferon therapy of chronic hepatitis C: results of a multicenter, randomized, controlled trial," Hepatology, vol. 31, no. 3, pp. 730–736, 2000.

60. J. Kato, K. Miyanishi, M. Kobune et al., "Long-term phlebotomy with low-iron diet therapy lowers risk of development of hepatocellular carcinoma from chronic hepatitis C," Journal of Gastroenterology, vol. 42, no. 10, pp. 830–836, 2007.

61. C. L. Mendenhall, T. E. Moritz, G. A. Roselle et al., "A study of oral nutritional support with oxandrolone in malnourished patients with alcoholic hepatitis: results of a Department of Veterans Affairs cooperative study," Hepatology, vol. 17, no. 4, pp. 564–576, 1993.

62. R. A. Richardson, H. I. Davidson, A. Hinds, S. Cowan, P. Rae, and O. J. Garden, "Influence of the metabolic sequelae of liver cirrhosis on nutritional intake," American Journal of Clinical Nutrition, vol. 69, no. 2, pp. 331–337, 1999.

63. B. Campillo, J. P. Richardet, E. Scherman, and P. N. Bories, "Evaluation of nutritional practice in hospitalized cirrhotic patients: results of a prospective study," Nutrition, vol. 19, no. 6, pp. 515–521, 2003.

64. M. Merli, "Nutritional status in cirrhosis," Journal of Hepatology, vol. 21, no. 3, pp. 317–325, 1994.

65. M. Tajika, M. Kato, H. Mohri et al., "Prognostic value of energy metabolism in patients with viral liver cirrhosis," Nutrition, vol. 18, no. 3, pp. 229–234, 2002.

66. O. E. Owen, F. A. Reichle, M. A. Mozzoli, et al., "Hepatic, gut, and renal substrate flux rates in patients with hepatic cirrhosis," Journal of Clinical Investigation, vol. 68, no. 1, pp. 240–252, 1981.

67. K. Nielsen, J. Kondrup, L. Martinsen, B. Stilling, and B. Wikman, "Nutritional assessment and adequacy of dietary intake in hospitalized patients with alcoholic liver cirrhosis," British Journal of Nutrition, vol. 69, no. 3, pp. 665–679, 1993.

68. B. Campillo, P. N. Bories, M. Leluan, B. Pornin, M. Devanlay, and P. Fouet, "Short-term changes in energy metabolism after 1 month of a regular oral diet in severely malnourished cirrhotic patients," Metabolism: Clinical and Experimental, vol. 44, no. 6, pp. 765–770, 1995.

69. Y. Muto, S. Sato, A. Watanabe et al., "Overweight and obesity increase the risk for liver cancer in patients with liver cirrhosis and long-term oral supplementation with branched-chain amino acid granules inhibits liver carcinogenesis in heavier patients with liver cirrhosis," Hepatology Research, vol. 35, no. 3, pp. 204–214, 2006.

70. K. Yasutake, M. Bekki, M. Ichinose, et al., "Assessing current nutritional status of patients with HCV-related liver cirrhosis in the compensated stage," Asia Pacific Journal of Clinical Nutrition, vol. 21, no. 3, pp. 400–405, 2012.

71. M. Plauth, E. Cabré, O. Riggio et al., "ESPEN guidelines on enteral nutrition: liver disease," Clinical Nutrition, vol. 25, no. 2, pp. 285–294, 2006.

72. M. Kato, Y. Miwa, M. Tajika, T. Hiraoka, Y. Muto, and H. Moriwaki, "Preferential use of branched-chain amino acids as an energy substrate in patients with liver cirrhosis," Internal Medicine, vol. 37, no. 5, pp. 429–434, 1998.

73. M. Shiraki, Y. Shimomura, Y. Miwa et al., "Activation of hepatic branched-chain α-keto acid dehydrogenase complex by tumor necrosis factor-α in rats," Biochemical and Biophysical Research Communications, vol. 328, no. 4, pp. 973–978, 2005.

74. G. R. Swart, M. C. Zillikens, J. K. Van Vuure, and J. W. O. Van den Berg, "Effect of a late evening meal on nitrogen balance in patients with cirrhosis of the liver," British Medical Journal, vol. 299, no. 6709, pp. 1202–1203, 1989.

75. M. C. Zillikens, J. W. O. Van Den Berg, J. L. D. Wattimena, T. Rietveld, and G. R. Swart, "Nocturnal oral glucose supplementation. The effects on protein metabolism in cirrhotic patients and in healthy controls," Journal of Hepatology, vol. 17, no. 3, pp. 377–383, 1993.

76. M. Yamauchi, K. Takeda, K. Sakamoto, M. Ohata, and G. Toda, "Effect of oral branched chain amino acid supplementation in the late evening on the nutritional state of patients with liver cirrhosis," Hepatology Research, vol. 21, no. 3, pp. 199–204, 2001.

77. M. Tsuchiya, I. Sakaida, M. Okamoto, and K. Okita, "The effect of a late evening snack in patients with liver cirrhosis," Hepatology Research, vol. 31, no. 2, pp. 95–103, 2005.

78. Y. Nakaya, K. Okita, K. Suzuki et al., "BCAA-enriched snack improves nutritional state of cirrhosis," Nutrition, vol. 23, no. 2, pp. 113–120, 2007.

79. K. Aoyama, M. Tsuchiya, K. Mori et al., "Effect of a late evening snack on outpatients with liver cirrhosis," Hepatology Research, vol. 37, no. 8, pp. 608–614, 2007.

80. W. K. Chang, Y. C. Chao, H. S. Tang, H. F. Lang, and C. T. Hsu, "Effects of extra-carbohydrate supplementation in the late evening on energy expenditure and substrate oxidation in patients with liver cirrhosis," Journal of Parenteral and Enteral Nutrition, vol. 21, no. 2, pp. 96–99, 1997.

81. H. Yamanaka-Okumura, T. Nakamura, H. Takeuchi et al., "Effect of late evening snack with rice ball on energy metabolism in liver cirrhosis," European Journal of Clinical Nutrition, vol. 60, no. 9, pp. 1067–1072, 2006.

82. Y. Miwa, M. Shiraki, M. Kato et al., "Improvement of fuel metabolism by nocturnal energy supplementation in patients with liver cirrhosis," Hepatology Research, vol. 18, no. 3, pp. 184–189, 2000.

83. H. Yatsuhashi, Y. Ohnishi, S. Nakayama, et al., "Anti-hypoalbuminemic effect of branched-chain amino acid granules in patients with liver cirrhosis is independent of dietary energy and protein intake," Hepatology Research, vol. 41, no. 11, pp. 1027–1035, 2011.

84. G. Marchesini, G. Bianchi, M. Merli et al., "Nutritional supplementation with branched-chain amino acids in advanced cirrhosis: a double-blind, randomized trial," Gastroenterology, vol. 124, no. 7, pp. 1792–1801, 2003.

85. R. T. P. Poon, W. C. Yu, S. T. Fan, and J. Wong, "Long-term oral branched chain amino acids in patients undergoing chemoembolization for hepatocellular carcinoma: a randomized trial," Alimentary Pharmacology and Therapeutics, vol. 19, no. 7, pp. 779–788, 2004.

86. A. Kato and K. Suzuki, "How to select BCAA preparations," Hepatology Research, vol. 30, pp. S30–S35, 2004.

87. E. Imano, T. Kanda, Y. Nakatani et al., "Impaired splanchnic and peripheral glucose uptake in liver cirrhosis," Journal of Hepatology, vol. 31, no. 3, pp. 469–473, 1999.

88. A. S. Petrides, T. Stanley, D. E. Matthews, C. Vogt, A. J. Bush, and H. Lambeth, "Insulin resistance in cirrhosis: prolonged reduction of hyperinsulinemia normalizes insulin sensitivity," Hepatology, vol. 28, no. 1, pp. 141–149, 1998.

89. H. Barkoukis, K. M. Fiedler, and E. Lerner, "A combined high-fiber, low-glycemic index diet normalizes glucose tolerance and reduces hyperglycemia and hyperinsulinemia in adults with hepatic cirrhosis," Journal of the American Dietetic Association, vol. 102, no. 10, pp. 1503–1507, 2002.

90. D. J. A. Jenkins, N. Shapira, G. Greenberg et al., "Low glycemic index foods and reduced glucose, amino acid, and endocrine responses in cirrhosis," American Journal of Gastroenterology, vol. 84, no. 7, pp. 732–739, 1989.

91. S. Gentile, S. Turco, G. Guarino et al., "Effect of treatment with acarbose and insulin in patients with non-insulin-dependent diabetes mellitus associated with non-alcoholic liver cirrhosis," Diabetes, Obesity and Metabolism, vol. 3, no. 1, pp. 33–40, 2001.

92. M. C. Zillikens, G. R. Swart, J. W. O. Van den Berg, and J. H. P. Wilson, "Effects of the glucosidase inhibitor acarbose in patients with liver cirrhosis," Alimentary Pharmacology and Therapeutics, vol. 3, no. 5, pp. 453–459, 1989.

93. G. Marchesini, E. Bugianesi, M. Ronchi, R. Flamia, K. Thomaseth, and G. Pacini, "Zinc supplementation improves glucose disposal in patients with cirrhosis," Metabolism: Clinical and Experimental, vol. 47, no. 7, pp. 792–798, 1998.

94. J. Córdoba, J. López-Hellín, M. Planas et al., "Normal protein diet for episodic hepatic encephalopathy: results of a randomized study," Journal of Hepatology, vol. 41, no. 1, pp. 38–43, 2004.

95. P. Sharma, B. C. Sharma, V. Puri, and S. K. Sarin, "An open-label randomized controlled trial of lactulose and probiotics in the treatment of minimal hepatic encephalopathy," European Journal of Gastroenterology and Hepatology, vol. 20, no. 6, pp. 506–511, 2008.

96. P. Reding, J. Duchateau, and C. Bataille, "Oral zinc supplementation improves hepatic encephalopathy. Results of a randomised controlled trial," Lancet, vol. 2, no. 8401, pp. 493–495, 1984.

97. Y. Takuma, K. Nousot, Y. Makino, M. Hayashi, and H. Takahashi, "Clinical trial: oral zinc in hepatic encephalopathy," Alimentary Pharmacology and Therapeutics, vol. 32, no. 9, pp. 1080–1090, 2010.

98. E. E. Calle, C. Rodriguez, K. Walker-Thurmond, and M. J. Thun, "Overweight, obesity, and mortality from cancer in a prospectively studied cohort of U.S. Adults," The New England Journal of Medicine, vol. 348, no. 17, pp. 1625–1638, 2003.

99. S. Nishitani, K. Takehana, S. Fujitani, and I. Sonaka, "Branched-chain amino acids improve glucose metabolism in rats with liver cirrhosis," American Journal of Physiology, vol. 288, no. 6, pp. G1292–G1300, 2005.

100. H. Fukushima, Y. Miwa, M. Shiraki et al., "Oral branched-chain amino acid supplementation improves the oxidized/ reduced albumin ratio in patients with liver cirrhosis," Hepatology Research, vol. 37, no. 9, pp. 765–770, 2007.

101. T. Ohno, Y. Tanaka, F. Sugauchi et al., "Suppressive effect of oral administration of branched-chain amino acid granules on oxidative stress and inflammation in HCV-positive patients with liver cirrhosis," Hepatology Research, vol. 38, no. 7, pp. 683–688, 2008.

This chapter was originally published under the Creative Common Attribution License. Yasutake, K., Kohjima, M., Nakashima, M., Katoh, K., Nakamuta, M., and Enjoji, M. Nutrition Therapy for Liver Diseases Based on the Status of Nutritional Intake. Gastroenterology Research and Practice. 2012; Article ID 859697, doi :10.1155/2012/859697.

CHAPTER 5

ROLE OF NUTRITION IN THE MANAGEMENT OF HEPATIC ENCEPHALOPATHY IN END-STAGE LIVER FAILURE

CHANTAL BÉMEUR, PAUL DESJARDINS, and ROGER F. BUTTERWORTH

5.1 INTRODUCTION

Malnutrition is a common complication of end-stage liver failure (cirrhosis) and is an important prognostic indicator of clinical outcome (survival rate, length of hospital stay, posttransplantation morbidity, and quality of life) in patients with cirrhosis. Several studies have evaluated nutritional status in patients with liver cirrhosis of different etiologies and varying degrees of liver insufficiency [1, 2] leading to a consensus of opinion that malnutrition is recognizable in all forms of cirrhosis [3] and that the prevalence of malnutrition in cirrhosis has been estimated to range from 65%–100% [4, 5]. The causes of malnutrition in liver disease are complex and multifactorial.

The present paper reviews the role of nutrition in relation to the management of hepatic encephalopathy (HE), a major neuropsychiatric complication of end-stage liver failure. Nutritional consequences of liver failure with the potential to cause central nervous system dysfunction are reviewed. In particular, the roles of dietary protein (animal versus vegetable), branched-chain amino acids, dietary fibre, probiotics, vitamins and antioxidants, minerals (zinc, magnesium) as well as L-carnitine in relation to HE are discussed. An update of the impact of nutritional supplementation on the management of HE is included.

5.2 MALNUTRITION IN LIVER DISEASE

The functional integrity of the liver is essential for nutrient supply (carbohydrates, fat, and proteins), and the liver plays a fundamental role in intermediary metabolism. For example, the liver regulates the synthesis, storage, and breakdown of glycogen, and hepatocytes express enzymes that enable them to synthesize glucose from various precursors such as amino acids, pyruvate, and lactate (gluconeogenesis). In addition, the liver is a major site of fatty acid breakdown and triglyceride synthesis. The breakdown of fatty acids provides an alternative source of energy when glucose is limited during, for example, fasting or starvation. The liver also plays a crucial role in the synthesis and degradation of protein. Protein synthesis by the liver is influenced by the nutritional state, as well as by hormones and alcohol.

The liver plays a central role in the regulation of nutrition by trafficking the metabolism of nutrients, and many factors disrupt this metabolic balance in end-stage liver failure. Consequently, when the liver fails, numerous nutritional problems occur (Table 1). Several factors contribute to malnutrition in liver failure including inadequate dietary intake of nutrients, reduction in their synthesis or absorption (diminished protein synthesis, malabsorption), increased protein loss, disturbances in substrate utilization, a hypermetabolic state as well as increased energy-protein expenditure and requirements. Because of decreased glycogen stores and gluconeogenesis [6], energy metabolism may shift from carbohydrate to fat oxidation [7] while insulin resistance may also develop. Consequently, liver cirrhosis frequently results in a catabolic state resulting in a lack of essential nutrients.

TABLE 1: Metabolic alterations leading to malnutrition in end-stage liver failure.

Protein	Carbohydrate	Fat
(i) Increased catabolism	(i) Decreased hepatic and skeletal muscle glycogen synthesis	(i) Increased lipolysis
(ii) Increased utilization of BCAAs	(ii) Increased gluconeogenesis	(ii) Enhanced turnover and oxidation of fatty acids
(iii) Decreased ureagenesis	(iii) Glucose intolerance and insulin resistance	(iii) Increased Ketogenesis

TABLE 2: Nutritional recommendations for the management of HE in end-stage liver failure.

Substrate	Recommendation
Energy	35–40 kcal/kg/day
Protein	1.2–1.5 g/kg of body weight/day*
BCAA	In severely protein-intolerant patients
Antioxidant and vitamins	Multivitamin supplements
Probiotics, prebiotics	Increasing use for ammonia-lowering and anti-inflammatory actions

In severely protein intolerant patients, protein may be reduced for short periods of time, particularly in grade III-IV hepatic encephalopathy.

It has been estimated that at least 25% of patients with liver cirrhosis experience HE during the natural history of the disease. HE is more frequent in patients with more severe liver insufficiency and in those with spontaneous or surgically created portal-systemic shunts. Whether or not malnourished patients are more prone to develop HE has not been clearly established, but could be anticipated based on several factors. Firstly, malnutrition tends to be more common in patients with advanced liver disease, and HE is more likely in this group. Secondly, nutritional deficits such as decreased lean body mass (muscle is important in ammonia uptake) and hypoalbuminemia (which increases free tryptophan levels) could promote HE [8].

5.3 FACTORS CONTRIBUTING TO MALNUTRITION IN CIRRHOSIS

A range of factors are known to contribute to malnutrition in cirrhosis. These factors include (Figure 1) the following.

5.3.1 INADEQUATE DIETARY INTAKE

Cirrhotic patients may unintentionally consume a low energy diet, an observation that is attributed to several factors including loss of appetite [9], anorexia, nausea, vomiting, early satiety, taste abnormalities, poor palatability of diets, reflux disease [10, 11], and impaired expansion capacity of the stomach [9].

5.3.2 INADEQUATE SYNTHESIS OR ABSORPTION OF NUTRIENTS

The cirrhotic liver may inadequately synthesize proteins and has diminished storage capacity and an impaired enterohepatic cycle. In addition, portal hypertensive enteropathy may lead to impaired absorption of essential nutrients. Moreover, pancreatic insufficiency, cholestasis, and drug-related diarrhea may all contribute to malabsorption in liver disease.

5.3.3 INCREASED PROTEIN LOSSES

Loss of proteins and minerals may result from complications of cirrhosis or from iatrogenic interventions such as the use of diuretics for the treatment of ascites and fluid retention as well as from the use of lactulose for the management of HE. Other potentially important causes of increased protein losses are blood loss from oesophageal and gastric varices and from the intestinal lumen due to ulcers or portal enteropathy.

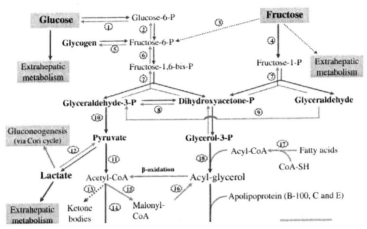

FIGURE 1: Factors contributing to malnutrition in end-stage liver failure.

5.3.4 HYPERMETABOLIC STATE/INCREASED ENERGY-PROTEIN EXPENDITURE AND REQUIREMENTS

The hyperdynamic circulation in cirrhosis leads to systemic vasodilation and an expanded intravascular blood volume. As a direct effect, a higher cardiac blood volume and therefore a greater use of macro- and micronutrients is a common cause of high energy expenditure and demand. Furthermore, the inability of the damaged liver to adequately clear activated proinflammatory mediators such as cytokines may promote the development of an inflammatory response with an increase in both energy expenditure and protein catabolism [12]. It has been suggested that elevated pro- and anti-inflammatory cytokine levels have the potential to result in hypermetabolism in cirrhosis [13, 14].

5.3.5 INSULIN RESISTANCE

Insulin resistance and diabetes mellitus are common in patients with liver cirrhosis [15, 16]. Hyperinsulinemia and hyperglucagonemia are frequently present in cirrhotic patients where glucagon is disproportionately increased resulting in an elevated glucagon/insulin ratio. There is also impairment of glucose homeostasis due to hepatic insulin resistance characterized by altered gluconeogenesis, low glycogen stores, and impaired glycogenolysis [15, 16].

5.3.6 GASTROINTESTINAL BLEEDING

Bleeding esophageal varices as a consequence of portal hypertension are frequent and severe complications of liver cirrhosis. Gastrointestinal bleeding is also a precipitating factor in HE and may accelerate progression of malnutrition in cirrhotic patients.

5.3.7 ASCITES

Impaired expansion capacity of the stomach due to the presence of clinically evident ascites may lead to an inadequate intake of nutrients [9], and cirrhotic patients with ascites often report early satiety and subsequent decreased oral intake which may result in significant weight loss [17].

5.3.8 INFLAMMATION/INFECTION

Malnourished patients with cirrhosis are prone to the development of inflammation and sepsis and their survival may be further shortened by these complications. There is a significant negative correlation between plasma levels of proinflammatory cytokines such as tumor necrosis factor-alpha (TNF-α) and nutrient intake [18]. In order to reduce intestinal bacterial translocation and to improve gut immune function, it has been proposed that pre- and probiotics be added to the diet [19].

5.3.9 HYPONATREMIA

Hyponatremia is a common complication of patients with advanced liver disease [20] and is an important predictor of short-term mortality. Hyponatremia is also an important pathogenic factor in patients with HE. Cirrhotic patients have abnormal sodium and water handling that may lead to refractory ascites. These patients retain sodium, and dilutional hyponatremia may develop, characterized by reduced serum sodium. In such situations, saline infusion should be avoided and it has been suggested that sodium intake should not exceed 2 g [21].

5.4 ASSESSMENT OF NUTRITIONAL STATUS IN END-STAGE LIVER FAILURE

The nutritional assessment of the cirrhotic patient begins with the dietary history that should focus on nutritional intake and assessment of recent weight loss. However, altered mental status may preclude obtaining a meaningful history, and interviewing family members may be helpful.

Liver disease may interfere with biomarkers of malnutrition such as albumin, making it difficult to identify subjects at risk of malnutrition and to evaluate the need for nutritional intervention. Furthermore, anthropometric and bioelectrical impedance analysis may be biased by the presence of edema or ascites associated with liver failure. Body mass index (BMI), an index of nutritional status, may also be overvalued in patients with edema and ascites. Careful interpretation of nutritional data using these techniques in the presence of these complications is therefore required.

Generally accepted methods for assessing the clinical status and severity of disease in cirrhotic patients are the Child-Pugh-Turcotte classification [22] and the model for end-stage liver disease (MELD) [23, 24]. Unfortunately, these systems do not include an assessment of nutritional status in spite of the fact that malnutrition plays an important role in morbidity and mortality in end-stage liver failure. The omission of nutritional assessment results no doubt from the heterogeneous nature of the nutritional deficits in this population.

Subjective Global Assessment (SGA) and anthropometric parameters are the methods that are frequently used to evaluate nutritional status in end-stage liver failure [25]. SGA collects clinical information through history-taking, physical examination, and recent weight change and is considered to be reliable since it is minimally affected by fluid retention or the presence of ascites. The use of anthropometric parameters which are not affected by the presence of ascites or peripheral edema has also been recommended [22, 25]. Such parameters include mid-arm muscle circumference (MAMC), mid-arm circumference (MAC), and triceps skin fold thickness (TST). Diagnosis of malnutrition is established by values of MAMC and/or TST below the 5th percentile in patients aged 18–74 years, or the 10th percentile in patients aged over 74 years [26].

BMI changes may afford a reliable indicator of malnutrition using different BMI cutoff values depending on the presence and severity of ascites [26]; patients with a BMI below 22 with no ascites, below 23 with mild ascites, or below 25 with tense ascites are considered to be malnourished. Hand-grip examination by dynamometer has also been proposed as a simple method to detect patients at risk for the development of malnutrition [27]. In an interesting new development, Morgan et al. [28] validated a method where BMI and MAMC are combined with details of dietary intake in a semistructured algorithmic construct to provide a method for nutritional assessment in patients with end-stage liver failure [28]. Despite these advances, a standardized simple and accurate method for evaluating malnutrition in cirrhosis remains to be established.

5.5 CONSEQUENCES OF CIRRHOSIS WITH A POTENTIAL TO IMPACT UPON NUTRITIONAL STATUS AND BRAIN FUNCTION

Cirrhosis results in multiple metabolic abnormalities and alterations in the synthesis, turnover, and elimination of a range of metal and micronutrients with the potential to alter nutritional status and consequently cerebral function. Such alterations include the following.

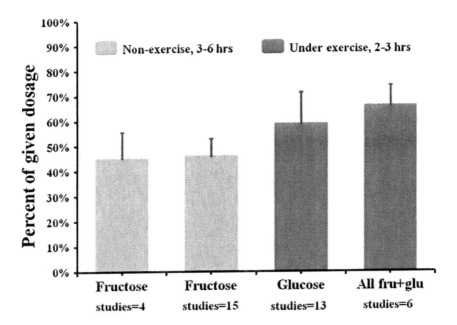

FIGURE 2: Inter-organ trafficking of ammonia in normal physiological conditions, in well-nourished patients with end-stage liver failure compared to malnourished end-stage liver failure patients.

5.5.1 HYPERAMMONEMIA

Under normal physiological conditions, ammonia is metabolized by the liver, brain, muscle, and kidney (Figure 2). In well-nourished cirrhotic patients, the affected liver has an impaired capacity for removal of ammonia in the form of urea, which may result in increased muscle glutamine synthetase in order to provide an alternative mechanism for ammonia removal as glutamine. Glutamine synthesis also increases to some extent in the brain of these patients. HE may develop as a consequence of increased circulating and cerebral ammonia in well-nourished cirrhotic patients. On the other hand, in malnourished cirrhotic patients, the loss of muscle mass, commonly seen as a consequence of malnutrition, can adversely affect this alternative route of ammonia removal. The brain being the main organ metabolizing ammonia in these conditions, severe HE is commonly diagnosed in malnourished cirrhotic patients.

Hyperammonemia may lead to increased uptake of tryptophan by the brain which may lead to increased synthesis and release of serotonin and anorexia. This symptom may render the patient prone to chronic catabolism and malnutrition, and in turn to increased ammonia load, resulting in a vicious cycle [29, 30]. In addition, hyperammonemia may be more prominent after gastrointestinal bleeding due to the absence of isoleucine [31]. Since haemoglobin molecule lacks the essential amino acid isoleucine, gastrointestinal bleed may stimulate the induction of net catabolism [32].

5.5.2 ZINC

Zinc is an essential trace element that plays an important role in the regulation of protein and nitrogen metabolism as well as in antioxidant defense. Reduced zinc content is common in cirrhotic patients, but zinc deficiency cannot be effectively diagnosed based upon serum concentrations since zinc is bound to albumin, which is also decreased in these patients [33, 34]. Among the mechanisms contributing to zinc deficiency, poor dietary intake [35], reduced intestinal absorption [36], reduced hepatointestinal extraction [37], portal-systemic shunting, and altered protein and amino acid metabolism have all been implicated [38]. Zinc deficiency may impair the activity of enzymes of the urea cycle as well as glutamine synthetase [39, 40], and decreased activity of these enzymes has the potential to lead to further increases in circulating and brain ammonia with the potential to cause worsening of HE. Not surprisingly, therefore, an inverse relationship between serum zinc and ammonia concentrations has been described [41, 42]. Zinc deficiency has been implicated in multiple complications of cirrhosis, including poor appetite, immune dysfunction, altered taste and smell, anorexia as well as altered protein metabolism [43, 44]. Surprisingly, in spite of evidence of hypozincemia in cirrhosis, zinc supplementation in the treatment of HE based on a small number of controlled trials has so far provided inconsistent results, a finding that may be attributable to variations in the nature and doses of zinc salts used and to duration of therapy [45].

5.5.3 SELENIUM

Decreased levels of selenium have been reported in cirrhotic patients [46, 47]. However, the relationship of diminished selenium to the pathogenesis of cirrhosis and its complications, including HE, has not been clearly established.

5.5.4 MANGANESE

In cirrhotic patients, the elimination of manganese is decreased secondary to impaired hepatobiliary function and portal-systemic shunting, which result in increased blood manganese levels and increased manganese deposition in basal ganglia structures of the brain, in particular in globus pallidus [48–52]. Manganese has also been correlated to increased brain glutamine levels [53] and changes in dopamine metabolism [49, 54] and may be related to other alterations in cirrhotic patients with HE, such as the characteristic astrocytic morphologic changes [55]. Toxic effects of manganese on central nervous system could be mediated by effects on the glycolytic enzyme glyceraldehyde-3-phosphate dehydrogenase (GAP-DH) [56]. It was also suggested that manganese-induced increases of "peripheral-type" benzodiazepine receptors (PTBRs) could contribute to the pathogenesis of HE [57].

5.5.5 L-CARNITINE

The liver is a major site for the production of ketone bodies from the oxidation of fatty acids. Fatty acids cannot penetrate the inner mitochondrial matrix and cross the mitochondrial membrane to undergo oxidation unless they are transported by a carrier process involving L-carnitine (3-hydroxy-4-trimethylammoniobutanoate). Carnitine is a cofactor for mitochondrial oxidation of fatty acids and prevents the body from using fats for energy production particularly during starvation. Carnitine deficiency may result in lethargy, somnolence, confusion, and encephalopathy. Studies of carnitine status in cirrhotic patients have yielded conflicting results; the source of this lack of consensus likely results from both the etiology of cirrhosis and the severity of liver disease. For example, Rudman et al. [58] reported reduced plasma and tissue carnitine concentrations in patients with alcoholic cirrhosis complicated by cachexia, whereas later studies by Fuller and Hoppel [59, 60] reported an increase of plasma carnitine in alcoholics with or without cirrhosis. De Sousa et al. [61] reported no such changes in a similar patient population. In a subsequent study by Amodio et al. [62], plasma carnitine levels were measured in cirrhotic patients and the relationship to nutritional status and severity of liver damage was assessed. Plasma carnitine levels did not differ between Child-Pugh class A, B, and C patients. Significantly higher levels of acetylcarnitine, short chain acylcarnitine, total esterified carnitine, and total carnitine were observed in cirrhotic patients independent of etiology of cirrhosis. The issue of carnitine in relation to liver disease was re-evaluated in 1997 by Krähenbühl and Reichen [63] who studied carnitine metabolism in 29 patients with chronic liver disease of varying degrees of severity and various etiologies. Patients with alcoholic cirrhosis manifested increased total plasma carnitine levels with a close correlation to serum bilirubin. Urinary carnitine excretion was not different between cirrhotic patients and controls with the exception of patients with primary biliary cirrhosis. It was concluded that patients with cirrhosis are not normally carnitine deficient and that patients with alcohol-induced cirrhosis manifest hypercarnitinemia which results primarily from increased carnitine synthesis due to increased skeletal muscle protein turnover [63].

5.5.6 VITAMIN B1 (THIAMINE)

Wernicke's Encephalopathy caused by vitamin B1 deficiency and characterized by a triad of neurological symptoms (ophthalmoplegia, ataxia, global confusional state) is common in cirrhotic patients. In a retrospective neuropathological study of sections from patients with end-stage liver failure who died in hepatic coma, 64% were found to manifest thalamic lesions typical of Wernicke's Encephalopathy [64]. None of the cases of Wernicke's Encephalopathy had been suspected based upon clinical symptoms during life, a finding which draws into question the classical textbook definition based upon symptomatology associated with the disorder [65].

Causes of vitamin B1 deficiency in cirrhosis include reduced dietary intake, impaired absorption, and loss of hepatic stores of the vitamin. Alcoholic cirrhotic patients manifest increased incidence of vitamin B1 deficiency compared to nonalcoholic cirrhotics [66]. Moreover, ethanol is known to impair both intestinal absorption of vitamin B1 [67] and to impair the transformation of the vitamin into its active (diphosphorylated) form [68]. It has been suggested that common pathophysiologic mechanisms exist in Wernicke's and hepatic encephalopathies, related to deficits of vitamin B1-dependent enzymes [69]. Vitamin B1 supplementation is highly recommended in patients with end-stage liver failure of either alcoholic or nonalcoholic etiologies.

5.6 NUTRITION, HE, AND LIVER TRANSPLANTATION

HE in end-stage liver failure may contribute to malnutrition in the pre-transplant period as a consequence of diminished food uptake [70]. Alterations in markers of nutritional status such as serum albumin are significant risk factors for both surgical [71] and postsurgical [72] complications of liver transplantation. Moreover, it has been suggested that nonabsorbable disaccharides (such as lactulose) administered for the management of HE may result in intestinal malabsorption in patients with end-stage liver failure with the potential to result in poor transplant outcome [73].

The negative impact of malnutrition on liver transplantation had been reported in early retrospective studies [74]. Both preoperative hypermetabolism and body cell mass depletion proved to be of prognostic value for transplantation outcome [75]. Malnutrition is known to lead to glycogen depletion, and this has been suggested to increase the plasma lactate:pyruvate ratio during the anhepatic phase and to induce an exacerbated proinflammatory cytokine response, thereby favouring the development of postoperative systemic inflammatory response syndrome and multiorgan failure in these patients [76]. To date, there are still insufficient data in the pretransplant period upon which to base specific recommendations. In the posttransplant period, nutritional therapy improves nitrogen balance, decreases viral infection, and shows a trend to shortened intensive care unit stays with lowering of hospitalisation costs [77, 78].

5.7 NUTRITIONAL RECOMMENDATIONS FOR HE IN END-STAGE LIVER FAILURE (TABLE 2)

5.7.1 GENERAL CONSIDERATIONS

Considering the high prevalence of malnutrition in cirrhotic patients together with the lack of simple and accurate methods of assessment of malnutrition in this patient population, it is reasonable to assume that malnutrition occurs in all patients. Nutritional requirements may vary according to the specific clinical situation. Multiple (5-6) small feedings with a carbohydrate-rich evening snack have been recommended with complex rather than simple carbohydrates used for calories. Lipids could provide 20%–40% of caloric needs. Long-term nutritional supplements may be necessary to provide recommended caloric and protein requirements. Additional studies are needed in order to formulate specific recommendations for nutrients such as zinc, selenium, and carnitine.

5.7.2 ENERGY REQUIREMENTS

The primary goal for a patient suffering from end-stage liver failure should be to avoid by all means possible intentional or unintentional weight loss and sustain a diet rich in nutrients. It has been suggested that patients with liver cirrhosis should receive 35–40 kcal/kg per day [25].

5.7.3 LOW PROTEIN DIET TO BE AVOIDED

Restriction of dietary protein was long considered a mainstay in the management of liver disease and HE [79, 80]. In particular, protein restriction (0–40 g protein/day) was shown to decrease encephalopathy grade in patients following surgical creation of a portal-systemic shunt, the only available therapy at one time for bleeding varices. Protein restriction (0–40 g protein/day) was later extended to include all patients with cirrhosis who developed encephalopathy. However, more recently, studies have shown that protein restriction in these patients has no impact on encephalopathy grade and that it may even worsen their nutritional status [81]. The increased awareness of the progressive deterioration of nutritional status in liver cirrhosis combined with a better understanding of metabolic alterations in the disorder has questioned the practice of prolonged protein restriction in the management of HE [82]. In fact, protein requirements are increased in cirrhotic patients, and high protein diets are generally well tolerated in the majority of patients. Moreover, the inclusion of adequate protein in the diets of malnourished patients with end-stage liver failure is often associated with a sustained improvement in their mental status. Furthermore, protein helps preserve lean body mass; this is crucial in patients with liver failure in whom skeletal muscle makes a significant contribution to ammonia removal. The consensus of opinion nowadays is that protein restriction be avoided in all but a small number of patients with severe protein intolerance and that protein be maintained between 1.2 and 1.5 g of proteins per kg of body weight per day. In severely protein intolerant patients, particularly in patients in grades III-IV HE, protein may be reduced for short periods of time [83–85].

5.7.4 VEGETABLE VERSUS ANIMAL PROTEINS

It has been suggested that vegetable proteins are better tolerated than animal proteins in patients with end-stage liver failure, a finding that has been attributed to either their higher content of branched-chain amino acids and/or because of their influence on intestinal transit [86, 87]. One study reported that a diet rich in vegetable protein (71 g/d) significantly improved the mental status of patients suffering from HE while increasing their nitrogen balance [88]. Vegetable proteins may also increase intraluminal pH and decrease gastric transit time. High dietary fibre diet has been recommended in order to abolish constipation which is an established precipitating factor for HE in patients with cirrhosis [89, 90]. A daily intake of 30–40 g vegetable protein has been found to be effective in the majority of patients [88].

5.7.5 BRANCHED-CHAIN AMINO ACIDS (BCAAS)

These amino acids (leucine, isoleucine, and valine) cannot be synthesized de novo but must be obtained from dietary sources and have a unique role in amino acid metabolism, regulating the intra- and interorgan exchange of nitrogen and amino acids by different tissues [91]. Chronic liver disease and portal-systemic shunting are characterized by a decrease in the plasma concentrations of BCAAs [92], whereas hyperammonemia increases their utilization. Since hyperammonemia results in increased utilization of BCAAs, which are largely metabolized by the muscle, it would be anticipated that providing BCAAs could facilitate ammonia detoxification by supporting muscle glutamine synthesis. Administration of BCAAs has been shown to stimulate hepatic protein synthesis; indeed, leucine stimulates the synthesis of hepatocyte growth factor by stellate cells [93]. Also, BCAAs reduce postinjury catabolism and improve nutritional status. Inadequate dietary protein intake or low levels of BCAAs may have a deleterious effect on HE [94], nutritional status [80], and clinical outcome [25, 81] in patients with end-stage liver failure. Clinical trials of BCAAs in the treatment of HE have yielded inconsistent findings. Several controlled clinical studies reported no efficacy of BCAAs on encephalopathy grade in patients with cirrhosis [95, 96]. However, other trials demonstrated that BCAAs were beneficial in similar patients [97, 98].

A double-blind, randomized clinical trial demonstrated that, in advanced cirrhosis, long-term nutritional supplementation with oral BCAA was useful to prevent progressive hepatic failure [99]. Furthermore, administration of solutions enriched with BCAAs has been shown to improve cerebral perfusion in cirrhotic patients [100]. Muto et al. [101] confirmed the beneficial effects of BCAAs using a more palatable granular formula. In a multicenter randomized study, it was also reported that long-term oral supplementation with a BCAA mixture improved the serum albumin level as well as cellular energy metabolism in cirrhotic patients [102].

The timing of BCAA supplementation in patients with end-stage liver failure may be crucial. This issue was addressed by a crossover study of 12 cirrhotic patients [103]. Daytime administration improved nitrogen balance and Fischer's ratio (ratio of BCAA/AAAs); however, both were further improved with nocturnal administration. At 3 months, a significant increase in serum albumin level was observed in patients administered nocturnal BCAAs, but not daytime BCAAs. It is possible that daytime BCAAs may be used primarily as calories, whereas nocturnal BCAAs may be preferentially used for protein synthesis. Furthermore, the long-term use of BCAAs in liver cirrhosis leads to an increase of serum protein of approximately 10% if given before bedtime [104]. Problems that limit the widespread use of BCAAs in the treatment of HE include their expense and unpalatability [105], both of which may result in poor patient compliance.

5.8 ANTIOXIDANTS

5.8.1 RATIONALE FOR USE OF ANTIOXIDANTS

Cirrhotic patients manifest evidence of increased expression of biomarkers of oxidative stress such as increased lipid peroxidation [106, 107], as well as impaired antioxidant defences. Decreased levels of antioxidant micronutrients, including zinc [33, 107], selenium [46, 47], and vitamin E [107, 108] have been described in patients with end-stage liver failure. The potential benefits of vitamin E have been investigated, but results are conflicting. One randomized, placebo-controlled trial of vitamin E supplementation revealed a significant amelioration in terms of liver inflammation and fibrosis in patients with nonalcoholic steatohepatitis [109], while other studies with biochemical end points did not demonstrate any significant beneficial effect of vitamin E supplements [110]. In an earlier placebo-controlled randomized trial, 1-year vitamin E supplementation to patients with end-stage liver failure led to increased serum alpha-tocopherol levels, but did not result in any improvement in survival or quality of life [111]. The benefits of vitamin E therapy in relation to HE have not been assessed.

5.8.2 N-ACETYLCYSTEINE

A widely used complementary medical therapy for acute liver failure is the glutathione prodrug, N-acetylcysteine (NAC) [112, 113]. Glutathione is a major component of the pathways by which cells are protected from oxidative stress. NAC is an antioxidant with a thiol-containing compound and is used to restore cytosolic glutathione and detoxify reactive oxygen species and free radicals. NAC has proven beneficial in patients with type I hepatorenal syndrome [112] but was inefficient in patients with hepatitis C [113]. While NAC is widely used to treat acetaminophen hepatotoxicity, its benefit in end-stage liver failure with specific reference to HE remains to be established. In this regard, NAC is known to cross the blood-brain barrier and to improve central antioxidant status in the brain in mice with acute liver failure due to azoxymethane-induced hepatotoxicity [114].

5.9 WATER-SOLUBLE AND FAT-SOLUBLE VITAMINS

Deficiencies in water-soluble vitamins (particularly the vitamin B complex) are common in end-stage liver failure [115]. A wide range of neuropsychiatric symptomatology associated with liver disease may be the consequence of water-soluble vitamin deficiencies. For example, peripheral neuropathy may result from pyridoxine, thiamine, or vitamin B12 deficiency. Confusion, ataxia and ocular disturbances are cardinal features of a lack of thiamine, and thiamine deficiency has been reported in patients with hepatitis C-related cirrhosis [116]. Deficiencies in vitamin B12, thiamine, and folic acid may develop faster in cirrhotic patients due to diminished hepatic storage.

Fat-soluble vitamins (A, D, and K) deficiencies are likely to arise from malabsorption associated with end-stage liver failure. Vitamin A supplementation may be considered since vitamin A deficiency results in nyctalopia and dry cornea, and is associated with increased risk of hepatocellular carcinoma in patients with end-stage liver disease [117, 118]. Prescription of vitamin D, especially in patients with cholestasis (in combination with calcium since osteoporosis may be a complication of end-stage liver failure), is advised [118, 119]. Also, supplementation of vitamin K in conditions with high risk of bleeding such as the presence of impaired prothrombin time and oesophageal varices, should be considered [118]. In view of these findings, administration of multivitamin preparations is recommended.

5.10 PROBIOTICS, PREBIOTICS, AND SYNBIOTICS

Probiotics are live microbiological dietary supplements with beneficial effects on the host beyond their nutritional properties. Prebiotics stimulate the growth and activity of beneficial bacteria within the intestinal flora. Synbiotics are a combination of pro- and prebiotics. Their mechanisms of action include the deprivation of substrates for potentially pathogenic bacteria, together with the provision of fermentation end products for potentially beneficial bacteria. Probiotic or prebiotic treatments aim at increasing the intestinal content of lactic acid-type bacteria at the expense of other species with more pathogenic potential.

The concept of treating HE with probiotics was already suggested several decades ago [120–122]. The therapeutic benefit of acidifying the gut lumen with synbiotics in cirrhotic patients with minimal HE was demonstrated by Liu et al. [123] who showed that synbiotic/probiotic supplementation ameliorates hepatic function as reflected by reduced bilirubin and albumin levels and prothrombin times [123]. Modulation of gut flora was also associated with a significant reduction in blood ammonia levels and a reversal of minimal HE in 50% of patients [123]; improved hepatic function and serum transaminase levels in patients with alcohol- and hepatitis C-related cirrhosis have also been reported [124]. Another group reported improvement in biochemical and neuropsychological tests in cirrhotic patients receiving probiotics [125, 126]. Furthermore, liver transplant recipients who received a synbiotic regimen developed significantly fewer bacterial infections [127]. In a subsequent clinical trial, the incidence of postoperative bacterial infection as well as the duration of antibiotic therapy was significantly reduced in liver transplant patients receiving prebiotics [128]. More recently, Bajaj et al. [129] demonstrated a significant rate of minimal HE reversal in cirrhotic patients after probiotic yogurt supplements. Probiotics may provide additional benefits over dietary supplementation in reducing episodes of infection. Given the efficacy of probiotics and their lack of side effects, they are increasingly being used in the management of HE.

5.11 CONCLUSION

Malnutrition is common in patients with end-stage liver failure and HE and adversely affects prognosis. Inadequate dietary intake, altered synthesis and absorption of nutrients, increased protein losses, hypermetabolism, and inflammation are among the factors contributing to malnutrition in this patient population. Although there are now several available methods to assess malnutrition, a standardized simple and accurate method for evaluating malnutrition in end-stage liver failure remains a challenge. Consequences of end-stage liver failure with a potential to impact upon nutritional status and brain function are numerous and include hyperammonemia, reduced zinc and selenium, manganese accumulation as well as deficiencies of carnitine and water-soluble vitamins, particularly thiamine. The primary goal for a patient with end-stage liver failure is to avoid by all means possible weight loss and sustain a diet rich in nutrients. A caloric intake of 35–40 kcal/kg/day is recommended. Low protein diets should be avoided and protein intake maintained at 1.2–1.5 g/kg/day. Particular attention should also be drawn to vegetable protein as well as to BCAAs which have proven beneficial in the treatment of HE. Antioxidants as well as probiotics are increasingly being employed in order to optimize the nutritional status in cirrhotic patients. Administration of multivitamin preparations, particularly thiamine, is recommended for patients with end-stage liver failure. Nutritional support to meet energy and substrate needs and to optimize the removal of circulating ammonia, reduce proinflammatory mechanisms, and improve antioxidant defenses has the potential to limit the progression of liver dysfunction, treat HE, and improve quality of life in patients with end-stage liver failure.

REFERENCES

1. Italian Multicentre Cooperative Project on Nutrition in Liver Cirrhosis, "Nutritional status in cirrhosis," Journal of Hepatology, vol. 21, no. 3, pp. 317–325, 1994.

2. M. J. Müller, "Malnutrition in cirrhosis," Journal of Hepatology, Supplement, vol. 23, no. 1, pp. 31–35, 1995.

3. L. Caregaro, F. Alberino, P. Amodio, et al., "Malnutrition in alcoholic and virus-related cirrhosis," American Journal of Clinical Nutrition, vol. 63, no. 4, pp. 602–609, 1996.

4. C. Mendenhall, G. A. Roselle, P. Gartside, and T. Moritz, "Relationship of protein calorie malnutrition to alcoholic liver disease: a reexamination of data from two Veteran Administration Cooperative Studies," Alcoholism: Clinical and Experimental Research, vol. 19, no. 3, pp. 635–641, 1995.

5. B. Campillo, J. P. Richardet, E. Scherman, and P. N. Bories, "Evaluation of nutritional practice in hospitalized cirrhotic patients: results of a prospective study," Nutrition, vol. 19, no. 6, pp. 515–521, 2003.

6. K. K. Changani, R. Jalan, I. J. Cox, M. Ala-Korpela, K. Bhakoo, S. D. Taylor-Robinson, and J. D. Bell, "Evidence for altered hepatic gluconeogenesis in patients with cirrhosis using in vivo 31-phosphorus magnetic resonance spectroscopy," Gut, vol. 49, no. 4, pp. 557–564, 2001.

7. B. Campillo, C. Chapelain, and C. Chapelain, "Hormonal and metabolic changes during exercise in cirrhotic patients," Metabolism, vol. 39, no. 1, pp. 18–24, 1990.

8. T. L. Sourkes, "Tryptophan in hepatic coma," Journal of Neural Transmission, Supplement, no. 14, pp. 79–86, 1978.

9. M. Plauth and E. T. Schütz, "Cachexia in liver cirrhosis," International Journal of Cardiology, vol. 85, no. 1, pp. 83–87, 2002.

10. F. Izbéki, I. Kiss, T. Wittmann, T. T. Várkonyi, P. Légrády, and J. Lonovics, "Impaired accommodation of proximal stomach in patients with alcoholic liver cirrhosis," Scandinavian Journal of Gastroenterology, vol. 37, no. 12, pp. 1403–1410, 2002.

11. B. A. Aqel, J. S. Scolapio, R. C. Dickson, D. D. Burton, and E. P. Bouras, "Contribution of ascites to impaired gastric function and nutritional intake in patients with cirrhosis and ascites," Clinical Gastroenterology and Hepatology, vol. 3, no. 11, pp. 1095–1100, 2005.

12. M. A. Boermeester, A. P. Houdijk, and A. P. Houdijk, "Liver failure induces a systemic inflammatory response: prevention by recombinant N-terminal bactericidal/permeability-increasing protein," American Journal of Pathology, vol. 147, no. 5, pp. 1428–1440, 1995.

13. H. Tilg, A. Wilmer, W. Vogel, M. Herold, B. Nolchen, G. Judmaier, and C. Huber, "Serum levels of cytokines in chronic liver diseases," Gastroenterology, vol. 103, no. 1, pp. 264–274, 1992.

14. V. von Baehr, W. D. Döcke, and W. D. Döcke, "Mechanisms of endotoxin tolerance in patients with alcoholic liver cirrhosis: role of interleukin 10, interleukin 1 receptor antagonist, and soluble tumour necrosis factor receptors as well as effector cell desensitisation," Gut, vol. 47, no. 2, pp. 281–287, 2000.

15. A. J. McCullough and A. S. Tavill, "Disordered energy and protein metabolism in liver disease," Seminars in Liver Disease, vol. 11, no. 4, pp. 265–277, 1991.

16. T. Nishida, S. Tsuji, and S. Tsuji, "Oral glucose tolerance test predicts prognosis of patients with liver cirrhosis," American Journal of Gastroenterology, vol. 101, no. 1, pp. 70–75, 2006.

17. J. S. Scolapio, A. Ukleja, K. McGreevy, O. L. Burnett, and P. C. O'Brien, "Nutritional problems in end-stage liver disease: contribution of impaired gastric emptying and ascites," Journal of Clinical Gastroenterology, vol. 34, no. 1, pp. 89–93, 2002.

18. C. Gerstner, T. Schuetz, V. von Baehr, et al., "Correlation between energy expenditure, nutrient intake, malnutrition and activation of the inflammatory system in patients with liver cirrhosis," Journal of Hepatology, vol. 34, supplement 1, pp. 195–196, 2001.

19. G. Bianchi, R. Marzocchi, C. Lorusso, V. Ridolfi, and G. Marchesini, "Nutritional treatment of chronic liver failure," Hepatology Research, vol. 38, no. 1, pp. S93–S101, 2008.

20. E. Bartoli, L. Castello, and P. P. Sainaghi, "Diagnosis and therapy of hyponatremia," Annali Italiani di Medicina Interna, vol. 18, no. 4, pp. 193–203, 2003.

21. N. Tözün, "Influence of the metabolic complications of liver cirrhosis on dietary intake," Medical Science Monitor, vol. 6, no. 6, pp. 1223–1226, 2000.

22. F. Gunsar, M. L. Raimondo, and M. L. Raimondo, "Nutritional status and prognosis in cirrhotic patients," Alimentary Pharmacology and Therapeutics, vol. 24, no. 4, pp. 563–572, 2006.

23. L. M. Forman and M. R. Lucey, "Predicting the prognosis of chronic liver disease: an evolution from child to MELD," Hepatology, vol. 33, no. 2, pp. 473–475, 2001.

24. L. Pagliaro, "MELD: the end of Child-Pugh classification?" Journal of Hepatology, vol. 36, no. 1, pp. 141–142, 2002.

25. M. Plauth, E. Cabré, and E. Cabré, "ESPEN Guidelines on Enteral Nutrition: liver disease," Clinical Nutrition, vol. 25, no. 2, pp. 285–294, 2006.

26. B. Campillo, J. P. Richardet, and P. N. Bories, "Enteral nutrition in severely malnourished and anorectic cirrhotic patients in clinical practice: benefit and prognostic

factors," Gastroenterologie Clinique et Biologique, vol. 29, no. 6-7, pp. 645–651, 2005.

27. M. R. Álvares-da-Silva and T. Reverbel da Silveira, "Comparison between handgrip strength, subjective global assessment, and prognostic nutritional index in assessing malnutrition and predicting clinical outcome in cirrhotic outpatients," Nutrition, vol. 21, no. 2, pp. 113–117, 2005.

28. M. Y. Morgan, A. M. Madden, C. T. Soulsby, and R. W. Morris, "Derivation and validation of a new global method for assessing nutritional status in patients with cirrhosis," Hepatology, vol. 44, no. 4, pp. 823–835, 2006.

29. C. Bachmann, O. Braissant, A. M. Villard, O. Boulat, and H. Henry, "Ammonia toxicity to the brain and creatine," Molecular Genetics and Metabolism, vol. 81, pp. S52–S57, 2004.

30. R. M. Cohn and K. S. Roth, "Hyperammonemia, bane of the brain," Clinical Pediatrics, vol. 43, no. 8, pp. 683–689, 2004.

31. C. H. Dejong, W. J. Meijerink, C. L. van Berlo, N. E. Deutz, and P. B. Soeters, "Decreased plasma isoleucine concentrations after upper gastrointestinal haemorrhage in humans," Gut, vol. 39, no. 1, pp. 13–17, 1996.

32. S. W. Olde Damink, C. H. Dejong, and R. Jalan, "Review article: hyperammonaemic and catabolic consequences of upper gastrointestinal bleeding in cirrhosis," Alimentary Pharmacology and Therapeutics, vol. 29, no. 8, pp. 801–810, 2009.

33. K. Kisters, C. Spieker, S. Q. Nguyen, H. P. Bertram, C. Muller, and W. Zidek, "Zinc concentrations in human liver tissue and in blood plasma in cirrhosis of the liver due to alcoholism," Trace Elements and Electrocytes, vol. 11, no. 3, pp. 101–103, 1994.

34. H. F. Goode, J. Kelleher, and B. E. Walker, "Relation between zinc status and hepatic functional reserve in patients with liver disease," Gut, vol. 31, no. 6, pp. 694–697, 1990.

35. L. Capocaccia, M. Merli, C. Piat, R. Servi, A. Zullo, and O. Riggio, "Zinc and other trace elements in liver cirrhosis," Italian Journal of Gastroenterology, vol. 23, no. 6, pp. 386–391, 1991.

36. K. Gohshi, S. Fujiyama, J. Shibata, T. Sato, A. Higashi, and I. Matsuda, "Zinc absorption and its correlation with results of oral zinc tolerance testing in non-alcoholic liver cirrhosis; kinetic study," Hepatogastroenterology, vol. 42, no. 5, pp. 487–491, 1995.

37. P. W. Keeling, W. Ruse, J. Bull, B Hannigan, and R. P. Thompson, "Direct measurement of the hepatointestinal extraction of zinc in cirrhosis and hepatitis," Clinical Science, vol. 61, no. 4, pp. 441–444, 1981.

38. E. Rocchi, P. Borella, A. Borghi, F. Paolillo, M. Pradelli, F. Farina, and G. Casalgrandi, "Zinc and magnesium in liver cirrhosis," European Journal of Clinical Investigation, vol. 24, no. 3, pp. 149–155, 1994.

39. O. Riggio, M. Merli, and M. Merli, "Zinc supplementation reduces blood ammonia and increases liver ornithine transcarbamylase activity in experimental cirrhosis," Hepatology, vol. 16, no. 3, pp. 785–789, 1992.

40. A. S. Prasad, P. Rabbani, A. Abbasii, E. Bowersox, and M. R. Fox, "Experimental zinc deficiency in humans," Annals of Internal Medicine, vol. 89, no. 4, pp. 483–490, 1978.

41. P. Reding, J. Duchateau, and C. Bataille, "Oral zinc supplementation improves hepatic encephalopathy. Results of a randomised controlled trial," Lancet, vol. 2, no. 8401, pp. 493–495, 1984.

42. K. Grüngreiff, H. J. Presser, D. Franke, B. Lössner, K. Abicht, and F. D. Kleine, "Correlations between zinc, amino acids and ammonia in liver cirrhosis," Zeitschrift fur Gastroenterologie, vol. 27, no. 12, pp. 731–735, 1989.

43. A. S. Prasad, "Effects of zinc deficiency on Th1 and Th2 cytokine shifts," Journal of Infectious Diseases, vol. 182, no. 3, pp. S62–S68, 2000.

44. G. Marchesini, A. Fabbri, G. Bianchi, M. Brizi, and M. Zoli, "Zinc supplementation and amino acid-nitrogen metabolism in patients with advanced cirrhosis," Hepatology, vol. 23, no. 5, pp. 1084–1092, 1996.

45. P. Marchetti, P. Amodio, L. Caregaro, and A. Gatta, "Zinc deficiency in liver cirrhosis: a curiosity or problem?" Annali Italiani di Medicina Interna, vol. 13, no. 3, pp. 157–162, 1998.

46. B. Dworkin, W. S. Rosenthal, R. H. Jankowski, G. G. Gordon, and D. Haldea, "Low blood selenium levels in alcoholics with and without advanced liver disease. Correlations with clinical and nutritional status," Digestive Diseases and Sciences, vol. 30, no. 9, pp. 838–844, 1985.

47. A. Van Gossum and J. Nève, "Low selenium status in alcoholic cirrhosis is correlated with aminopyrine breath test: preliminary effects of selenium supplementation," Biological Trace Element Research, vol. 47, no. 1–3, pp. 201–207, 1995.

48. G. Pomier-Layrargues, L. Spahr, and R. F. Butterworth, "Increased manganese concentrations in pallidum of cirrhotic patients," Lancet, vol. 345, no. 8951, p. 735, 1995.

49. R. F. Butterworth, L. Spahr, S. Fontaine, and G. P. Layrargues, "Manganese toxicity, dopaminergic dysfunction and hepatic encephalopathy," Metabolic Brain Disease, vol. 10, no. 4, pp. 259–267, 1995.

50. L. Spahr, R. F. Butterworth, and R. F. Butterworth, "Increased blood manganese in cirrhotic patients: relationship to pallidal magnetic resonance signal hyperintensity and neurological symptoms," Hepatology, vol. 24, no. 5, pp. 1116–1120, 1996.

51. C. Rose, R. F. Butterworth, and R. F. Butterworth, "Manganese deposition in basal ganglia structures results from both portal-systemic shunting and liver dysfunction," Gastroenterology, vol. 117, no. 3, pp. 640–644, 1999.

52. G. P. Layrargues, D. Shapcott, L. Spahr, and R. F. Butterworth, "Accumulation of manganese and copper in pallidum of cirrhotic patients: role in the pathogenesis of hepatic encephalopathy?" Metabolic Brain Disease, vol. 10, no. 4, pp. 353–356, 1995.

53. S. Montes, M. Alcaraz-Zubeldia, P. Muriel, and C. Rios, "Role of manganese accumulation in increased brain glutamine of the cirrhotic rat," Neurochemical Research, vol. 28, no. 6, pp. 911–917, 2003.

54. S. C. Sistrunk, M. K. Ross, and N. M. Filipov, "Direct effects of manganese compounds on dopamine and its metabolite Dopac: an in vitro study," Environmental Toxicology and Pharmacology, vol. 23, no. 3, pp. 286–296, 2007.

55. R. F. Butterworth, "Complications of cirrhosis. III. Hepatic encephalopathy," Journal of Hepatology, vol. 32, no. 1, pp. 171–180, 2000.

56. A. S. Hazell, P. Desjardins, and R. F. Butterworth, "Increased expression of glyceraldehyde-3-phosphate dehydrogenase in cultured astrocytes following exposure to manganese," Neurochemistry International, vol. 35, no. 1, pp. 11–17, 1999.

57. A. S. Hazell, P. Desjardins, and R. F. Butterworth, "Chronic exposure of rat primary astrocyte cultures to manganese results in increased binding sites for the 'peripheral-type' benzodiazepine receptor ligand H3-PK 11195," Neuroscience Letters, vol. 271, no. 1, pp. 5–8, 1999.

58. D. Rudman, C. W. Sewell, and J. D. Ansley, "Deficiency of carnitine in cachectic cirrhotic patients," Journal of Clinical Investigation, vol. 60, no. 3, pp. 716–723, 1977.

59. R. K. Fuller and C. L. Hoppel, "Elevated plasma carnitine in hepatic cirrhosis," Hepatology, vol. 3, no. 4, pp. 554–558, 1983.

60. R. K. Fuller and C. L. Hoppel, "Plasma carnitine in alcoholism," Alcoholism: Clinical and Experimental Research, vol. 12, no. 5, pp. 639–642, 1988.

61. C. De Sousa, N. W. Leung, R. A. Chalmers, and T. J. Peters, "Free and total carnitine and acylcarnitine content of plasma, urine, liver and muscle of alcoholics," Clinical Science, vol. 75, no. 4, pp. 437–440, 1988.

62. P. Amodio, P. Angeli, C. Merkel, F. Menon, and A. Gatta, "Plasma carnitine levels in liver cirrhosis: relationship with nutritional status and liver damage," Journal of Clinical Chemistry and Clinical Biochemistry, vol. 28, no. 9, pp. 619–626, 1990.

63. S. Krähenbühl and J. Reichen, "Carnitine metabolism in patients with chronic liver disease," Hepatology, vol. 25, no. 1, pp. 148–153, 1997.

64. J. J. Kril and R. F. Butterworth, "Diencephalic and cerebellar pathology in alcoholic and nonalcoholic patients with end-stage liver disease," Hepatology, vol. 26, no. 4, pp. 837–841, 1997.

65. C. G. Harper and R. F. Butterworth, "Nutritional and metabolic disorders," in Greenfield's Neuropathology, pp. 601–655, Hodder Arnold, 6th edition, 1997.

66. U. Laforenza, C. Patrini, G. Gastaldi, and G. Rindi, "Effects of acute and chronic ethanol administration on thiamine metabolizing enzymes in some brain areas and in other organs of the rat," Alcohol and Alcoholism, vol. 25, no. 6, pp. 591–603, 1990.

67. A. D. Thomson, H. Baker, and C. M. Leevy, "Patterns of S-thiamine hydrochloride absorption in the malnourished alcoholic patient," The Journal of Laboratory and Clinical Medicine, vol. 76, no. 1, pp. 34–45, 1970.

68. G. Rindi, L. Imarisio, and C. Patrini, "Effects of acute and chronic ethanol administration on regional thiamin pyrophosphokinase activity of the rat brain," Biochemical Pharmacology, vol. 35, no. 22, pp. 3903–3908, 1986.

69. R. F. Butterworth, "Thiamine deficiency-related brain dysfunction in chronic liver failure," Metabolic Brain Disease, vol. 24, no. 1, pp. 189–196, 2009.

70. A. S. Henkel and A. L. Buchman, "Nutritional support in patients with chronic liver disease," Nature Clinical Practice Gastroenterology and Hepatology, vol. 3, no. 4, pp. 202–209, 2006.

71. S. A. McCluskey, K. Karkouti, and K. Karkouti, "Derivation of a risk index for the prediction of massive blood transfusion in liver transplantation," Liver Transplantation, vol. 12, no. 11, pp. 1584–1593, 2006.

72. G. Fusai, P. Dhaliwal, and P. Dhaliwal, "Incidence and risk factors for the development of prolonged and severe intrahepatic cholestasis after liver transplantation," Liver Transplantation, vol. 12, no. 11, pp. 1626–1633, 2006.

73. L. W. Teperman and V. P. Peyregne, "Considerations on the impact of hepatic encephalopathy treatments in the pretransplant setting," Transplantation, vol. 89, no. 7, pp. 771–778, 2010.

74. B. W. Shaw, R. P. Wood, R. D. Gordon, S. Iwatsuki, W. P. Gillquist, and T. E. Starzl, "Influence of selected patient variables and operative blood loss on six-month survival following liver transplantation," Seminars in Liver Disease, vol. 5, no. 4, pp. 385–393, 1985.

75. O. Selberg, J. Böttcher, G. Tusch, R. Pichlmayr, E. Henkel, and M. J. Müller, "Identification of high- and low-risk patients before liver transplantation: a prospective cohort study of nutritional and metabolic parameters in 150 patients," Hepatology, vol. 25, no. 3, pp. 652–657, 1997.

76. C. Miki, K. Iriyama, A. D. Mayer, J. A. C. Buckels, J. D. Harrison, H. Suzuki, and P. McMaster, "Energy storage and cytokine response in patients undergoing liver transplantation," Cytokine, vol. 11, no. 3, pp. 244–248, 1999.

77. J. M. Hasse, L. S. Blue, and L. S. Blue, "Early enteral nutrition support in patients undergoing liver transplantation," Journal of Parenteral and Enteral Nutrition, vol. 19, no. 6, pp. 437–443, 1995.

78. J. Reilly, R. Mehta, and R. Mehta, "Nutritional support after liver transplantation: a randomized prospective study," Journal of Parenteral and Enteral Nutrition, vol. 14, no. 4, pp. 386–391, 1990.

79. S. Sherlock, "Hepatic encephalopathy," in Diseases of the Liver and Biliary System, pp. 109–110, Blackwell Scientific, Oxford, UK, 8th edition, 1989.

80. A. Donaghy, "Issues of malnutrition and bone disease in patients with cirrhosis," Journal of Gastroenterology and Hepatology, vol. 17, no. 4, pp. 462–466, 2002.

81. J. K. Heyman, C. J. Whitfield, K. E. Brock, G. W. McCaughan, and A. J. Donaghy, "Dietary protein intakes in patients with hepatic encephalopathy and cirrhosis: current practice in NSW and ACT," Medical Journal of Australia, vol. 185, no. 10, pp. 542–543, 2006.

82. K. D. Mullen and S. Dasarathy, "Protein restriction in hepatic encephalopathy: necessary evil or illogical dogma?" Journal of Hepatology, vol. 41, no. 1, pp. 147–148, 2004.

83. M. Plauth, M. Merli, J. Kondrup, A. Weimann, P. Ferenci, and M. J. Müller, "ESPEN guidelines for nutrition in liver disease and transplantation," Clinical Nutrition, vol. 16, no. 2, pp. 43–55, 1997.

84. M. Plauth, M. Merli, and J. Kondrup, "Management of hepatic encephalopathy," New England Journal of Medicine, vol. 337, no. 26, pp. 1921–1922, 1997.

85. M. Merli and O. Riggio, "Dietary and nutritional indications in hepatic encephalopathy," Metabolic Brain Disease, vol. 24, no. 1, pp. 211–221, 2009.

86. N. J. Greenberger, J. Carley, S. Schenker, I. Bettinger, C. Stamnes, and P. Beyer, "Effect of vegetable and animal protein diets in chronic hepatic encephalopathy," American Journal of Digestive Diseases, vol. 22, no. 10, pp. 845–855, 1977.

87. A. Keshavarzian, J. Meek, C. Sutton, V. M. Emery, E. A. Hughes, and H. J. Hodgson, "Dietary protein supplementation from vegetable sources in the management

of chronic portal systemic encephalopathy," American Journal of Gastroenterology, vol. 79, no. 12, pp. 945–949, 1984.

88. G. P. Bianchi, G. Marchesini, A. Fabbri, A. Rondelli, E. Bugianesi, M. Zoli, and E. Pisi, "Vegetable versus animal protein diet in cirrhotic patients with chronic encephalopathy. A randomized cross-over comparison," Journal of Internal Medicine, vol. 233, no. 5, pp. 385–392, 1993.

89. D. K. Podolsky and K. J. Isselbacher, "Maladie alcoolique du foie et cirrhoses," in Harrison Médecine Interne, pp. 1483–1495, 13th edition, 1995.

90. S. Sherlock, Diseases of the Liver and Biliary System, Blackwell Scientific, 9th edition, 1993.

91. P. Felig and J. Wahren, "Protein turnover and amino acid metabolism in the regulation of gluconeogenesis," Federation Proceedings, vol. 33, no. 4, pp. 1092–1097, 1974.

92. P. B. Soeters and J. E. Fischer, "Insulin, glucagon, aminoacid imbalance, and hepatic encephalopathy," Lancet, vol. 2, no. 7991, pp. 880–882, 1976.

93. T. Tomiya, Y. Inoue, and Y. Inoue, "Leucine stimulates the secretion of hepatocyte growth factor by hepatic stellate cells," Biochemical and Biophysical Research Communications, vol. 297, no. 5, pp. 1108–1111, 2002.

94. J. Córdoba, J. López-Hellín, and J. López-Hellín, "Normal protein diet for episodic hepatic encephalopathy: results of a randomized study," Journal of Hepatology, vol. 41, no. 1, pp. 38–43, 2004.

95. L. S. Eriksson, A. Persson, and J. Wahren, "Branched-chain amino acids in the treatment of chronic hepatic encephalopathy," Gut, vol. 23, no. 10, pp. 801–806, 1982.

96. J. Wahren, J. Denis, P. Desurmont, et al., "Is intravenous administration of branched chain amino acids effective in the treatment of hepatic encephalopathy? A multi-center study," Hepatology, vol. 3, no. 4, pp. 475–480, 1983.

97. E. H. Egberts, H. Schomerus, W. Hamster, and P. Jürgens, "Branched chain amino acids in the treatment of latent portosystemic encephalopathy. A double-blind placebo-controlled crossover study," Gastroenterology, vol. 88, no. 4, pp. 887–895, 1985.

98. M. Plauth, E. H. Egberts, and E. H. Egberts, "Long-term treatment of latent porto-systemic encephalopathy with branched-chain amino acids. A double-blind placebo-controlled crossover study," Journal of Hepatology, vol. 17, no. 3, pp. 308–314, 1993.

99. G. Marchesini, G. Bianchi, and G. Bianchi, "Nutritional supplementation with branched-chain amino acids in advanced cirrhosis: a double-blind, randomized trial," Gastroenterology, vol. 124, no. 7, pp. 1792–1801, 2003.

100. M. Iwasa, K. Matsumura, and K. Matsumura, "Improvement of regional cerebral blood flow after treatment with branched-chain amino acid solutions in patients with cirrhosis," European Journal of Gastroenterology and Hepatology, vol. 15, no. 7, pp. 733–737, 2003.

101. Y. Muto, S. Sato, and S. Sato, "Effects of oral branched-chain amino acid granules on event-free survival in patients with liver cirrhosis," Clinical Gastroenterology and Hepatology, vol. 3, no. 7, pp. 705–713, 2005.

102. Y. Nakaya, K. Okita, and K. Okita, "BCAA-enriched snack improves nutritional state of cirrhosis," Nutrition, vol. 23, no. 2, pp. 113–120, 2007.

103. H. Fukushima, Y. Miwa, and Y. Miwa, "Nocturnal branched-chain amino acid administration improves protein metabolism in patients with liver cirrhosis: comparison

with daytime administration," Journal of Parenteral and Enteral Nutrition, vol. 27, no. 5, pp. 315–322, 2003.

104. G. Bianchi, R. Marzocchi, F. Agostini, and G. Marchesini, "Update on nutritional supplementation with branched-chain amino acids," Current Opinion in Clinical Nutrition and Metabolic Care, vol. 8, no. 1, pp. 83–87, 2005.

105. S. Khanna and S. Gopalan, "Role of branched-chain amino acids in liver disease: the evidence for and against," Current Opinion in Clinical Nutrition and Metabolic Care, vol. 10, no. 3, pp. 297–303, 2007.

106. P. Clot, M. Tabone, S. Aricò, and E. Albano, "Monitoring oxidative damage in patients with liver cirrhosis and different daily alcohol intake," Gut, vol. 35, no. 11, pp. 1637–1643, 1994.

107. S. Moscarella, A. Duchini, and G. Buzzelli, "Lipoperoxidation, trace elements and vitamin E in patients with liver cirrhosis," European Journal of Gastroenterology and Hepatology, vol. 6, no. 7, pp. 633–636, 1994.

108. A. Nagita and M. Ando, "Assessment of hepatic vitamin E status in adult patients with liver disease," Hepatology, vol. 26, no. 2, pp. 392–397, 1997.

109. S. A. Harrison, S. Torgerson, P. Hayashi, J. Ward, and S. Schenker, "Vitamin E and vitamin C treatment improves fibrosis in patients with nonalcoholic steatohepatitis," American Journal of Gastroenterology, vol. 98, no. 11, pp. 2485–2490, 2003.

110. M. Kugelmas, D. B. Hill, B. Vivian, L. Marsano, and C. J. McClain, "Cytokines and NASH: a pilot study of the effects of lifestyle modification and vitamin E," Hepatology, vol. 38, no. 2, pp. 413–419, 2003.

111. M. P. de la Maza, M. Petermann, D. Bunout, and S. Hirsch, "Effects of long-term vitamin E supplementation in alcoholic cirrhotics," Journal of the American College of Nutrition, vol. 14, no. 2, pp. 192–196, 1995.

112. S. Holt, D. Goodier, and D. Goodier, "Improvement in renal function in hepatorenal syndrome with N-acetylcysteine," Lancet, vol. 353, no. 9149, pp. 294–295, 1999.

113. G. Idéo, A. Bellobuono, and A. Bellobuono, "Antioxidant drugs combined with alpha-interferon in chronic hepatitis C not responsive to alpha-interferon alone: a randomized, multicentre study," European Journal of Gastroenterology and Hepatology, vol. 11, no. 11, pp. 1203–1207, 1999.

114. C. Bémeur, J. Vaquero, P. Desjardins, and R. F. Butterworth, "N-acetylcysteine attenuates cerebral complications of non-acetaminophen-induced acute liver failure in mice: antioxidant and anti-inflammatory mechanisms," Metabolic Brain Disease, vol. 25, no. 2, pp. 241–249, 2010.

115. E. Cabré and M. A. Gassull, "Nutritional aspects of chronic liver disease," Clinical Nutrition, vol. 12, no. 1, pp. S52–S63, 1993.

116. S. Lévy, C. Hervé, E. Delacoux, and S. Erlinger, "Thiamine deficiency in hepatitis C virus and alcohol-related liver diseases," Digestive Diseases and Sciences, vol. 47, no. 3, pp. 543–548, 2002.

117. P. N. Newsome, I. Beldon, Y. Moussa, T. E. Delahooke, G. Poulopoulos, P. C. Hayes, and J. N. Plevris, "Low serum retinol levels are associated with hepatocellular carcinoma in patients with chronic liver disease," Alimentary Pharmacology and Therapeutics, vol. 14, no. 10, pp. 1295–1301, 2000.

118. F. Gundling, N. Teich, H. M. Strebel, W. Schepp, and C. Pehl, "Nutrition in liver cirrhosis," Medizinische Klinik, vol. 102, no. 6, pp. 435–444, 2007.

119. S. Masuda, T. Okano, K. Osawa, M. Shinjo, T. Suematsu, and T. Kobayashi, "Concentrations of vitamin D-binding protein and vitamin D metabolites in plasma of patients with liver cirrhosis," Journal of Nutritional Science and Vitaminology, vol. 35, no. 4, pp. 225–234, 1989.

120. W. A. Macbeth, E. N. Kass, and W. V. Mcdermott Jr., "Treatment of hepatic encephalopathy by alteration of intestinal flora with Lactobacillus acidophilus," The Lancet, vol. 285, no. 7382, pp. 399–403, 1965.

121. C. Loguercio, C. Del Vecchio Blanco, and M. Coltorti, "Enterococcus lactic acid bacteria strain SF68 and lactulose in hepatic encephalopathy: a controlled study," Journal of International Medical Research, vol. 15, no. 6, pp. 335–343, 1987.

122. C. Loguercio, R. Abbiati, M. Rinaldi, A. Romano, C. Del Vecchio Blanco, and M. Coltorti, "Long-term effects of Enterococcus faecium SF68 versus lactulose in the treatment of patients with cirrhosis and grade 1-2 hepatic encephalopathy," Journal of Hepatology, vol. 23, no. 1, pp. 39–46, 1995.

123. Q. Liu, Z. P. Duan, D. K. Ha, S. Bengmark, J. Kurtovic, and S. M. Riordan, "Synbiotic modulation of gut flora: effect on minimal hepatic encephalopathy in patients with cirrhosis," Hepatology, vol. 39, no. 5, pp. 1441–1449, 2004.

124. C. Loguercio, A. Federico, C. Tuccillo, F. Terracciano, M. V. D'Auria, C. De Simone, and C. Del Vecchio Blanco, "Beneficial effects of a probiotic VSL#3 on parameters of liver dysfunction in chronic liver diseases," Journal of Clinical Gastroenterology, vol. 39, no. 6, pp. 540–543, 2005.

125. M. Malaguarnera, F. Greco, G. Barone, M. P. Gargante, M. Malaguarnera, and M. A. Toscano, "Bifidobacterium longum with fructo-oligosaccharide (FOS) treatment in minimal hepatic encephalopathy: a randomized, double-blind, placebo-controlled study," Digestive Diseases and Sciences, vol. 52, no. 11, pp. 3259–3265, 2007.

126. M. Malaguarnera, M. P. Gargante, and M. P. Gargante, "Bifidobacterium combined with fructo-oligosaccharide versus lactulose in the treatment of patients with hepatic encephalopathy," European Journal of Gastroenterology and Hepatology, vol. 22, no. 2, pp. 199–206, 2010.

127. N. Rayes, D. Seehofer, and D. Seehofer, "Early enteral supply of Lactobacillus and fiber versus selective bowel decontamination: a controlled trial in liver transplant recipients," Transplantation, vol. 74, no. 1, pp. 123–128, 2002.

128. N. Rayes, D. Seehofer, and D. Seehofer, "Supply of pre- and probiotics reduces bacterial infection rates after liver transplantation—a randomized, double-blind trial," American Journal of Transplantation, vol. 5, no. 1, pp. 125–130, 2005.

129. J. S. Bajaj, K. Saeian, and K. Saeian, "Probiotic yogurt for the treatment of minimal hepatic encephalopathy," American Journal of Gastroenterology, vol. 103, no. 7, pp. 1707–1715, 2008.

This chapter was originally published under the Creative Commons Attribution License. Bémeur, C., Desjardins, P., and Butterworth, R. F. Role of Nutrition in the Management of Hepatic Encephalopathy in End-Stage Liver Failure . Journal of Nutrition and Metabolism 2010. doi:10.1155/2010/489823.

PARENTERAL NUTRITION COMBINED WITH ENTERAL NUTRITION FOR SEVERE ACUTE PANCREATITIS

AKANAND SINGH, MING CHEN, TAO LI, XIAO-LI YANG, JIN-ZHENG LI, and JIAN-PING GONG

6.1 INTRODUCTION

Acute pancreatitis (AP) is an acute inflammation process of the pancreas with variable involvement of other tissue or remote organ systems ranging from a mild, self-limited course requiring only brief hospitalization to a rapidly progressive, fulminant illness resulting in the multiple organ dysfunction syndromes with or without accompanying sepsis. Severe acute pancreatitis (SAP) is a common disease with emergency situation involving organ failure and/or local complications such as necrosis, abscess, or pseudocysts having mortality of up to 30 percent. Despite improvements in intensive care treatment during the past few decades, the rate of death from SAP has not significantly declined [1]. The pathogenesis of acute pancreatitis relates to inappropriate conversion of trypsinogen to trypsin and a lack of prompt elimination of active trypsin inside pancreas [2].

SAP includes a hyper catabolic state leading to protein catabolism and increased resting energy requirements [3]. As premorbid malnutrition is frequent, nutritional therapy is now recognized as an important component of SAP management [4]. The traditional approach to nutritional therapy in SAP was to rest the pancreas by way of a nil-by-mouth regimen and to deliver parenteral nutrition (PN) to meet the nutritional requirement. However, the recent studies show merits of early EN over PN [5–8]. The European Society for Clinical Nutrition and Metabolism guidelines suggest that "all patients who are not expected to be on normal nutrition within 3 days should receive PN within 24 to 48 h if EN is contraindicated or if they cannot tolerate EN" [9]. The American Society for Parenteral and Enteral Nutrition guidelines in collaboration with the Society of Critical Care Medicine state: "If early EN is not feasible or available during the first seven days following admission to the ICU, no nutrition support therapy should be provided" [10].

PN has been associated with gut mucosal atrophy, overfeeding, hyperglycemia, increased risk of infectious complications, and increased mortality rate [11, 12]. EN may be associated with high gastric residue, bacterial colonization of stomach, and increased risk of aspiration pneumonia [13]. Several studies have reported failure to deliver adequate energy intake in clinical practice [14–18], and in practice, it commonly takes up to 7 days to achieve nutritional goal by EN [19]. Nutrition in SAP has been discussed and researched over the years and still there is dominance of providing treatment which the doctors think rather than following protocols and evidence. The role of early EN is well established in SAP and should be implemented earlier. However the role of PN too cannot be ignored in SAP [20]. Since 2002, we began to use progressive combined nutritional support to cure SAP in which PN is combined to EN and we achieved good results. To discuss the mechanisms of progressive combined nutritional support in the treatment of SAP we studied retrospectively two groups of patients with two different treatments for nutritional support and compared the advantages and disadvantages of both nutritional supports.

6.2 MATERIALS AND METHODS

This study is approved by the Review Board of the Second Affiliated Hospital of Chongqing Medical University, China. Total of 130 patients with severe acute pancreatitis having similar severity index, treated at The Second Affiliated Hospital of Chongqing Medical University, Chongqing, China, between January 1998 and June 2008, were retrospectively selected in to two groups, which include 58 males and 72 females with the median age of 49 ranging from 20 to 85 years old. The diagnostic criteria of severe acute pancreatitis include: clinical features, hyperamylasemia/hyperlipasemia (three times the normal upper limit); radiological evidence of severe acute pancreatitis (contrast enhanced CT scan); evidence of organ failure and/or local complications such as pancreatic necrosis; pseudocyst, abscess; computed tomography severity index (CTSI) equal to or greater than 7; Ranson score ≥ 3 and APACHE II score ≥ 8.

Group I includes 59 patients from January 1998 to December 2001 out of whom 27 were male and 32 were female whose age was between 20 to 82 years old. The median age was 51 years. More detailed characteristics of study patients are presented in Table 1. At the time of admission, the average APACHE II score was 12.21 ± 2.56 (markers of the disease at the time of admission and during the hospital stay are shown in Table 2). Group I adopted comprehensive treatment which included anti-shock therapy to maintain water, electrolyte, and acid-base; to stabilize internal environment, rational use of broad-spectrum antibiotics, sedative therapy, peritoneal lavage, organ support treatment; and treatment for the etiology of primary disease. Nutritional support was parenteral route and strictly followed by formula; Actual Energy Expenditure (AEE) = BMR × AF × IF × TF (BMR = Basic Metabolic Rate, AF = Activity Factor, IF = Injury Factor, TF = Thermal Factor).

TABLE 1: Characteristics of study patients.

	Group I n = 59	Group II n = 71	P value
Age in years (average)	51	52.5	
Male	27	31	
Female	32	40	
Etiology			
Gallstones	25 (49.01%)	34 (47.88%)	
Alcohol	21 (41.17%)	28 (39.43%)	
Idiopathic	3 (5.88%)	6 (8.45%)	
Drug Induced	2 (3.92%)	3 (4.22%)	
Duration of symptom of disease at the time of admission (days in mean ± SD and range)	2.63 ± 0.73 (1–5)	2.77 ± 1.01 (1–5)	0.247[a]

[a]Mann-Whitney U-Test.

TABLE 2: Markers of disease at the time of admission and during the hospital stay.

	Group I	Group II	P value
	Mean ± SD (range)	Mean ± SD (range)	Group I versus Group II[a]
APACHE-II Score			
Day 0	12.21 ± 2.57	12.47 ± 3.71	0.363
Day 4	11.59 ± 5.12	11.45 ± 4.31	0.276
Day 7	11.53 ± 4.49	10.29 ± 4.21	0.010
Day 14	10.78 ± 4.77	09.07 ± 4.97	0.009
IL-6			
Day 0	434.43 ± 187.29 ng/L	429.57 ± 179.61 ng/L	0.755
Day 4	397.50 ± 124.15 ng/L	382.21 ± 135.73 ng/L	0.716
Day 7	387.50 ± 165.92 ng/L	285.69 ± 199.17 ng/L	0.016
Day 14	385.50 ± 194.52 ng/L	180.33 ± 143.38 ng/L	0.006
Serum Albumin Level			
Day 0	28.6 ± 3.7 g/L	30.03 ± 6.2 g/L	0.963
Day 4	29.36 ± 4.6 g/L	28.8 ± 5.3 g/L	0.865
Day 7	29.64 ± 5.1 g/L	29.3 ± 4.6 g/L	0.872
Day 14	29.7 ± 4.2 g/L	30.01 ± 5.7 g/L	0.987

[a]*Mann-Whitney U-test.*

Group II include 71 patients from January 2002 to June 2008 out of whom 31 were males and 40 were females. The patients were 20 to 85 years in age and the median age was 52.5 years. APACHE II score at the time of admission at hospital was 12.47 ± 3.71. Group II adopted progressive supportive treatment in which different course period of the disease have different nutritional supports. The first stage (up to day 3-4), the energy is calculated by formula 1/2 to 1/3 of BMR in which only glucose is administered by single parenteral route. At the second stage (from day 4 to day 7), the energy is calculated by 2/3 to 1 of BMR in which glucose accounted for 40–50 percent and fat for 50–60 percent. Both the enteral route plus parenteral route were used to achieve 100 percent target. At the third stage (day 7–10 later), the energy supplied was increased on basic requirement and strictly followed the formula AEE. At this stage the glucose accounts for 50–70 percent, fat for 30–50 percent, and the way was both the enteral and parenteral nutrition.

In this study, the nutritional therapy period is defined as the time from enrolment until the first day the patient received more than 70 per cent of their estimated nutritional requirements through volitional oral intake. PN was the provision of intravenous nutrients with the exception of ≤5% dextrose solutions. EN was defined as the provision of a nutritionally complete formula into gastrointestinal tract through a mechanical tube (gastric or small bowel tubes). EN was delivered into the jejunum distally to the ligament of Treitz. Oral intake was food taken orally by mouth. The proportion of the daily target volume of either PN or EN was calculated by dividing the delivered volume by the target volume.

At the time of hospital admission, there was no significant difference between the two groups of patients in clinical data and APACHE II score ($t_0 = -0.352$, $P = 0.726$, $P > 0.05$).

In both the groups, we analyzed APACHE-II score, IL-6 level, serum protein level, complication rate, mortality, cure rate, length of hospital stay, and average hospital cost. Results for normally distributed outcomes are reported using medians and interquartile ranges (IQRs). A non-parametric Mann-Whitney -test was used to compare the values between the two groups. All the data used SPSS 11.0 for statistical analysis. A two-sided P value of <0.05 was considered statically significant.

6.3 RESULTS

6.3.1 APACHE-II SCORE

In Group I, the APACHE II scores on days 4, 7, and 14 were 11.59 ± 5.12, 11.53 ± 4.49, 10.78 ± 4.77 and respectively. In Group II, on day 4, it was 11.45 ± 4.31 which shows no significant difference compared to day 4 of the Group I, $P > 0.05$. However, on day 7 and 14 after the treatment in Group II, the APACHE-II scores were 10.29 ± 4.21 and 9.07 ± 4.97, respectively, which is significantly lower than Group I, $P < 0.05$ (Figure 1).

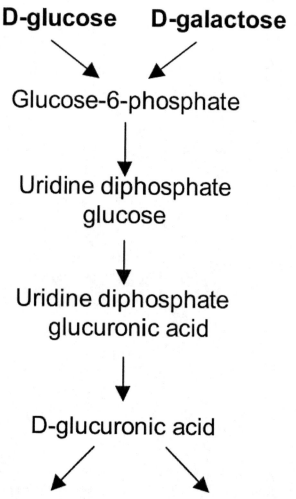

FIGURE 1: Comparison of APACHE II score on days 0, 4, 7, and 14 between Group I and Group II. #P > 0.05, which is not significant different between Group I and Group II on Day 1 and Day 4. However, *P < 0.05, which is statically significant between group I and Group II on Day 7 and Day 14.

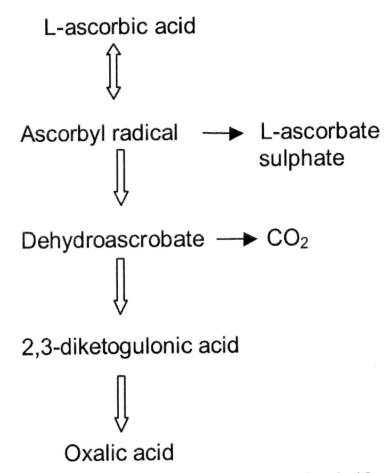

FIGURE 2: Comparison of IL-6 level on days 0, 4, 7, and 14 between Group I and Group II. #P > 0.05, which is not significant different between Group I and Group II on Day 1 and Day 4. However, *P < 0.05, which is statically significant between group I and Group II on Day 7 and Day 14.

6.3.2 IL-6 LEVEL

Before the treatment, the IL-6 level was 434.43 ± 187.29 ng/L in Group I. After 4, 7, and 14 day of treatment, the IL-6 levels were 397.50 ± 124.15 ng/L, 387.5 ± 165.92 ng/L and 385.50 ± 194.52 ng/L, respectively. In group II, the level of IL-6 before the treatment and after 4 days of treatment was 429.57 ± 179.61 ng/L and 382.21 ± 135.73 ng/L, respectively. Comparing with Group I show no significant difference ($t_0 = -0.320$, $P = 0.755$, $P > 0.05$; $t_{4d} = -0.320$, $P = 0.755$, $P > 0.50$). However, 7 and 14 day after the treatment, the IL-6 levels of Group II were 258.69 ± 199.17 ng/L and 180.33 ± 143.38 ng/L, respectively, which is significantly lower than group I ($t_{7d} = 2.877$, $P = 0.016$, $P < 0.05$; $t_{14d} = 3.436$, $P = 0.006$, $P < 0.05$) (Figure 2).

6.3.3 SERUM ALBUMIN LEVEL

14 day after the treatment, the serum albumin in Group I and Group II was 29.7 ± 4.2 g/L and 30.01 ± 5.7 g/L, respectively, which is not significant between the two Groups ($t_{14d} = -0.016$, $P = 0.987$, $P > 0.05$) (Figure 3).

6.3.4 COMPLICATION RATE

The complication rate of Group II is 39.4 percent which is significantly less than Group I which has 66.1 percent ($X^2 = 9.173$, $P = 0.010$, $P < 0.05$) (Figure 4).

6.3.5 MORTALITY

The mortality of Group II was 12.7 percent which is significantly less than the mortality of Group I which has mortality 30.5 percent ($X^2 = 6.227$, $P = 0.044$, $P < 0.05$) (Table 3).

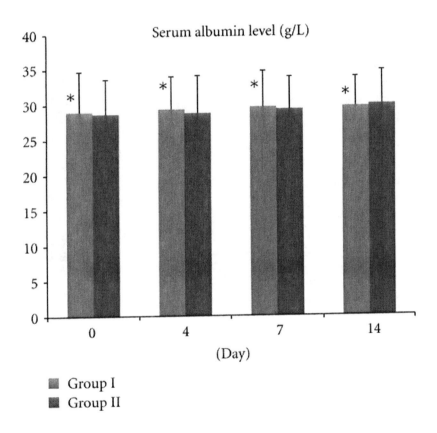

FIGURE 3: Comparison of serum albumin concentrations on days 0, 4, 7, and 14 between Group I and Group II. *P > 0.05 Group I versus Group II, which is not significant.

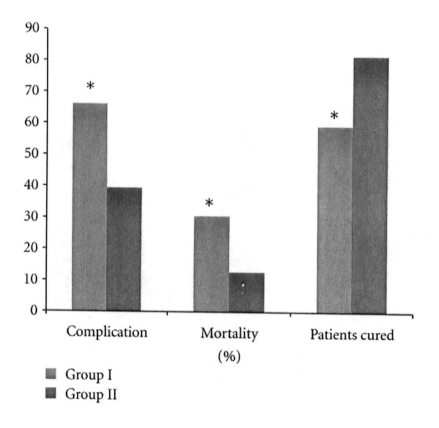

FIGURE 4: Comparison of complications, mortality, and patients-cured between Group I and Group II. *P < 0.05 Group I versus Group II, which is significant.

Table 3: Outcome in the two groups.

	Group I	Group II	Pvalue
Complication rate	66.1%	39.4%	0.010[a]
Mortality	30.5%	12.7%	0.044[a]
Cure rate	59.3%	81.7%	0.019[a]
Length of hospitalization	51 ± 8 days	32 ± 9 days	0.005[b]
Treatment cost	¥ 45534 ± 3031.5	¥ 30869 ± 12794.6	0.001[b]

[a]*Mann-Whitney U-test.*
[b]*Fisher's exact test.*

6.3.6 CURE RATE

In Group II, the cure rate is 81.7 percent which is significantly higher than 59.3 percent in Group I ($X^2 = 7.918$, P = 0.019, P < 0.05) (Table 3).

6.3.7 LENGTH OF HOSPITALIZATION

The length of hospitalization in Group II was 32 ± 9 days which is significantly shorter than the days in Group I (t = 2.881, P = 0.005, P < 0.05) (Table 3).

6.3.8 TREATMENT COST

For the Group II, it is 30869 ± 12794.6 Chinese Yuan which is significantly less than Chinese Yuan in Group I. (t = -3.475, P = 0.001, P < 0.05) (Table 3).

6.4 DISCUSSION

Severe acute pancreatitis (SAP) is acute pancreatitis associated with complications that are either local (e.g., peripancreatic fluid collection,

necrosis, abscess, pseudocyst) or systemic (e.g., organ dysfunction). According to the Atlanta Classification, SAP can be divided into two phas-
es. The first phase of about 7–10 days start with aseptic inflammation,
systemic inflammation response syndrome (SIRS), sepsis, multi organs
failure (MOF), and even death [21]. The second phase usually after the
second week of the disease, the circumscribed complications such as pancreatic necrosis began to appear. During this period, the lives of these
patients are still in serious threat of necrotizing pancreas, complication,
and death which is due to inflammatory immune response of pancreatic
necrosis and infection [22]. In SAP, basal metabolic rate (BMR) increases
due to inflammation and acute stress reaction thereby increase the overall
energy consumption. Eighty percent of patients with severe necrotizing
pancreatitis are overcatabolic and everyday lose more than 40 g of proteins
which give negative balance and is adverse to the disease recovery [4, 23,
24]. Therefore, nutrition support must be guaranteed; if not in time, denu-
trition will get the condition worse [23]. Over the past, number of medical institutions used Harris-Benedict equation measured by resting energy
expenditure (REE) of patients with SAP, but at the time when body is at
stress due to the disease, there might be high metabolic decompensating
state and hence exogenous nutrients may have refractoriness. Cerra et al.
has proposed the concept of metabolic support which advocates, providing
the necessary nutrients substrate for the body; we must also take another
fact into account that it should not increase the load of the body's organs
[25]. Lugli et al. has proposed the principles of the nutrition support treatment for acute pancreatitis: (a) asses the nutritional status of patients; (b)
according to the severity of the disease to take the nutrition therapy; (c)
confirm the patients with indications of the special nutritional support to
give special way nutrition therapy [26]. All the nutritional support should
supply the energy as much as possible to meet the need of body under
the premise of not stimulating pancreatic exocrine function [27]. At present, very few researches about gradually combined treatment of parenteral
nutrition with enteral nutrition for severe acute pancreatitis have been reported. We think this research will be interesting to the readers.

　　This study compares the result of two groups of SAP patients to explore the nutrition requirements of various stages of SAP and to propose

the method of Gradually Combined Treatment of Nutrition Support for SAP.

In the course duration of SAP, the need for nutrients varies with the change of the duration. In order to comply with metabolism of the body in SAP, we should take the right amount of progressive nutrition support. The body's requirements for the amount of nutrients based on the balance of the body metabolic rate (BMR) and body's stress response to the inflammation of pancreatitis. At the period of stress response, the body itself is in the stage of macrophages. At this stage, the patients exhibits higher basal metabolic and catabolic rates as well as impaired metabolic capability to use exogenous amino acid and energy. As the disease goes on, the body adapts to the trauma and the tissues and organs are recovered. At this time, the body's requirements for nutritional substrate are gradually reduced and finally become close to BMR. With the stress response reduced, body's repair to trauma and anabolic enhanced, exogenous nutritional substrate requirement is gradually increased. In this stage, the energy requirement is equal to acute energy expenditure (AEE).

Till days 3-4 of the onset of SAP, a serious Systemic Inflammatory Response Syndrome (SIRS) may occur. The body is in the high catabolic stage and in stress, which represents macrophages to itself and metabolic disturbance. The principal contraindication of this phase is to improve the intracellular environment and microcirculation. Intravenous perfusion of the high calories and high viscosity nutrients solution will increase the imbalance in the intracellular environment and microcirculation. Therefore the amount of substrate required by nutritional support should be reduced, the amount should be equivalent to half of the BMR, the energy should be supplied by monosaccharide, which mainly provide to the tissue and cells rely solely, such as the brain, RBSs, and others.

After the comprehensive treatment, the maintenance of the intracellular environment and microcirculation of most patients are improved. The differences between decomposition and synthesis of metabolic in the body reduced, the phenomenon of self-macrophages gradually improved, the demand for the non-protein calories began to increase to half of BMR and requires the energy of fats as well as glucose. However, the body is still in the stress state, the intracellular environment has not fully recovered, and cells' anabolism lack vitality; high nutritional supplements will increase the burden of tissue and organ, leading to variety of metabolic complications. When SAP entered the second stage of about 7–10 days, most patients have successfully recovered through the stress period, the environment and microcirculation improved, assimilation is enhanced, demand of exogenous nutrients substrate increased. After 2 weeks, the energy demand basically reached AEE.

In this study, we analyzed APACHE-II score and IL-6 levels. After being admitted in hospital, APACHE-II score is one of the best predictor to assess the severity of pancreatitis [28]. Also the IL-6 is important parameter to show the prognostic of SAP and IL-6 > 1000 ng/L prompted a higher mortality rate [29–31]. As the time course of treatment increased, APACHE-II score and IL-6 level of both the groups were decreased. However, differences between Group I and Group II were significant on day 7 and day 14 of the admission. Also the complications, mortality, length of hospitalization, and the average cost of treatment in Group II were lower than Group I. The cure rate in Group II was higher than the Group I. On day 14 of the treatment, the serum albumin level between the two Groups was not significantly different. This is because the plasma protein levels are not a good indicator for nutrition status during inflammation due to many factors such as the acute-phase response, concomitant diseases, and the long half-life of albumin.

Patients with SAP are frequently hypercatabolic; timely institution of feeding is important if malnutrition is to be avoided or treated. Local complications of pancreatitis might cause upper gastrointestinal tract obstruction, making enteral nutrition problematic. There are also concerns that enteral nutrition may exacerbate the severity of SAP through further pancreatic stimulation and enzyme release. These considerations have led to a widespread reliance on parenteral nutrition as the main nutritional support modality in SAP.

Many evidences suggest that there are several potential benefits to enteral nutrition compared with parenteral nutrition including a reduction in microbial translocation, improvements in gut blood flow, and preservation of gut mucosal surface immunity. Furthermore, since altered gut microbiological flora and barrier function may contribute to the development of infected pancreatic necrosis, there are theoretical advantages to enteral feeding in SAP.

About the timing of nutritional support for the patients with SAP, in most of the studies, both parenteral nutrition and enteral nutrition begin within 48 h; parenteral nutrition is started later than enteral nutrition, more likely an assistant method of enteral nutrition [32]. Although enteral nutrition is a more beneficial nutrition support, it is not easy to implement at early time and has high risk [33]. In Group II, parenteral nutrition was used at the first stage in order to avoid excessive irritation in severe stress period. In the second and third stages, parenteral and enteral nutrition were used together to make up for each other's deficiencies.

6.5 CONCLUSION

In severe acute pancreatitis, evaluation of body's metabolism should be the first consideration and then gradually combined treatment of parenteral nutrition with enteral nutrition should be used as routine therapy. This cannot only improve the natural history of pancreatitis but also can reduce the incidence of complication and mortality.

REFERENCES

1. C. J. McKay and C. W. Imrie, "The continuing challenge of early mortality in acute pancreatitis," British Journal of Surgery, vol. 91, no. 10, pp. 1243–1244, 2004.
2. D. C. Whitcomb, "Value of genetic testing in the management of pancreatitis," Gut, vol. 53, no. 11, pp. 1710–1717, 2004.
3. Working Party of the British Society of Gastroenterology, Association of Surgeons of Great Britain and Ireland; Pancreatic Society of Great Britain and Ireland, and Association of Upper GI Surgeons of Great Britain and Ireland, "UK guidelines for the management of acute pancreatitis," Gut, vol. 54, supplement 3, pp. iii1–iii9, 2005.
4. R. Meier, J. Ockenga, M. Pertkiewicz et al., "ESPEN guidelines on enteral nutrition: pancreas," Clinical Nutrition, vol. 25, no. 2, pp. 275–284, 2006.
5. F. Kalfarentzos, J. Kehagias, N. Mead, K. Kokkinis, and C. A. Gogos, "Enteral nutrition is superior to parenteral nutrition in severe acute pancreatitis: results of a randomized prospective trial," British Journal of Surgery, vol. 84, no. 12, pp. 1665–1669, 1997.

6. S. Abou-Assi, K. Craig, and S. J. D. O'Keefe, "Hypocaloric jejunal feeding is better than total parenteral nutrition in acute pancreatitis: results of a randomized comparative study," American Journal of Gastroenterology, vol. 97, no. 9, pp. 2255–2262, 2002.

7. A. Oláah, G. Pardavi, T. Beláagyi, A. Nagy, Á. Issekutz, and G. E. Mohamed, "Early nasojejunal feeding in acute pancreatitis is associated with a lower complication rate," Nutrition, vol. 18, no. 3, pp. 259–262, 2002.

8. P. E. Marik and G. P. Zaloga, "Meta-analysis of parenteral-nutrition versus enteral nutrition in patients with acute pancreatitis," British Medical Journal, vol. 328, no. 7453, pp. 1407–1410, 2004.

9. P. Singer, M. M. Berger, G. Van den Berghe et al., "ESPEN guidelines on parenteral nutrition: intensive care," Clinical Nutrition, vol. 28, no. 4, pp. 387–400, 2009.

10. S. A. McClave, R. G. Martindale, V. W. Vanek et al., "Guidelines for the provision and assessment of nutrition support therapy in the adult critically ill patient: society of critical care medicine (SCCM) and American society for parenteral and enteral nutrition (A.S.P.E.N.)," Journal of Parenteral and Enteral Nutrition, vol. 33, no. 3, pp. 277–316, 2009.

11. K. A. Kudsk, M. A. Croce, T. C. Fabian et al., "Enteral versus parenteral feeding: effects on septic morbidity after blunt and penetrating abdominal trauma," Annals of Surgery, vol. 215, no. 5, pp. 503–513, 1992.

12. D. K. Heyland, S. MacDonald, L. Keefe, and J. W. Drover, "Total parenteral nutrition in the critically Ill patient: a meta- analysis," Journal of the American Medical Association, vol. 280, no. 23, pp. 2013–2019, 1998.

13. J. Rello, E. Quintana, V. Ausina et al., "Incidence, etiology, and outcome of nosocomial pneumonia in mechanically ventilated patients," Chest, vol. 100, no. 2, pp. 439–444, 1991.

14. S. Adam and S. Batson, "A study of problems associated with the delivery of enteral feed ill critically ill patients in five ICUs is the UK," Intensive Care Medicine, vol. 23, no. 3, pp. 261–266, 1997.

15. N. P. Woodcock, D. Zeigler, M. D. Palmer, P. Buckley, C. J. Mitchell, and J. MacFie, "Enteral versus parenteral nutrition: a pragmatic study," Nutrition, vol. 17, no. 1, pp. 1–12, 2001.

16. C. L. Reid, I. T. Campbell, and R. A. Little, "Muscle wasting and energy balance in critical illness," Clinical Nutrition, vol. 23, no. 2, pp. 273–280, 2004.

17. C. Weissman, M. Kemper, and J. Askanazi, "Resting metabolic rate of the critically ill patient: measured versus predicted," Anesthesiology, vol. 64, no. 6, pp. 673–679, 1986.

18. B. De Jonghe, C. Appere-De-Vechi, M. Fournier et al., "A prospective survey of nutritional support practices in intensive care unit patients: what is prescribed? What is delivered?" Critical Care Medicine, vol. 29, no. 1, pp. 8–12, 2001.

19. P. Bauer, C. Charpentier, C. Bouchet, L. Nace, F. Raffy, and N. Gaconnet, "Parenteral with enteral nutrition in the critically ill," Intensive Care Medicine, vol. 26, no. 7, pp. 893–900, 2000.

20. P. Amin, "Nutritional support in acute pancreatitis: the saga continues!," Critical Care Medicine, vol. 39, no. 3, pp. 587–588, 2011.

21. I. Poves Prim, J. Fabregat Prous, F. J. García Borobia, R. Jorba Martí, J. Figueras
     Felip, and E. Jaurrieta Mas, "Early onset of organ failure is the best predictor of
     mortality in acute pancreatitis," Revista Espanola de Enfermedades Digestivas, vol.
     96, no. 10, pp. 705–713, 2004.
22. M. Casas, J. Mora, E. Fort et al., "Total enteral nutrition vs. total parenteral nutri-
     tion in patients with severe acute pancreatitis," Revista Espanola de Enfermedades
     Digestivas, vol. 99, no. 5, pp. 264–269, 2007.
23. R. F. Meier and C. Beglinger, "Nutrition in pancreatic diseases," Best Practice and
     Research, vol. 20, no. 3, pp. 507–529, 2006.
24. S. J. O'Keefe and S. A. McClave, "Feeding the injured pancreas," Gastroenterology,
     vol. 129, no. 3, pp. 1129–1130, 2005.
25. F. B. Cerra, P. A. Alden, F. Negro et al., "Sepsis and exogenous lipid modulation,"
     Journal of Parenteral and Enteral Nutrition, vol. 12, supplement 6, pp. 63S–68S,
     1988.
26. A. K. Lugli, F. Carli, and L. Wykes, "The importance of nutrition status assess-
     ment: the case of severe acute pancreatitis," Nutrition Reviews, vol. 65, no. 7, pp.
     329–334, 2007.
27. O. Ioannidis, A. Lavrentieva, and D. Botsios, "Nutrition support in acute pancreati-
     tis," Journal of the Pancreas, vol. 9, no. 4, pp. 375–390, 2008.
28. D. C. Whitcomb, "Acute pancreatitis," The New England Journal of Medicine, vol.
     354, no. 20, pp. 2142–2150, 2006.
29. I. A. Al Mofleh, "Severe acute pancreatitis: pathogenetic aspects and prognostic fac-
     tors," World Journal of Gastroenterology, vol. 14, no. 5, pp. 675–684, 2008.
30. G. Sathyanarayan, P. K. Garg, H. K. Prasad, and R. K. Tandon, "Elevated level of in-
     terleukin-6 predicts organ failure and severe disease in patients with acute pancreati-
     tis," Journal of Gastroenterology and Hepatology, vol. 22, no. 4, pp. 550–554, 2007.
31. F. G. Brivet, D. Emilie, and P. Galanaud, "Pro- and anti-inflammatory cytokines dur-
     ing acute severe pancreatitis: an early and sustained response, although unpredict-
     able of death," Critical Care Medicine, vol. 27, no. 4, pp. 749–755, 1999.
32. A. Kumar, N. Singh, S. Prakash, A. Saraya, and Y. K. Joshi, "Early enteral nutrition
     in severe acute pancreatitis: a prospective randomized controlled trial comparing
     nasojejunal and nasogastric routes," Journal of Clinical Gastroenterology, vol. 40,
     no. 5, pp. 431–434, 2006.
33. A. Thomson, "Nutritional support in acute pancreatitis," Current Opinion in Clinical
     Nutrition & Metabolic Care, vol. 11, no. 3, pp. 261–266, 2008.

This chapter was originally published under the Creative Commons Attribution License. Sineh, A.,
Chen, M., Li, T., Yang, X-L, Li, J-Z, and Gong, J-P. Parenteral Nutrition Combined with Enteral
Nutrition for Severe Acute Pancreatitis. ISRN Gastroentogy, vol. 2012, Article ID 791383. 2012.
doi:10.5402/2012/791383.

CHAPTER 7

DIETARY PROTEIN INTAKE AND RENAL FUNCTION

WILLIAM F. MARTIN, LAWRENCE E. ARMSTRONG, and NANCY R. RODRIGUEZ

7.1 DIETARY PROTEIN INTAKE AND RENAL FUNCTION

Dietary protein intake can modulate renal function [1] and its role in renal disease has spawned an ongoing debate in the literature. At the center of the controversy is the concern that habitual consumption of dietary protein in excess of recommended amounts promotes chronic renal disease through increased glomerular pressure and hyperfiltration [2,3]. Media releases often conclude that, "too much protein stresses the kidney" [4]. The real question, however, is whether research in healthy individuals supports this notion. In fact, studies suggest that hyperfiltration in response to various physiological stimuli is a normal adaptative mechanism [5-10].

The purpose of this paper is to review the available evidence regarding the effects of protein intake on renal function with particular emphasis on renal disease. This review will consider research regarding the role of dietary protein in chronic kidney disease, normal renal function and kidney stone formation and evaluate the collective body of literature to ascertain whether habitual consumption of dietary protein in excess of what is recommended warrants a health concern in terms of the initiation and promotion of renal disease. In the following review, high protein (HP) diets will be defined as a daily consumption of greater than or equal to 1.5 g/kg/day, which is almost twice the current Recommended Dietary Allowance but within the range of current Dietary Reference Intakes (DRIs) for protein [11]. The Institute of Medicine DRI report concluded that there was insufficient scientific evidence for recommendations of an upper limit of protein intake but suggested an acceptable macronutrient distribution range of 10–35% of total energy for protein intake [11].

While the optimal ratio of macronutrient intake for adults has typically focused on fat and carbohydrate [12], contemporary discussions include the role of dietary protein [13-15]. This is particularly true given the recent popularity of high protein diets in weight management [16]. Although the efficacy of these diets with regard to weight loss is still subject to debate, several studies have demonstrated favorable physiological effects [12,16-24]. This has led to a substantial increase in protein intake by individuals adhering to contemporary weight loss plans. As a result, the safety of habitually consuming dietary protein in excess of the Recommended Daily Allowance (RDA) has been questioned.

7.2 AN OVERVIEW OF CHRONIC KIDNEY DISEASE

Chronic Kidney Disease (CKD) is defined as either kidney damage or a decline in renal function as determined by decreased glomerular filtration rate (GFR) for three or more months [25]. It is estimated that 1 in 9 adults in the United States meet this criteria, while an additional 1 in 9 adults are at increased risk for CKD [26]. In the general population, a decline in renal function is considered an independent risk factor for both cardiovascular disease and all-cause mortality [27]. However, the extent to which a mild diminution in renal function influences this risk is not known [28].

According to the National Kidney Foundation guidelines, CKD is classified into five stages, each of which directly correlates with the severity of the disease [25]. As one progresses from stage 1 to 5 there is a concomitant decline in GFR and thus renal function. The final stage, known as end stage renal disease, represents the most severe manifestation of CKD [29]. This classification system provides a universal standard for application of clinical treatment guidelines.

Hypertension is the second leading cause of CKD and accounts for approximately 30% of all cases in the U.S. [30,31]. In one study, hypertension was associated with a premature decline in renal function in men with normal kidney function [32]. Although, initial estimates of CKD prevalence in hypertensive individuals were about 2%, recent evidence suggests that prevalence rates may be significantly higher [33]. Blood pressure control is of particular importance in hypertensive individuals with CKD. This point has been demonstrated in several trials in which antihypertensive therapy slowed the progression of CKD [34-36].

Race, gender, age and family history are four risk factors for CKD [37-40]. Recent findings suggest that modifiable lifestyle risk factors (i.e., physical inactivity, smoking, obesity) are also associated with CKD. Limited data exist regarding the role of dietary protein intake as an independent risk factor for either the initiation or progression of renal disease but population studies have consistently demonstrated an inverse relationship between dietary protein intake and systemic blood pressure [41,42]. In a randomized control trial [43], dietary protein and fiber had additive effects in lowering 24-hour and awake systolic blood pressure in a group of 36 hypertensives. While these findings suggest that high protein diets may be beneficial to hypertensive individuals, additional research is warranted since increased protein intakes often result in increased consumption of certain micronutrients known to impact blood pressure (e.g., potassium, magnesium, calcium) [44].

7.3 DIETARY PROTEIN AND RENAL FUNCTION

The relationship between dietary protein and renal function has been studied for over half a century [1]. In 1923, Addis and Drury [45] were among the first to observe a relationship between level of dietary protein and rates of urea excretion. Soon after, it was established that increased protein intake elevated rates of creatinine and urea excretion in the dog model [46]. The common mechanism underlying increased excretion rates was eventually attributed to changes in GFR [47,48] and Van Slyke et al. [49] demonstrated that renal blood flow was the basis for GFR mediated changes in clearance rates in response to increased protein intake. Clearly dietary protein effects GFR [50], with both acute and chronic increases in protein consumption elevating GFR [50,51].

7.4 DIETARY PROTEIN AND THE PROGRESSION OF RENAL DISEASE

Observational data from epidemiological studies provide evidence that dietary protein intake may be related to the progression of renal disease [52]. In the Nurses' Health Study, protein intake, assessed with a semi-quantitative food frequency questionnaire, was compared to the change in estimated GFR over an 11-year span in individuals with pre-existing renal disease [53]. Regression analysis showed an association between increased consumption of animal protein and a decline in renal function suggesting that high total protein intake may accelerate renal disease leading to a progressive loss of renal capacity. However, no association between protein intake and change in GFR was found in a different cohort of 1,135 women with normal renal function (Figure 1.). The latter finding led the authors to conclude that there were no adverse effects of high protein intakes on kidney function in healthy women with normal renal status.

Research by Johnson et al. [54], showed protein intake as a possible risk factor for progressive loss of remaining renal function in dialysis patients. Indeed, dietary protein restriction is a common treatment modality for patients with renal disease [55,56] and practice guidelines exist regarding reduced dietary protein intakes for individuals with chronic renal disease in which proteinuria is present [57]. The National Kidney Foundation (NKF) has extensive recommendations with regard to protein intake, which are a byproduct of the Dialysis Outcome Quality Initiative [58]. Again, it is important to note that these recommendations are not indicated for individuals with normal renal function nor are they intended to serve as a prevention strategy to avoid developing CKD. Despite the clarity of these guidelines, their mere existence has resulted in concern regarding

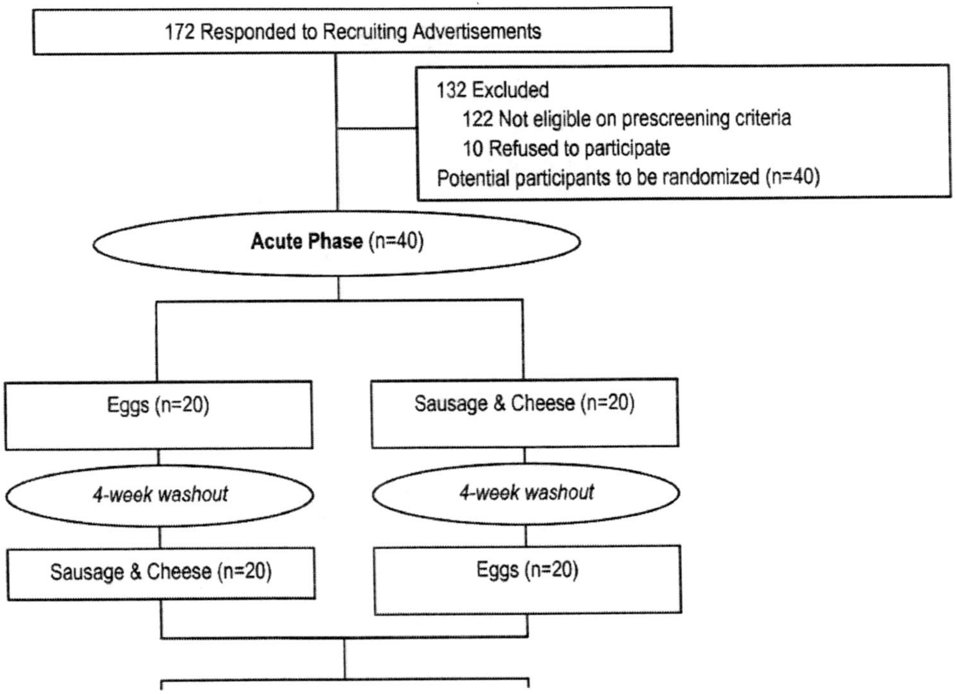

FIGURE 1: This figure is a plot of multivariate linear regression for change in estimated GFR according to quintile of total protein intake*
in participants with normal renal function (n = 1135). Data are taken from Knight et al., Ann Intern Med 2003 Mar 18;138(6):460-7 [53].

the role of dietary protein in the onset or progression of renal disease in the general population [59].

7.5 DIETARY PROTEIN AND RENAL DISEASE

Allen and Cope's observation that increased dietary protein induced renal hypertrophy in dogs [60] led to speculation that dietary protein intake may have deleterious effects on the kidney. Later research in the rat model produced evidence supporting earlier observations from canine research [61-63]. Recently, Hammond and Janes [64] demonstrated an independent effect of increased protein intake on renal hypertrophy in mice. In this study, changes in renal function (i.e., increased glomerular filtration rate and renal hypertrophy) were observed.

Currently, a combination of hormonal interactions and renal processes are thought to explain protein-induced hyperfiltration [65]. Increased glucagon secretion in response to protein administration induced hyperfiltration [66] subsequent to a cascade of events referred to as the"pancreato-hepatorenal cascade" [67]. It has been hypothesized that cAMP works in concert with glucagon to mediate GFR [68]. To date, however, this hypothesis has not been tested and other competing hypotheses suggest other novel mechanisms of protein-induced hyperfiltration [69].

While the effect of hyperfiltration on renal function in those individuals with pre-existing renal disease is well documented [52], the application of these observations to healthy persons with normal renal function is not appropriate. To date, scientific data linking protein-induced renal hypertrophy or hyperfiltration to the initiation or progression of renal disease in healthy individuals is lacking. The possibility that protein-induced changes in renal function are a normal physiological adaptation to nitrogen load and increased demands for renal clearance is supported by changes noted in renal structure and function during pregnancy [70]. GFR increases by as much as 65% in healthy women [8] during pregnancy, typically returning to nonpregnant levels by three months postpartum [7]. Despite these changes in renal function, pregnancy is not a risk factor for developing CKD [6].

The renal hypertrophy and accompanying improvements in renal function in the contralateral kidney that occur subsequent to unilateral nephrectomy also suggest these processes are an adaptive, and possibly beneficial, response [5]. Studies show, despite prolonged hyperfiltration, remnant kidney function remained normal and did not deteriorate during long-term (> 20 yrs) follow-up in nephrectomized patients [9,10]. Thus, compensatory hyperfiltration appears to be a biological adaptation to a variety of renal challenges that is not associated with increased risk of chronic kidney disease in healthy individuals.

7.6 THE BRENNER HYPOTHESIS

Perhaps the most consistently cited reference with regard to the potentially harmful effects of dietary protein intake on renal function is that of Brenner et al. [3]. In brief, the Brenner Hypothesis states that situations associated with increased glomerular filtration and glomerular pressure cause renal injury, ultimately compromise renal function, and potentially increase the risk for or progression of renal disease. Brenner proposed that habitual consumption of excessive dietary protein negatively impacted kidney function by a sustained increased in glomerular pressure and renal hyperfiltration [3]. Since the majority of scientific evidence cited by the authors was generated from animal models and patients with co-existing renal disease, extension of this relationship to healthy individuals with normal renal function is inappropriate. Indeed, a relationship between increased glomerular pressure or hyperfiltration and the onset or progression of renal disease in healthy individuals has not been clearly documented in the scientific literature. Rather, findings from individuals with compensatory hyperfiltration during pregnancy and following unilateral nephrectomy suggest otherwise [9].

The Modification of Diet in Renal Disease (MDRD) study was the largest randomized multicenter, controlled trial undertaken to evaluate the effect of dietary protein restriction on the progression of renal disease [71]. Several variables, including GFR, were measured in patients with chronic renal disease at baseline and throughout the approximately

2 year follow-up period. Patients with renal disease randomized to the very low-protein diet group had slightly slower decline in GFR decline compared with patients randomized to the low-protein diet group. Further data analyses showed patients with lower total protein intake would have a longer time to renal failure and suggested that a lower protein intake postponed the progression of advanced renal disease. Using meta-analysis to assess the efficacy of dietary protein restriction in previously published studies of diabetic and nondiabetic renal diseases, including the MDRD Study, Pedrini et al. concluded that the progression of both nondiabetic and diabetic renal disease could be effectively delayed with restriction of dietary protein [56]. Indeed, current clinical guidelines for the management of patients with renal disease continue to be based on the premise that protein intake greater than that recommended or which results in a renal solute load in excess of the kidney's excretory capabilities will contribute to progressive renal failure in persons with compromised renal function. However, of significance to this review, is the fact that imposing these guidelines on healthy individuals with normal renal function is overzealous given the current status of the scientific literature in this area.

7.7 DIETARY PROTEIN AND RENAL STRAIN

Concerns about level of dietary protein and renal function are often presented in public health guidelines [59]. In addition to the claims that high protein intake causes renal disease, some studies have suggested that renal function may be negatively affected by routine consumption of high protein diets [72-75]. Although high protein diets cause changes in renal function (i.e., increased GFR) and several related endocrine factors [1,76,77] that may be harmful to individuals with renal disease [52,53], there is not sufficient research to extend these findings to healthy individuals with normal renal function at this time.

The lay public is often told that high protein diets "overwork" the kidney and may negatively impact renal function over time [78]. In addition, a number of highly regarded organizations appear to support this line of reasoning [79] given the physiological processes required for excretion of protein-related metabolic waste products to maintain homeostasis following consumption of protein at levels in excess of recommended amounts. Increased consumption of dietary protein is linearly related to the production of urea [80] and urea excretion is controlled by the kidney. These processes are of significant energetic cost to the kidney and represent the physiological "strain" associated with increased protein intake [81].

The word "strain" is misleading given its negative connotation. In a press release [82], one group asserted that increased dietary protein "strains" the kidney via increased urea production, and causes dehydration and accumulation of blood urea nitrogen. This press release also suggested that these events synergistically overwork the kidney and predispose humans to CKD. Scientific research is often misrepresented in this context. Research from our laboratory [83] which is cited in the press release, does not support these contentions. Rather, we found that habitual consumption of a high protein diet minimally affected hydration indices. Changes in total body water and renal function were not measured.

The concept that increased dietary protein leads to dehydration may have originated from an unsubstantiated extension of a 1954 review of the nitrogen balance literature [84]. This review focused on the design of survival rations for military operations in the desert or at sea, when water supply and energy intake are limited. Since the excretion of 1 gram of urea nitrogen requires 40 – 60 mL of additional water, increased protein intakes in the study translated into an increased water requirement (i.e., +250 mL water per 6 grams of dietary nitrogen in a 500 Kcal diet) for excretion of urea nitrogen. This increased fluid requirement is situation specific and is not necessarily applicable to individuals whose calorie and water intakes are adequate. Presently, we know of no studies executed in healthy individuals with normal renal function which demonstrate a clear relation between increased dietary protein intake and dehydration or a detrimental "strain" on the kidney. Therefore, claims that a high protein diet promotes dehydration or adversely "strains" the kidney remain speculative.

7.8 EVIDENCE IN HEALTHY INDIVIDUALS

Although the efficacy of high protein diets for weight loss has been evaluated, there have been no reports of protein-induced diminutions in renal function despite subject populations that are generally at risk for kidney disease (e.g., dyslipidemia, obesity, hypertension) [14,15,22,85-87]. A randomized comparison of the effects of high and low protein diets on renal function in obese individuals suggested that high protein diets did not present a health concern with regard to renal function their study population [65]. In this study, 65 overweight, but otherwise healthy, subjects adhered to a low or high protein diet for six months. In the high protein group, both kidney size and GFR were significantly increased from that measured at baseline. No changes in albumin excretion were noted for either group and the authors concluded that, despite acute changes in renal function and size, high protein intake did not have detrimental effects on renal function in healthy individuals. Similar findings were recently reported by Boden et al. [88] in a study of 10 subjects who consumed their typical diet for 7 days followed by strict adherence to a high protein diet for 14 days. No significant changes were noted in serum or urinary creatinine and albumin excretion, suggesting no ill-effects of a high protein diet on renal function.

Athletes, particularly in sports requiring strength and power, consume high levels of dietary protein [89,90]. In fact, many athletes habitually consume protein in excess of 2.0 g/kg/day [91]. Supplementation with amino acids will further increase dietary protein levels in these individuals [92]. Yet there is no evidence that this population is at greater risk for kidney disease or losses in renal function [90]. Poortsmans and Dellalieux [93] found that protein intakes in the range of ~1.4–1.9 g/kg/day or 170–243% of the recommended dietary allowance did not impair renal function in a group of 37 athletes. We found no data in the scientific literature to link high protein intakes to increased risk for impaired kidney function in healthy, physically active men and women.

7.9 DIETARY PROTEIN AND RENAL FUNCTION IN ANIMAL MODELS

Although there is limited research regarding the long-term effects of high protein intakes on renal function in humans, animal models have provided insight into this quandary. Mammals fed acute and chronic high protein diets exhibit increases in GFR and renal blood flow [94]. These changes, which are comparable to those observed in humans, led to the hypothesis that high protein intakes are associated with progressive glomeruloscle-rosis in the rat. Recently, Lacroix et al. [95] studied the effects of a diet containing 50% protein on renal function in Wistar rats and noted no ab-normalities in renal function or pathology. Collins et al. [96] also reported no adverse effects of long-term consumption of high protein diets on renal function when two years of a diet containing 60% protein failed to evoke changes in the percentage of sclerotic glomeruli in rats. Robertson et al., [97] studied the effect of increased protein intake on hyperperfusion and the progression of glomerulosclerosis in dogs that were 75% nephrecto-mized. After four years of feeding diets that were either 56, 27 or 19% protein, no association between diet and structural changes in the kidney were observed.

To the best of our knowledge, there has been only one report of a po-tentially toxic effect of excessive protein intake on renal function in the rat. Stonard et al. [98] found a diet containing 33% protein produced tu-bular damage in a specific strain of female rats. However, findings from this study are limited by the fact that damage was induced by a bacterial single-cell protein (Pruteen).

In summary, studies documenting high protein intake as a cause of re-nal disease in any animal model have not been done. Rather, studies have typically focused on the interaction between protein intake and renal func-tion in the diseased state. As a result, findings from these investigations should not be used as a basis for dietary recommendations for humans. Studies designed to characterize the effects of dietary protein intake on renal function in healthy subjects are warranted.

7.10 DIETARY PROTEIN AND KIDNEY STONES

The role of high protein diets in kidney stone formation has received considerable attention. Excessive protein intake increases excretion of potentially lithogenic substances such as calcium and uric acid [99,100]. Reddy et al. [101] noted that consumption of a high protein diet for six weeks was associated aciduria and urinary calcium and claimed

that this constituted increased risk of stone formation in ten healthy subjects although none of the ten subjects developed renal stones. The severe
carbohydrate restriction imposed in this study may have increased keto-
acid production thereby contributing acid formation. Since consumption
of fruits and vegetables usually produces a marked base load [102], restriction of these foods subsequent to the diet intervention may have also
contributed to the net acid load.

Studies that claim an increased propensity for stone formation as a result of increased protein intake should be taken at face value because propensity is a surrogate marker and does not represent actual stone formation. Further, randomized control trials have not been done to test whether
an increased tendency for stone formation is enhanced with consumption
of a high protein diet.

Epidemiological studies provide conflicting evidence with regard to the
association between protein intake and the predisposition for kidney stone
formation. In a prospective study of over 45,000 men, researchers found a
direct correlation between animal protein intake and risk of stone formation [103]. However, findings in women are difficult to interpret due to conflicting reports in the literature. While some studies have shown a direct
relationship between animal protein intake and risk of stone formation in
women [104,105], other work suggests an inverse relationship exists [106].

Conflicting findings regarding the role of dietary protein in kidney
stone formation limit the development of universal guidelines with regard
to a recommended protein intake for individuals at increased risk for stone
formation [107]. It is not likely that diet alone causes kidney stone formation [108]. Rather, metabolic abnormalities are typically the underlying
cause [109]. For example, Nguyen et al. [110] found that high intakes of
animal protein adversely affected markers of stone formation in those afflicted with a stone causing disorder, while no changes were observed in
healthy individuals. It has been suggested that one must have a preexisting
metabolic dysfunction before dietary protein can exert an effect relative to
stone formation [108]. This notion has been coined the "powderkeg and
tinderbox" theory of renal stone disease by Jaeger [111]. This theory as-
serts that dietary excesses, such as high protein intake, serve as a tinderbox
which, only in tandem with a metabolic abnormality (the powderkeg), can

bring about stone formation. At the present time, however, evidence showing that a high protein intake is an inherent cause of this renal abnormality or is consistently associated with increased kidney stone formation does not exist.

7.11 CONCLUSION

Although excessive protein intake remains a health concern in individuals with pre-existing renal disease, the literature lacks significant research demonstrating a link between protein intake and the initiation or progression of renal disease in healthy individuals. More importantly, evidence suggests that protein-induced changes in renal function are likely a normal adaptative mechanism well within the functional limits of a healthy kidney. Without question, long-term studies are needed to clarify the scant evidence currently available regarding this relationship. At present, there is not sufficient proof to warrant public health directives aimed at restricting dietary protein intake in healthy adults for the purpose of preserving renal function.

REFERENCES

1. King AJ, Levey AS: Dietary protein and renal function. J Am Soc Nephrol 1993, 3(11):1723-1737.
2. Metges CC, Barth CA: Metabolic consequences of a high dietary-protein intake in adulthood: assessment of the available evidence. J Nutr 2000, 130(4):886-889.
3. Brenner BM, Meyer TW, Hostetter TH: Dietary protein intake and the progressive nature of kidney disease: the role of hemodynamically mediated glomerular injury in the pathogenesis of progressive glomerular sclerosis in aging, renal ablation, and intrinsic renal disease. N Engl J Med 1982, 307(11):652-659.
4. The University of Pennsylvania Health System: Media Review: mouth to mouth. 1999. Janurary, 1999
5. Sugaya K, Ogawa Y, Hatano T, Koyama Y, Miyazato T, Naito A, Yonou H, Kagawa H: Compensatory renal hypertrophy and changes of renal function following nephrectomy. Hinyokika Kiyo 2000, 46(4):235-240.
6. Calderon JL, Zadshir A, Norris K: A survey of kidney disease and risk-factor information on the World Wide Web. MedGenMed 2004, 6(4):3.

7. Lindheimer MD, Katz AI: Physiology and Pathophysiology . In Renal physiology and disease in pregnancy. 2nd edition. Edited by Seldin DW, Giebisch G. New York, Raven Press ; 1992::3371–3431.

8. Conrad KP: Mechanisms of renal vasodilation and hyperfiltration during pregnancy. J Soc Gynecol Investig 2004, 11(7):438-448.

9. Higashihara E, Horie S, Takeuchi T, Nutahara K, Aso Y: Long-term consequence of nephrectomy. J Urol 1990, 143(2):239-243.

10. Regazzoni BM, Genton N, Pelet J, Drukker A, Guignard JP: Long-term followup of renal functional reserve capacity after unilateral nephrectomy in childhood. J Urol 1998, 160(3 Pt 1):844-848.

11. Food and Nutrition Board, Institute of Medicine: Macronutrient and Healthful Diets. In Dietary Reference Intakes for Energy, Carbohydrate, Fiber, Fat, Fatty Acids, Cholesterol, Protein, and Amino Acids (Macronutrients). Washington, D.C. , The National Academies Press; 2002::609-696.

12. Layman DK, Boileau RA, Erickson DJ, Painter JE, Shiue H, Sather C, Christou DD: A Reduced Ratio of Dietary Carbohydrate to Protein Improves Body Composition and Blood Lipid Profiles during Weight Loss in Adult Women. J Nutr 2003, 133(2):411-417.

13. Piatti PM, Monti F, Fermo I, Baruffaldi L, Nasser R, Santambrogio G, Librenti MC, Galli-Kienle M, Pontiroli AE, Pozza G: Hypocaloric high-protein diet improves glucose oxidation and spares lean body mass: comparison to hypocaloric high-carbohydrate diet. Metabolism 1994, 43(12):1481-1487.

14. Luscombe ND, Clifton PM, Noakes M, Farnsworth E, Wittert G: Effect of a high-protein, energy-restricted diet on weight loss and energy expenditure after weight stabilization in hyperinsulinemic subjects. Int J Obes Relat Metab Disord 2003, 27(5):582-590.

15. Brinkworth GD, Noakes M, Keogh JB, Luscombe ND, Wittert GA, Clifton PM: Long-term effects of a high-protein, low-carbohydrate diet on weight control and cardiovascular risk markers in obese hyperinsulinemic subjects. Int J Obes Relat Metab Disord 2004, 28(5):661-670.

16. Fine EJ, Feinman RD: Thermodynamics of weight loss diets. Nutr Metab (Lond) 2004, 1(1):15.

17. Parker B, Noakes M, Luscombe N, Clifton P: Effect of a High-Protein, High-Monounsaturated Fat Weight Loss Diet on Glycemic Control and Lipid Levels in Type 2 Diabetes . Diabetes Care 2002, 25(3):425-430.

18. Layman DK: Protein quantity and quality at levels above the RDA improves adult weight loss. J Am Coll Nutr 2004, 23(6 Suppl):631S-636S.

19. Wolfe RR, Chinkes D, Baba H, Rosenblatt J, Zhang XJ: Response of phosphoenolpyruvate cycle activity to fasting and to hyperinsulinemia in human subjects. Am J Physiol Endocrinol Metab 1996, 271(1):E159-176.

20. Sharman MJ, Volek JS: Weight loss leads to reductions in inflammatory biomarkers after a very-low-carbohydrate diet and a low-fat diet in overweight men. Clin Sci (Lond) 2004, 107(4):365-369.

21. Yancy WSJ, Olsen MK, Guyton JR, Bakst RP, Westman EC: A low-carbohydrate, ketogenic diet versus a low-fat diet to treat obesity and hyperlipidemia: a randomized, controlled trial. Ann Intern Med 2004, 140(10):769-777.

22. Johnston CS, Tjonn SL, Swan PD: High-Protein, Low-Fat Diets Are Effective for Weight Loss and Favorably Alter Biomarkers in Healthy Adults. J Nutr 2004, 134(3):586-591.
23. Foster GD, Wyatt HR, Hill JO, McGuckin BG, Brill C, Mohammed BS, Szapary PO, Rader DJ, Edman JS, Klein S: A randomized trial of a low-carbohydrate diet for obesity. N Engl J Med 2003, 348(21):2082-2090.
24. Skov AR, Toubro S, Ronn B, Holm L, Astrup A: Randomized trial on protein vs carbohydrate in ad libitum fat reduced diet for the treatment of obesity. Int J Obes Relat Metab Disord 1999, 23(5):528-536.
25. Levey AS, Coresh J, Balk E, Kausz AT, Levin A, Steffes MW, Hogg RJ, Perrone RD, Lau J, Eknoyan G: National Kidney Foundation practice guidelines for chronic kidney disease: evaluation, classification, and stratification. Ann Intern Med 2003, 139(2):137-147.
26. Coresh J, Byrd-Holt D, Astor BC, Briggs JP, Eggers PW, Lacher DA, Hostetter TH: Chronic Kidney Disease Awareness, Prevalence, and Trends among U.S. Adults, 1999 to 2000. J Am Soc Nephrol 2005, 16(1):180-188.
27. Muntner P, He J, Hamm L, Loria C, Whelton PK: Renal insufficiency and subsequent death resulting from cardiovascular disease in the United States. J Am Soc Nephrol 2002, 13(3):745-753.
28. Coresh J, Astor BC, Greene T, Eknoyan G, Levey AS: Prevalence of chronic kidney disease and decreased kidney function in the adult US population: Third National Health and Nutrition Examination Survey. Am J Kidney Dis 2003, 41(1):1-12.
29. Johnson CA: Creating practice guidelines for chronic kidney disease: an insider's view. Am Fam Physician 2004, 70(5):823-824.
30. Palmer BF: Disturbances in renal autoregulation and the susceptibility to hypertension-induced chronic kidney disease. Am J Med Sci 2004, 328(6):330-343.
31. National Kidney Foundation: Chronic Kidney Diseases. [http://www.kidneynca.org/WhatsNew_Campaigns_KidneyUrologicDisease.asp]
32. Vupputuri S, Batuman V, Muntner P, Bazzano LA, Lefante JJ, Whelton PK, He J: Effect of blood pressure on early decline in kidney function among hypertensive men. Hypertension 2003, 42(6):1144-1149.
33. Segura J, Campo C, Gil P, Roldan C, Vigil L, Rodicio JL, Ruilope LM: Development of chronic kidney disease and cardiovascular prognosis in essential hypertensive patients. J Am Soc Nephrol 2004, 15(6):1616-1622.
34. Wright JTJ, Bakris G, Greene T, Agodoa LY, Appel LJ, Charleston J, Cheek D, Douglas-Baltimore JG, Gassman J, Glassock R, Hebert L, Jamerson K, Lewis J, Phillips RA, Toto RD, Middleton JP, Rostand SG: Effect of blood pressure lowering and antihypertensive drug class on progression of hypertensive kidney disease: results from the AASK trial. Jama 2002, 288(19):2421-2431.
35. Kasiske BL, Kalil RS, Ma JZ, Liao M, Keane WF: Effect of antihypertensive therapy on the kidney in patients with diabetes: a meta-regression analysis. Ann Intern Med 1993, 118(2):129-138.
36. Peterson JC, Adler S, Burkart JM, Greene T, Hebert LA, Hunsicker LG, King AJ, Klahr S, Massry SG, Seifter JL: Blood pressure control, proteinuria, and the progression of renal disease. The Modification of Diet in Renal Disease Study. Ann Intern Med 1995, 123(10):754-762.

37. Tarver-Carr ME, Powe NR, Eberhardt MS, LaVeist TA, Kington RS, Coresh J, Brancati FL: Excess risk of chronic kidney disease among African-American versus white subjects in the United States: a population-based study of potential explanatory factors. J Am Soc Nephrol 2002, 13(9):2363-2370.
38. Zheng F, Plati AR, Banerjee A, Elliot S, Striker LJ, Striker GE: The molecular basis of age-related kidney disease. Sci Aging Knowledge Environ 2003, 2003(29):PE20.
39. Brown WW, Sandberg K: Introduction: gender and kidney disease. Adv Ren Replace Ther 2003, 10(1):1-2.
40. Satko SG, Freedman BI: The importance of family history on the development of renal disease. Curr Opin Nephrol Hypertens 2004, 13(3):337-341.
41. Zhou BF, Wu XG, Tao SQ, Yang J, Cao TX, Zheng RP, Tian XZ, Lu CQ, Miao HY, Ye FM, et al.: Dietary patterns in 10 groups and the relationship with blood pressure. Collaborative Study Group for Cardiovascular Diseases and Their Risk Factors. Chin Med J (Engl) 1989, 102(4):257-261.
42. He J, Klag MJ, Whelton PK, Chen JY, Qian MC, He GQ: Dietary macronutrients and blood pressure in southwestern China. J Hypertens 1995, 13(11):1267-1274.
43. Burke V, Hodgson JM, Beilin LJ, Giangiulioi N, Rogers P, Puddey IB: Dietary Protein and Soluble Fiber Reduce Ambulatory Blood Pressure in Treated Hypertensives. Hypertension 2001, 38(4):821-826.
44. St. Jeor ST, Howard BV, Prewitt TE, Bovee V, Bazzarre T, Eckel RH: Dietary Protein and Weight Reduction: A statement for healthcare professionals from the nutrition committee of the council on nutrition, physical Activity, and metabolism of the american heart association. Circulation 2001, 104(15):1869-1874.
45. Addis T, Drury DR: The Rate of Urea Excretion. VII. The effect of various other factors than blood urea concentration on the rate of urea excretion. J Biol Chem 1923, 55(4):629-638.
46. Jolliffe N, Smith HW: The Excretion of Urine In The Dog: I. The Urea and Creatinine Clearances on a Mixed Diet. Am J Physiol 1931, 98(4):572-577.
47. Shannon JA, Jolliffe N, Smith HW: The Excretion of Urine in The Dog: VI. The Filtration and Secretion of Exogenous Creatinine. Am J Physiol 1932, 102(3):534-550.
48. Herrin RC, Rabin A, Feinstein RN: The influence of diet upon urea clearance in dogs. Am J Physiol 1937, 119(1):87-92.
49. Van Slyke DD, Rhoads CP, Hiller A, Alving A: The relationship of the urea clearance to the renal blood flow. Am J Physiol 1934, 110(2):387-391.
50. Tuttle KR, Puhlman ME, Cooney SK, Short RA: Effects of amino acids and glucagon on renal hemodynamics in type 1 diabetes. Am J Physiol Renal Physiol 2002, 282(1):F103-12.
51. Bilo HJ, Schaap GH, Blaak E, Gans RO, Oe PL, Donker AJ: Effects of chronic and acute protein administration on renal function in patients with chronic renal insufficiency. Nephron 1989, 53(3):181-187.
52. Lentine K, Wrone EM: New insights into protein intake and progression of renal disease. Curr Opin Nephrol Hypertens 2004, 13(3):333-336.
53. Knight EL, Stampfer MJ, Hankinson SE, Spiegelman D, Curhan GC: The Impact of Protein Intake on Renal Function Decline in Women with Normal Renal Function or Mild Renal Insufficiency. Ann Intern Med 2003, 138(6):460-467.

54. Johnson DW, Mudge DW, Sturtevant JM, Hawley CM, Campbell SB, Isbel NM, Hollett P: Predictors of decline of residual renal function in new peritoneal dialysis patients. Perit Dial Int 2003, 23(3):276-283.

55. Meloni C, Tatangelo P, Cipriani S, Rossi V, Suraci C, Tozzo C, Rossini B, Cecilia A, Di Franco D, Straccialano E, Casciani CU: Adequate protein dietary restriction in diabetic and nondiabetic patients with chronic renal failure. J Ren Nutr 2004, 14(4):208-213.

56. Pedrini MT, Levey AS, Lau J, Chalmers TC, Wang PH: The effect of dietary protein restriction on the progression of diabetic and nondiabetic renal diseases: a meta-analysis. Ann Intern Med 1996, 124(7):627-632.

57. Franz MJ, Wheeler ML: Nutrition therapy for diabetic nephropathy. Curr Diab Rep 2003, 3(5):412-417.

58. Beto JA, Bansal VK: Medical nutrition therapy in chronic kidney failure: integrating clinical practice guidelines. Journal of the American Dietetic Association 2004, 104(3):404-409.

59. Krauss RM, Eckel RH, Howard B, Appel LJ, Daniels SR, Deckelbaum RJ, Erdman JWJ, Kris-Etherton P, Goldberg IJ, Kotchen TA, Lichtenstein AH, Mitch WE, Mullis R, Robinson K, Wylie-Rosett J, St Jeor S, Suttie J, Tribble DL, Bazzarre TL: AHA Dietary Guidelines: revision 2000: A statement for healthcare professionals from the Nutrition Committee of the American Heart Association. Stroke 2000, 31(11):2751-2766.

60. Allen FM, Cope OM: Influence of Diet on Blood Pressure and Kidney Size in Dogs. J Urol 1942, 47:751.

61. Osborne TB, Mendel LB, Park EA, Winternitz MC, With the cooperation of Helen C. Cannon and Deborah Jackson: Physiological effectgs of diets unusually rich in protein or inorganic salts. J Biol Chem 1927, 71(2):317-350.

62. Wilson HE: An Investigation of the Cause of Renal Hypertrophy in Rats Fed on a High Protein Diet. Biochem J 1933, 27:1348.

63. Addis T, MacKay EM, MacKay LL: The effect on the kidney of the long continued administration of diets containing an excess of certain food elements. II. Excess of acid and alkali. J Biol Chem 1926, 71(1):157-166.

64. Hammond KA, Janes DN: The effects of increased protein intake on kidney size and function. J Exp Biol 1998, 201 (Pt 13):2081-2090.

65. Skov AR, Toubro S, Bulow J, Krabbe K, Parving HH, Astrup A: Changes in renal function during weight loss induced by high vs low-protein low-fat diets in overweight subjects. Int J Obes Relat Metab Disord 1999, 23(11):1170-1177.

66. Gorin E, Dickbuch S: Release of cyclic AMP from chicken erythrocytes. Horm Metab Res 1980, 12(3):120-124.

67. Bankir L, Martin H, Dechaux M, Ahloulay M: Plasma cAMP: a hepatorenal link influencing proximal reabsorption and renal hemodynamics? Kidney Int Suppl 1997, Suppl 59:S50-6.

68. Bankir L, Ahloulay M, Devreotes PN, Parent CA: Extracellular cAMP inhibits proximal reabsorption: are plasma membrane cAMP receptors involved? Am J Physiol Renal Physiol 2002, 282(3):F376-392.

69. Slomowitz LA, Gabbai FB, Khang S, Satriano J, Thareau S, Deng A, Thomson SC, Blantz RC, Munger KA: Protein intake regulates the vasodilatory function of the kidney and the NMDA receptor expression. Am J Physiol Regul Integr Comp Physiol 2004, :R1184-9.

70. Conrad KP, Novak J, Danielson LA, Kerchner LJ, Jeyabalan A: Mechanisms of renal vasodilation and hyperfiltration during pregnancy: current perspectives and potential implications for preeclampsia. Endothelium 2005, 12(1-2):57-62.

71. Klahr S: The modification of diet in renal disease study. N Engl J Med 1989, 320(13):864-866.

72. Consumer Reports on Health: Feature Report; Is your diet up-to-date? (New recommendations have changed the standard advice). 2003, :4-6.

73. Time: How to Eat Smarter; In a world that is raining food, making healthy choices about what and how to eat is not easy. Here are some rules to live by. 2003, :48.

74. CNBC: Diet Dangers; Debate on the dangers of high protein-low carb diets after Physicians Committee for Responsible Medicine came to warn about health risks. Capital Report , Video Monitoring Services of America; 2003.

75. Fox News Channel: Diet; People who do the low carb diet will get hurt. The O'Reilly Factor , Video Monitoring Services of America; 2004.

76. Schaffer SW, Lombardini JB, Azuma J: Interaction between the actions of taurine and angiotensin II. Amino Acids 2000, 18(4):305-318.

77. Brandle E, Sieberth HG, Hautmann RE: Effect of chronic dietary protein intake on the renal function in healthy subjects. Eur J Clin Nutr 1996, 50(11):734-740.

78. USA Today: High-protein diets gaining support. 1999.

79. Taubes G: What if It's All Been a Big Fat Lie? The New York Times Magazine 2002.

80. Young VR, El-Khoury AE, Raguso CA, Forslund AH, Hambraeus L: Rates of urea production and hydrolysis and leucine oxidation change linearly over widely varying protein intakes in healthy adults. J Nutr 2000, 130(4):761-766.

81. Bankir L, Bouby N, Trinh-Trang-Tan MM, Ahloulay M, Promeneur D: Direct and indirect cost of urea excretion. Kidney Int 1996, 49(6):1598-1607.

82. AtkinsExposed.org   [http://www.atkinsexposed.org/atkins/79/American_Kidney_Fund.htm]

83. Martin WF, Bolster DR, Gaine PC, Hanley LJ, Pikosky MA, Bennett BT, Maresh CM, Armstrong LE, Rodriguez NR: Increased Dietary Protein Affects Hydration Indices in Runners [in press]. J Am Diet Assoc 2006., 106(1)

84. Calloway DH, Spector H: Nitrogen balance as related to caloric and protein intake in active young men. Am J Clin Nutr 1954, 2(6):405-412.

85. Layman DK, Baum JI: Dietary Protein Impact on Glycemic Control during Weight Loss. J Nutr 2004, Suppl 4:968S-973.

86. Due A, Toubro S, Skov AR, Astrup A: Effect of normal-fat diets, either medium or high in protein, on body weight in overweight subjects: a randomised 1-year trial. Int J Obes Relat Metab Disord 2004, 28(10):1283-1290.

87. Stern L, Iqbal N, Seshadri P, Chicano KL, Daily DA, McGrory J, Williams M, Gracely EJ, Samaha FF: The effects of low-carbohydrate versus conventional weight loss diets in severely obese adults: one-year follow-up of a randomized trial. Ann Intern Med 2004, 140(10):778-785.

88. Boden G, Sargrad K, Homko C, Mozzoli M, Stein TP: Effect of a Low-Carbohydrate Diet on Appetite, Blood Glucose Levels, and Insulin Resistance in Obese Patients with Type 2 Diabetes. Ann Intern Med 2005, 142(6):403-411.

89. Fern EB, Bielinski RN, Schutz Y: Effects of exaggerated amino acid and protein supply in man. Experientia 1991, 47(2):168-172.

90. Lemon PW: Is increased dietary protein necessary or beneficial for individuals with a physically active lifestyle? Nutr Rev 1996, 54(4 Pt 2):S169-75.

91. Chen JD, Wang JF, Li KJ, Zhao YW, Wang SW, Jiao Y, Hou XY: Nutritional problems and measures in elite and amateur athletes. Am J Clin Nutr 1989, 49(5 Suppl):1084-1089.

92. Chromiak JA, Antonio J: Use of amino acids as growth hormone-releasing agents by athletes. Nutrition 2002, 18(7-8):657-661.

93. Poortmans JR, Dellalieux O: Do regular high protein diets have potential health risks on kidney function in athletes? Int J Sport Nutr Exerc Metab 2000, 10(1):28-38.

94. Singer MA: Dietary protein-induced changes in excretory function: a general animal design feature. Comparative Biochemistry and Physiology Part B: Biochemistry and Molecular Biology 2003, 136(4):785-801.

95. Lacroix M, Gaudichon C, Martin A, Morens C, Mathe V, Tome D, Huneau JF: A long-term high-protein diet markedly reduces adipose tissue without major side effects in Wistar male rats. Am J Physiol Regul Integr Comp Physiol 2004, 287(4):R934-42.

96. Collins DMCTRJBKPRTMCPEK: Chronic high protein feeding does not produce glomerulosclerosis or renal insufficiency in the normal rat. J Am Soc Nephrol 1990, 1:624.

97. Robertson JL, Goldschmidt M, Kronfeld DS, Tomaszewski JE, Hill GS, Bovee KC: Long-term renal responses to high dietary protein in dogs with 75% nephrectomy. Kidney Int 1986, 29(2):511-519.

98. Stonard MD, Samuels DM, Lock EA: The pathogenesis and effect on renal function of nephrocalcinosis induced by different diets in female rats. Food Chem Toxicol 1984, 22(2):139-146.

99. Wasserstein AG, Stolley PD, Soper KA, Goldfarb S, Maislin G, Agus Z: Case-control study of risk factors for idiopathic calcium nephrolithiasis. Miner Electrolyte Metab 1987, 13(2):85-95.

100. Robertson WG, Heyburn PJ, Peacock M, Hanes FA, Swaminathan R: The effect of high animal protein intake on the risk of calcium stone-formation in the urinary tract. Clin Sci (Lond) 1979, 57(3):285-288.

101. Reddy ST, Wang CY, Sakhaee K, Brinkley L, Pak CY: Effect of low-carbohydrate high-protein diets on acid-base balance, stone-forming propensity, and calcium metabolism. Am J Kidney Dis 2002, 40(2):265-274.

102. Cordain L, Eaton SB, Sebastian A, Mann N, Lindeberg S, Watkins BA, O'Keefe JH, Brand-Miller J: Origins and evolution of the Western diet: health implications for the 21st century. Am J Clin Nutr 2005, 81(2):341-354.

103. Curhan GC, Willett WC, Rimm EB, Stampfer MJ: A prospective study of dietary calcium and other nutrients and the risk of symptomatic kidney stones. N Engl J Med 1993, 328(12):833-838.

104. Breslau NA, Brinkley L, Hill KD, Pak CY: Relationship of animal protein-rich diet to kidney stone formation and calcium metabolism. J Clin Endocrinol Metab 1988, 66(1):140-146.
105. Curhan GC, Willett WC, Speizer FE, Spiegelman D, Stampfer MJ: Comparison of dietary calcium with supplemental calcium and other nutrients as factors affecting the risk for kidney stones in women. Ann Intern Med 1997, 126(7):497-504.
106. Curhan GC, Willett WC, Knight EL, Stampfer MJ: Dietary factors and the risk of incident kidney stones in younger women: Nurses' Health Study II. Arch Intern Med 2004, 164(8):885-891.
107. Meschi T, Schianchi T, Ridolo E, Adorni G, Allegri F, Guerra A, Novarini A, Borghi L: Body weight, diet and water intake in preventing stone disease. Urol Int 2004, Suppl 1:29-33.
108. Hess B: Nutritional aspects of stone disease. Endocrinol Metab Clin North Am 2002, 31(4):1017-30, ix-x.
109. Raj GV, Auge BK, Assimos D, Preminger GM: Metabolic abnormalities associated with renal calculi in patients with horseshoe kidneys. J Endourol 2004, 18(2):157-161.
110. Nguyen QV, Kalin A, Drouve U, Casez JP, Jaeger P: Sensitivity to meat protein intake and hyperoxaluria in idiopathic calcium stone formers. Kidney Int 2001, 59(6):2273-2281.
111. Jaeger P: Renal stone disease in the 1990s: the powder keg and tinderbox theory. Curr Opin Nephrol Hypertens 1992, 1(1):141-148.

This chapter was originally published under the Creative Commons Attribution License. Martin, W. F., Armstrong. L. E., and Rodriguez, N. R. Dietary Protein Intake and Renal Function. Nutrition & Metabolism 2005: 2(25). doi:10.1186/1743-7075-2-25.

CHAPTER 8

PHOSPHORUS AND NUTRITION IN CHRONIC KIDNEY DISEASE

EMILIO GONZÁLEZ-PARRA, CAROLINA GRACIA-IGUACEL,
JESÚS EGIDO, and ALBERTO ORTIZ

8.1 INTRODUCTION

Daily phosphorus ingestion is approximately 1200 mg, of which 950 mg are absorbed. Around 29% of body phosphorus is located in bone, and less than 1% is in the blood, which is the phosphorus that is quantified in clinical practice. Most phosphorus (70%) is located intracellularly and is interchangeable. Phosphorus is removed by two systems, the gastrointestinal tract, (150 mg/day) and the urine (800 mg/day) [1]. Ingestion of phosphorus by an individual with normal renal function results in immediate phosphaturia probably mediated by phosphatonins of intestinal origin [2]. A positive phosphorus balance recruits other phosphatonins. The first one, faster and transient, is parathyroid hormone (PTH) and the second one, slower and lasting, is Fibroblast Growth Factor 23 (FGF23).

Patients with renal impairment progressively lose the ability to excrete phosphorus. Decreased glomerular filtration of phosphorus is initially compensated by decreased tubular reabsorption regulated by PTH and FGF 23. This compensation leads to a normal urinary excretion of phosphorus in 24 h and in maintenance of normal serum phosphorus [3]. However, the adequacy of 24 h urinary phosphorus excretion is difficult to interpret, since we do not know the phosphorus ingested, and, as renal function deteriorates, a positive phosphorus balance results.

FGF23 is a 251 amino acid phosphatonin, which promotes phosphaturia by decreasing phosphorus reabsorption through inhibition of Na/P cotransporter type II activity in proximal tubules and by decreasing phosphorus absorption in the gut by inhibiting generation of active vitamin D in proximal tubules through inhibition of renal 1 alpha hydroxylase. Reduced active vitamin D facilitates PTH secretion, which further promotes renal phosphorus excretion [4–6]. FGF23 is released by bone generating the concept of an osteo-renal axis for phosphorus balance control that has changed traditional paradigms [4].

8.2 PROTEIN INTAKE AND PHOSPHORUS

There is a close relationship between protein and phosphorus intake [7]. Proteins are rich in phosphorus so most of the scientific societies recommend reducing protein intake from early stages in patients with chronic renal failure, to reduce the input of phosphorus. One gram of protein has 13–15 mg of phosphorus of which 30–70% is absorbed through the intestine. Thus, an intake of 90 g of proteins a day results in absorption of 600–700 mg of phosphorus daily. In hemodialysis the net positive phosphorus balance in 48 hours is 1200–1400 mg/day, of which dialysis only removes 500–600 mg/session. Thus, there are two good reasons to restrict protein intake in chronic renal disease. On one side, a low dietary protein content slows the progression of kidney disease, especially in patients with proteinuria [8]. In addition,a protein-restricted diet decreases the supply of phosphorus, which has been directly related with progression of kidney disease and with patient survival. A restricted protein diet has additional advantages (Table 1). In advanced chronic kidney disease (CKD) most guidelines recommend a diet containing 0.6 to 0.8 g protein/kg/day based on meta-analysis demonstrating its efficacy [9]. This restriction is safe nutritionally and metabolically [10].

TABLE 1: Consequences of dietary protein restriction in advanced chronic kidney disease.

Reduces proteinuria.
Improves lipid control
Reduces uremic toxins and acids
Reduces oxidative stress
Improves insulin resistance
Reduces phosphorus load

After initiating dialysis the dietary protein intake should be increased. Hemodialysis patients with higher protein intake have improved survival, despite higher phosphorus intake [11]. In a post hoc analysis of the HEMO study patients without dietary protein restriction have a better survival than those eating a protein-restricted diet [12]. However, a high protein intake is associated with a high intake of phosphorus and the latter is associated with increased cardiovascular mortality. This relationship holds even when adjusted for serum phosphorus, type and dose of phosphorus binders, and protein and energy intake [13]. For this reason an adequate protein intake should be associated with a restriction of dietary phosphorus.

The Food and Nutrition Board of the Institute of Medicine recommends a diet with 700 mg/day of phosphorus in healthy people, and 1250 mg/day in children and pregnant women [14]. However, a lower intake is recommended in the renal patient to reduce. The same recommendations advise restricting food additives containing phosphorus.

8.3 PHOSPHORUS ABSORPTION AND PROTEIN OF DIFFERENT ORIGINS

Phosphorus in foods is found in different forms. Organic phosphorus associates with proteins has a low absorption. By contrast absorption of inorganic phosphorus found in additives and preservatives is very high, above 90%. A large amount of phosphate are added to foods as preservatives as well as from common beverages such cola, with a high phosphate content

[15]. However, organic phosphorus from plant protein has a lower absorption than phosphorus from animal protein, ranging from 40 to 50%. The reason is that phosphorus from plants is in the form of phytates and mammals lack phytases. Phosphorus in animal protein is in the form of organic phosphate, which is readily hydrolyzed and absorbed [16].

In rats with slowly progressive renal failure fed a casein-based or a grain-based protein diet, both of which with equivalent total phosphorus contents had the same serum phosphorous levels. However, the casein-fed animals had increased urinary phosphorus excretion and elevated serum FGF23 compared to the grain-fed rats [17].

In a crossover trial 11 patients with CKD stages 3-4 ingested a diet with animal or vegetable protein for 7 days. Animal protein intake increased serum phosphorus and FGF23 more than vegetable protein intake [18]. The simple recommendation is to reduce preservatives and additives in the first place, favor foods rich in vegetables, reduce meat, and avoid convenience foods.

However, not all animal proteins and vegetables have the same proportion of phosphorus in their composition. There are tables and graphics depicting the amount of phosphorus contained in various foods [19]. Adequate labeling of food requires showing the ratio of phosphorus (in mg) to protein (in grams). The ratio ranges from <10 to >65 mg/g. Cheese and soft drinks have a high ratio. This ratio is recommended by KDOQI guidelines and has several advantages [19].

(a) It is independent of the portion of food served.
(b) It simultaneously represents the contribution of phosphorus, and protein.
(c) It draws attention to the phosphorus-rich foods, especially soft drinks and additives and are not proteins.

However, this ratio does not provide information on the bioavailability of phosphorus from different sources. Patients with CKD should be prescribed a low phosphorus, low inorganic phosphorus and low phosphorus/protein ratio diet, and with a proper protein content to improve the attractiveness of food.

The Mediterranean diet, until recently widespread in Spain, has a low phosphorous content and has been shown to reduce plasma homocysteine, serum phosphorus, microalbuminuria, and cardiovascular risk [20]. Food additives and preservatives are rich in phosphorus [21]. Additives account for about 1000 mg/day of phosphorus on average in the American diet. This amount is important in patients on hemodialysis [22]. Cheese and soft drinks have a high content of phosphoric acid, in addition to a high phosphorus-to-protein ratio [23].

Phosphorus intake is now a hallmark of poor quality food. Individuals with lower socioeconomic status and a lower income have higher serum phosphorus possibly due to the abuse of preprepared meals and fast food containing additives [24].

8.4 LOW-PROTEIN DIET AND MALNUTRITION

The diet in patients with advanced-stage CKD has been controversial throughout the history of Nephrology. CKD is associated with protein calorie malnutrition [25]. A diet with a too low-protein content can favor malnutrition and increase morbidity and mortality [7]. However a low-protein diet can slow the progression of renal disease. While normoproteic or high-protein diet may increase uremic symptoms and hyperphosphatemia. A delicate balance should be sought. A low-protein diet in CKD has the following potential advantages (Table 1): decreases uremic symptoms [11], improves phosphorus control [11], delays initiation of dialysis [9], does not increase the risk of protein malnutrition if accompanied by essential amino acid supplement [26], does not increase mortality in patients with low-protein diet after starting dialysis [27], and protects against oxidative stress which may aggravate progression of CKD [28].

In dialysis, protein intake should not be restricted despite a higher intake of phosphorus, since the risk of protein malnutrition and mortality exceeds that of hyperphosphatemia [11]. When dialysis patients are prescribed a low-protein intake, actual protein intake is frequently lower than expected, possibly because of the difficulty in implementing the diet. Thus, a recommended intake of 0.3–0.6 g/kg/day protein is estimated to result in an actual intake of 0.48–0.84 g/kg/day [26, 29]. Implementation of a low-protein diet requires a dedicated staff, with nurses, dietitians, and a close monitoring by nephrologists. However, in hemodialysis patients net phosphorus balance on a normoproteic diet is positive even after deducting the phosphorus removed during the dialysis session. Hemodialysis removes 800 mg phosphorus/session (2400 mg/week). Thus, a protein intake of 1 g/kg BW/day as recommended will result in an estimated weekly net balance of phosphorus of 2000 mg.

Savica el al. suggest to the patients undergoing periodic HD that they must ingest a quantity of protein of 1,2–1,4 gr per Kg of body weight in the day and in other hand that they must ingest a quantity of phosphate no more than 800 mg per day. So 1,2–1,4 gr of protein correspond to 1.450 mg–1600 mg of phosphate and 800 mg of phosphate correspond to 0.6 mg per Kg b.w. per day. If the patients follow the suggestion to ingest no more 800 mg of phosphate in the day they are at high risk for malnutrition. In fact both dialysis treatment and phosphate binders are unable to remove the phosphate ingested [15]. We report that 74% of CKD pts ingest beverages and if we considere this evidence we can calculate a weekly net positive balance of phosphate of about 2.800 mg. This weekly quantity of phosphate is very dangerous for calcification in CKD pts [30].

The association between low-protein intake and increased mortality in dialysis patients suggests that alternative methods are needed to reduce phosphorus absorption, since high phosphorus is associated with mortality. There are two main alternatives. One is the use of specific nutritional supplements high in energy and protein content, but low in phosphorus. This diet allows maintaining an adequate nutritional status, without altering the serum phosphorus, and without need for higher phosphorus binders [31]. The second alternative is nutritional education of the patient. This includes greater attention to additives and preservatives, to the contribution of phosphorus from different protein foods, so that the diet is based on low phosphorus/protein ratio ingredients, as well as the proper and early use of phosphorus binders [11].

8.5 PHOSPHORUS BINDERS

In a major retrospective study patients treated with phosphorus binders before entering dialysis and phosphate above 3.7 mg/dL, had a better long-term survival than those in whom binders were initiated after initiation of dialysis. Similar results were obtained when binder use in the first 90 days of dialysis was compared with later initiation of binders [32]. The authors speculated that the observation might be explained by modulation of direct effect of phosphorus or compensatory mechanisms such as FGF23 on patient survival [33]. However, this reduction in mortality was not observed in incident dialysis patients treated with calcium-containing binders, either calcium acetate or calcium carbonate [34]. Phosphorus binders lower serum phosphorus and also lower FGF23 levels. Indeed in early CKD binders may result in reduced FGF23 levels in the absence of changes in serum phosphorus [35].

The purpose of therapy with usual phosphate binders is either to limit the absorption of dietary phosphorous intake and to maintain phosphatemia in normal range. Mostly of them act by binding phosphate in gut and eliminating it in the stool. Authors have observed that the salivary phosphorous ratio in hemodialysis patients is more than doubled compared with healthy controls [36, 37]. Same authors have demonstrated that salivary phosphate binders, like chitosan-loaded chewing gum, reduced serum phosphate [38].

8.6 DIFFERENT EFFICACY AND TOLERANCE BETWEEN CAPTORS: BINDING TO BILE SALTS

There are different phosphorus binders for clinical use, which have different binding power and side effects. In addition, the binding power and side effects may differ between individuals and impact on efficacy [39]. The main side effects relate to digestive tolerance in around 15–20% of patients. [40, 41]. In case of intolerance, modification of the prescribed binders may reduce the side effects and decrease the absorption of phosphorus. Lanthanum carbonate has been successfully used in controlling hyperphosphatemia in patients with intolerance to other binders [42].

To better understand the causes of reduced efficiency and digestive intolerance, we must understand the peculiarities of the digestive tract in uremic patients. CKD patients frequently have intestinal dysbacteriosis, which may be multifactorial [43] (Table 2).

TABLE 2: Causes of CKD patients intestinal dysbacteriosis.

Dialysis patients eat less fiber than healthy individuals, in part because dietary restrictions that includes the reduction of fruit and vegetables to avoid an overload of potassium.

Uremia results in intestinal acidification.

Certain drugs, such as antibiotics and phosphate binders alter the intestinal flora.

Bowel dysfunction may cause constipation or increased intestinal transit time.

The metabolism and absorption of proteins is altered and this may lead to malnutrition.

Disbacteriosis promotes the release of products of bacterial metabolism that may enter the blood and originate uremic toxins such as phenols, indoles, and amines. Uremic toxins may contribute to an increased risk of cardiovascular and bone disease.

Uremic patients may have a poor digestion and malabsorption of protein, carbohydrates, and fats [44]. Potential causes are bacterial overgrowth or disorders of the exocrine pancreas or biliary function. Indeed, uremia is associated with high plasma levels of peptides such as secretin, pancreatic secretagogues and gastrin, and an abnormal composition of pancreatic secretion, including low bicarbonate and amylase levels.

Some phosphate binders bind to bile salts. Ten out of 49 dialysis patients studied had bacterial overgrowth as assessed by the lactulose test, and this was associated with dyspepsia [44]. Sevelamer exacerbated dyspepsia, but supplementation of oral pancreatic enzymes improved symptoms and the phosphate binder effectiveness. This highlights the interaction between intestinal dysbacteriosis, phosphate binder efficacy and patient tolerance to the binder.

Phosphorus binders binding to bile salts may interfere with soluble molecules that require biliary salts for absorption. In this sense sevelamer binding to bile salts results in reduced cholesterol absorption and lower serum LDL-cholesterol and in reduced vitamin D absorption [45].

8.7 CONCLUSIONS

Phosphate overload and hyperphosphatemia have emerged as risk factors for vascular calcification, cardiovascular mortality, left ventricular hypertrophym and progression of chronic kidney disease. Normoprotein or high-protein diet may increase uremic symptoms and hyperphosphatemia, but low protein intake and increased mortality in dialysis patients suggests that alternative methods are needed to reduce phosphorus absorption. An adequate nutritional status includes greater attention to additives and preservatives, to the contribution of phosphorus from different protein foods, a diet based on low phosphorus/protein ratio ingredients as well as the proper and early use of phosphorus binders.

REFERENCES

1. K. A. Hruska, S. Mathew, R. Lund, P. Qiu, and R. Pratt, "Hyperphosphatemia of chronic kidney disease," Kidney International, vol. 74, no. 2, pp. 148–157, 2008.
2. T. Isakova, O. M. Gutierrez, Y. Chang et al., "Phosphorus binders and survival on hemodialysis," Journal of the American Society of Nephrology, vol. 20, no. 2, pp. 388–396, 2009.
3. L. Craver, M. P. Marco, I. Martínez et al., "Mineral metabolism parameters throughout chronic kidney disease stages 1–5—achievement of K/DOQI target ranges," Nephrology Dialysis Transplantation, vol. 22, no. 4, pp. 1171–1176, 2007.
4. J. Danziger, "The bone-renal axis in early chronic kidney disease: an emerging paradigm," Nephrology Dialysis Transplantation, vol. 23, no. 9, pp. 2733–2737, 2008.
5. F. Takemoto, T. Shinki, K. Yokoyama, et al., "Gene expression of vitamin D hydroxylase in the remnant kidney of nephrectomized rats," Kidney International, vol. 71, pp. 31–38, 2003.

6. J. B. Wetmore and L. D. Quarles, "Calcimimetics or vitamin D analogs for suppressing parathyroid hormone in end-stage renal disease: time for a paradigm shift?" Nature Clinical Practice Nephrology, vol. 5, no. 1, pp. 24–33, 2009.

7. D. Fouque, S. Pelletier, D. Mafra, and P. Chauveau, "Nutrition and chronic kidney disease," Kidney International, vol. 80, pp. 348–357, 2011.

8. A. S. Levey, T. Greene, G. J. Beck et al., "Dietary protein restriction and the progression of chronic renal disease: what have all of the results of the MDRD study shown? Modification of diet in renal disease study group," Journal of the American Society of Nephrology, vol. 10, no. 11, pp. 2426–2439, 1999.

9. D. Fouque and M. Laville, "Low protein diets for chronic kidney disease in non diabetic adults," Cochrane Database of Systematic Reviews, no. 3, Article ID CD001892, 2009.

10. J. Bernhard, B. Beaufrère, M. Laville, and D. Fouque, "Adaptive response to a low-protein diet in predialysis chronic renal failure patients," Journal of the American Society of Nephrology, vol. 12, no. 6, pp. 1249–1254, 2001.

11. C. S. Shinaberger, S. Greenland, J. D. Kopple et al., "Is controlling phosphorus by decreasing dietary protein intake beneficial or harmful in persons with chronic kidney disease?" The American Journal of Clinical Nutrition, vol. 88, no. 6, pp. 1511–1518, 2008.

12. K. E. Lynch, R. Lynch, G. C. Curhan, and S. M. Brunelli, "Prescribed dietary phosphate restriction and survival among hemodialysis patients," Clinical Journal of the American Society of Nephrology, vol. 6, no. 3, pp. 620–629, 2011.

13. N. Noori, K. Kalantar-Zadeh, C. P. Kovesdy, R. Bross, D. Benner, and J. D. Kopple, "Association of dietary phosphorus intake and phosphorus to protein ratio with mortality in hemodialysis patients," Clinical Journal of the American Society of Nephrology, vol. 5, no. 4, pp. 683–692, 2010.

14. Food and Nutrition Board, "Phosphorus," in Dietary Reference Intakes: Calcium, Phosphorus, Magnesium, Vitamin D and Fluoride, pp. 146–189, edited by Institute of Medicine, National Academy Press, Washington, DC, USA, 1997.

15. V. Savica, G. Bellinghieri, and L. A. Calò, "Association of serum phosphorus concentration with cardiovascular risk," American Journal of Kidney Diseases, vol. 54, no. 2, p. 389, 2009.

16. M. Fukagawa, H. Komaba, and K. I. Miyamoto, "Source matters: from phosphorus load to bioavailability," Clinical Journal of the American Society of Nephrology, vol. 6, no. 2, pp. 239–240, 2011.

17. S. M. Moe, N. X. Chen, M. F. Seifert et al., "A rat model of chronic kidney disease-mineral bone disorder," Kidney International, vol. 75, no. 2, pp. 176–184, 2009.

18. S. M. Moe, M. P. Zidehsarai, M. A. Chambers et al., "Vegetarian compared with meat dietary protein source and phosphorus homeostasis in chronic kidney disease," Clinical Journal of the American Society of Nephrology, vol. 6, no. 2, pp. 257–264, 2011.

19. K. Kalantar-Zadeh, L. Gutekunst, R. Mehrotra et al., "Understanding sources of dietary phosphorus in the treatment of patients with chronic kidney disease," Clinical Journal of the American Society of Nephrology, vol. 5, no. 3, pp. 519–530, 2010.

20. A. De Lorenzo, A. Noce, M. Bigioni et al., "The effects of Italian Mediterranean Organic Diet (IMOD) on health status," Current Pharmaceutical Design, vol. 16, no. 7, pp. 814–824, 2010.

21. C. Sullivan, S. S. Sayre, J. B. Leon et al., "Effect of food additives on hyperphosphatemia among patients with end-stage renal disease: a randomized controlled trial," JAMA, vol. 301, no. 6, pp. 629–635, 2009.

22. J. Uribarri, "Phosphorus additives in food and their effect in dialysis patients," Clinical Journal of the American Society of Nephrology, vol. 4, no. 8, pp. 1290–1292, 2009.

23. M. Karalis and L. Murphy-Gutekunst, "Patient education. Enhanced foods: hidden phosphorus and sodium in foods commonly eaten," Journal of Renal Nutrition, vol. 16, no. 1, pp. 79–81, 2006.

24. O. M. Gutiérrez, C. Anderson, T. Isakova et al., "Low socioeconomic status associates with higher serum phosphate irrespective of race," Journal of the American Society of Nephrology, vol. 21, no. 11, pp. 1953–1960, 2010.

25. I. de Brito-Ashurst, M. Varagunam, M. J. Raftery, and M. M. Yaqoob, "Bicarbonate supplementation slows progression of CKD and improves nutritional status," Journal of the American Society of Nephrology, vol. 20, no. 9, pp. 2075–2084, 2009.

26. M. Aparicio, P. Chauveau, V. De Précigout, J. L. Bouchet, C. Lasseur, and C. Combe, "Nutrition and outcome on renal replacement therapy of patients with chronic renal failure treated by a supplemented very low protein diet," Journal of the American Society of Nephrology, vol. 11, no. 4, pp. 708–716, 2000.

27. G. Brunori, B. F. Viola, G. Parrinello et al., "Efficacy and safety of a very-low-protein diet when postponing dialysis in the elderly: a prospective randomized multicenter controlled study," American Journal of Kidney Diseases, vol. 49, no. 5, pp. 569–580, 2007.

28. E. Peuchant, M. C. Delmas-Beauvieux, L. Dubourg et al., "Antioxidant effects of a supplemented very low protein diet in chronic renal failure," Free Radical Biology and Medicine, vol. 22, no. 1-2, pp. 313–320, 1997.

29. F. Locatelli, D. Alberti, G. Graziani, G. Buccianti, B. Redaelli, and A. Giangrande, "Prospective, randomised, multicentre trial of effect of protein restriction on progression of chronic renal insufficiency. Northern Italian Cooperative Study Group," The Lancet, vol. 337, no. 8753, pp. 1299–1304, 1991.

30. L. A. Calò, V. Savica, P. A. Davis, et al., "Phosphate content of beverages in addition to food phoaphate additives :real and insidious danger for renal patients," Journal of Renal Nutrition, vol. 22, no. 2, pp. 292–293, 2012.

31. D. Fouque, J. McKenzie, R. de Mutsert et al., "Use of a renal-specific oral supplement by haemodialysis patients with low protein intake does not increase the need for phosphate binders and may prevent a decline in nutritional status

and quality of life," Nephrology Dialysis Transplantation, vol. 23, no. 9, pp. 2902–2910, 2008.

32. T. Isakova, O. M. Gutiérrez, Y. Chang et al., "Phosphorus binders and survival on hemodialysis," Journal of the American Society of Nephrology, vol. 20, no. 2, pp. 388–396, 2009.

33. O.M. Gutiérrez, M. Mannstadt, T. Isakova et al., "Fibroblast growth factor 23 and mortality among patients undergoing hemodialysis," The New England Journal of Medicine, vol. 359, no. 6, pp. 584–592, 2008.

34. W. C. Winkelmayer, J. Liu, and B. Kestenbaum, "Comparative effectiveness of calcium-containing phosphate binders in incident U.S. dialysis patients," Clinical Journal of the American Society of Nephrology, vol. 6, no. 1, pp. 175–183, 2011.

35. E. Gonzalez-Parra, M. L. Gonzalez-Casaus, A. Galán et al., "Lanthanum carbonate reduces FGF23 in chronic kidney disease Stage 3 patients," Nephrology Dialysis Transplantation, vol. 26, no. 8, pp. 2567–2571, 2011.

36. G. Bellinghieri, D. Santoro, and V. Savica, "Emerging drugs for hyperphosphatemia," Expert Opinion on Emerging Drugs, vol. 12, no. 3, pp. 355–365, 2007.

37. V. Savica, L. A. Calò, D. Santoro et al., "Salivary glands: a new player in phosphorus metabolism," Journal of Renal Nutrition, vol. 21, no. 1, pp. 39–42, 2011.

38. V. Savica, L. A. Calò, P. Monardo et al., "Salivary phosphate-binding chewing gum reduces hyperphosphatemia in dialysis patients," Journal of the American Society of Nephrology, vol. 20, no. 3, pp. 639–644, 2009.

39. J. T. Daugirdas, W. F. Finn, M. Emmett, G. M. Chertow, and Frequent Hemodialysis Network Trial Group, "The phosphate binder equivalent dose," Seminars in Dialysis, vol. 24, no. 1, pp. 41–49, 2011.

40. J. Delmez, G. Block, J. Robertson et al., "A randomized, double-blind, crossover design study of sevelamer hydrochloride and sevelamer carbonate in patients on hemodialysis," Clinical Nephrology, vol. 68, no. 6, pp. 386–391, 2007.

41. W. F. Finn, M. S. Joy, and LAM-308 Study Group, "A long-term, open-label extension study on the safety of treatment with lanthanum carbonate, a new phosphate binder, in patients receiving hemodialysis," Current Medical Research and Opinion, vol. 21, no. 5, pp. 657–664, 2005.

42. W. L. Chan, K. Rounsley, E. Chapman et al., "Lanthanum carbonate is an effective hypophosphatemic agent for hemodialysis patients intolerant of other phosphate binders," Journal of Renal Nutrition, vol. 20, no. 4, pp. 270–277, 2010.

43. P. Evenepoel, B. K. I. Meijers, B. R. M. Bammens, and K. Verbeke, "Uremic toxins originating from colonic microbial metabolism," Kidney International, vol. 76, supplement 114, pp. S12–S19, 2009.

44. A. Aguilera, M. A. Bajo, M. Espinoza et al., "Gastrointestinal and pancreatic function in peritoneal dialysis patients: their relationship with malnutrition and peritoneal membrane abnormalities," American Journal of Kidney Diseases, vol. 42, no. 4, pp. 787–796, 2003.

45. D. Pierce, S. Hossack, L. Poole et al., "The effect of sevelamer carbonate and lanthanum carbonate on the pharmacokinetics of oral calcitriol," Nephrology Dialysis Transplantation, vol. 26, no. 5, pp. 1615–1621, 2011.

This chapter was originalty published under the Creative Commons Attribution License. Gonzáles-Parra, E., Garcia-Iguacel, C., Egido, J., and Ortiz, A. Phosphorus and Nutrition in Chronic Kidney Disease. International Journal of Nephrology, vol. 2012, Article ID 597605.doi:10.1155/2012/597605.

PART III

DIETARY TREATMENTS FOR OBESITY AND TYPE 2 DIABETES

CHAPTER 9

KETOGENIC ENTERAL NUTRITION AS A TREATMENT FOR OBESITY: SHORT TERM AND LONG TERM RESULTS FROM 19,000 PATIENTS

GIANFRANCO CAPPELLO, ANTONELLA FRANCESCHELLI, ANNALISA CAPPELLO, and PAOLO DE LUCA

9.1 BACKGROUND

Obesity is a 21st century epidemic, and its relentless spreading is due to many different reasons. One reason is that the classic treatment, a long term hypocaloric diet, is unsuited to the spirit of our century that always aims for fast results. Dieters want instant weight loss and do not want to lose "only" a few pounds each week. Finding a fast and safe weight loss treatment could be the crucial battle to win in the war on obesity.

We know that weight loss is a consequence of negative caloric balance and the more negative the caloric balance the more rapid the weight reduction will be. Given this logic, total fasting should be the most rapid way to lose weight but it is impractical for two reasons:

1. It would cause extreme hunger [1].
2. It would entail loss of lean body mass (LBM), which can be unsafe for the patient [2]. Total fasting also causes neutropenia [3], lowers renal creatinine clearence [4] and increases levels of serum bilirubin [5]. The total nitrogen loss after 3 to 4 weeks of total starvation would be approximately 200 g, corresponding to 1,250 g of protein and equivalent to a loss of some 6 kg of muscle tissue [6,7]. The obese patient will lose body mass in the wrong places (e.g. thighs, limbs, chest) generating a cachectic appearance. Furthermore he will rapidly regain all the lost weight as the body works to rebuild its LBM [8]. Thus, optimal weight loss must be achieved through reducing fat mass.

An important experiment by Blackburn and colleagues in 1973 [9] demonstrated that, during fasting, a continuous intravenous infusion of an amino acid solution could greatly reduce protein loss. Because the treatment was able to totally prevent loss of LBM during fasting, it was said to have a protein sparing (PS) effect. Blackburn explained the PS effect through the action of insulin, the main regulator of energetic fuels, by reasoning that the infusion of amino acids during fasting reduced insulin levels and therefore prevented muscle catabolism while at the same time a strong lipolytic effect was promoted with high serum ketone bodies (KB) [10]. Increased serum KB will not harm the patient because high serum KB will eventually increase insulin secretion, modulating the lipolytic effect [11,12]. Furthermore high serum KB will reduce or eliminate hunger [13,14].

Blackburn et al. immediately realized the importance of the PS effect for the treatment of obesity. They invented a very low calorie protein diet [15], the protein sparing modified fast (PSMF), but their subsequent studies on obese patients were based on an oral protein diet which had two main drawbacks: (1) glucose intake could not be reduced to zero and (2) protein intake stopped during the night. Normally overnight fasting does not entail muscle catabolism because hepatic glycogen sustains the patient's energy requirement [16-18], but after one day of a high protein diet glycogen deposits are greatly reduced [16] and overnight fasting will entail muscle catabolism. As a result the lipolytic effect of the PSMF is reduced and many weeks of the diet are needed to obtain a 10% weight loss [15].

To add to the concerns about the PSMF, it was reported that the diet was suspected of causing severe cardiac arrhythmias [19-23]. A loss of cardiac protein content was supposed to be the mechanism the cardiac complications [24]. Other researchers [19,25,26] attributed the effect to the low quality of protein used in the PSMF, however the diet is thought to be safe for treatments not longer than 10 days [22,23].

Around the time of the original report published by Blackburn and colleagues, our Nutrition Unit at the University of Rome was using a PS diet (via 24 h IV infusion of strictly amino acids, minerals and vitamins) on our obese surgical patients. While the aim of our treatment was to improve our surgical results, we also noted that we confirmed Blackburn et al.'s findings with regards to weight loss [27].

In the 1980s, when enteral nutrition took the place of parenteral nutrition, we had the same results with a 24 h enteral infusion of a solution of only proteins, electrolytes and vitamins. Those results were not published. Enteral protein sparing was generally used for obese patients who needed nutritional support for postoperative complications or acute pancreatitis. Obesity was never the main indication for the enteral protein sparing treatment. They were all hospitalized patients. Nitrogen balance showed an acceptable level of nitrogen losses and blood samples showed good tolerance of the treatment with normal blood urea and electrolyte levels. No cardiac complications were ever documented.

Six years ago the young, obese daughter of one of our enteral protein sparing patients (with a postoperative colon fistula) asked to be treated only for her obesity. She underwent a home treatment and lost 15 kg of weight. Since then, thousands of patients have come to the University of Rome from all over Italy to be treated and they had all heard of us only by word of mouth. They signed a formal consent and were given a standard apparatus for enteral nutrition (a small nasogastric tube and a portable pump) for a 24 h infusion of protein to be administered in cycles of 10 days.

In a preliminary study we found that the infusion of 50–65 g/day of high biological value protein (whey protein) caused a mild ketonemia

(100–120 mg%), eliminated hunger and greatly reduced the loss of lean body mass while patients were losing weight rapidly. We named this approach Ketogenic Enteral Nutrition (KEN).

The aim of this study is to determine the feasibility of KEN therapy for a large population of overweight or obese patients and to assess its clinical results from a retrospective analysis of the records of all patients who underwent at least one cycle of KEN treatment. We also wanted to compare the results from KEN treatment to the results from other PSMF studies in which protein intake was given orally and was suspended during the night. Long term results have been as well investigated.

9.2 METHODS

The study was performed at the University La Sapienza in Rome within the Clinical Nutrition Service (CNS) of the Department of Surgery Paride Stefanini and included overweight and obese patients who did not have success with previous dietetic treatments for obesity.

Patients with type 1 diabetes, renal failure, heart failure, hepatic failure, history of severe cardiac arrhythmias, severe eating disorders or who were pregnant or lactating were excluded. Young patients under 14 were included only if their body mass index (BMI) was over 40 and they had undergone a series of dietary treatments without success. The patients were self-referred and each patient had to sign an informed consent release before the beginning of the treatment. The procedures were in accordance with the Helsinki Declaration of 1975 (as revised in 1983).

In a period of 5 years (from 2006 to 2011) 19,036 patients underwent at least one cycle of KEN treatment. The patients' ages varied from 10 to 78 (average 44.3 years). The male:female ratio was 2:5. The average weight at the start of the treatment was 101.4 kg, and was higher for men than women (118.9 kg vs 94.9 kg, respectively). The mean BMI was 36.5 kg/m^2 (in the limit for class 1 and class 2 of obesity) and was also higher in men than women (38.2 vs 35.8, respectively).

Each patient came to the CNS and received a medical checkup before the beginning of treatment and a 50 Hz impedance test for body composition analysis (Handy 3000; DS Medica, Italy). The body composition was

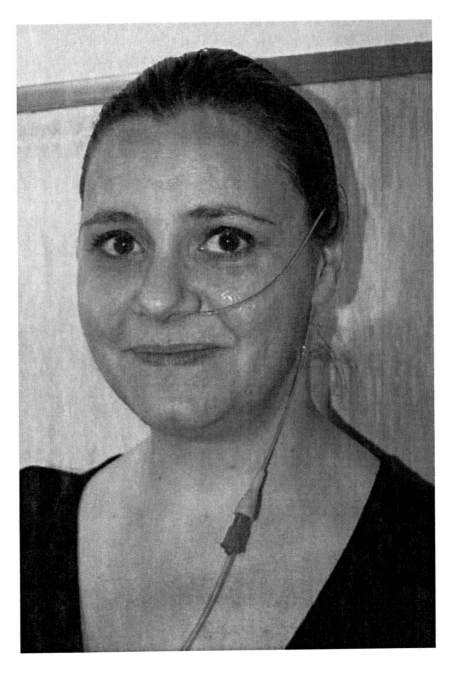

FIGURE 1: 6-French polyurethane tubes are almost invisible and very well tolerated.

calculated by a computerized program which was provided by the manu-facturer, according to the three-compartment model [28].

As shown in Table 1 at the start of the treatment men had a very high body cell mass (BCM; 42.7 kg vs 27.4) while the average fat mass (FM) was 40.9 kg and did not differ between men and women (40.0 kg vs 41.7).

TABLE 1: Patients' baseline data before KEN (n = 19,036)

Total	M	F	
Cases	19,036	5,148	13,888
Age	44.3 ± 13.0	44.7 ± 12.4	44.2 ± 13.2
Initial weight (kg)	101.4 ± 22.9	118.9 ± 22.9	94.9 ± 19.2
BMI (kg/m²)	36.5 ± 7.1	38.2 ± 6.8	35.8 ± 7.1
BCM (kg)	31.6 ± 8.7	42.7 ± 7.2	27.4 ± 4.6
FM (kg)	40.9 ± 12.8	40.0 ± 12.6	41.7 ± 12.8
TBW (kg)	43.5 ± 10.9	57.4 ± 9.2	38.3 ± 5.7

Table 1 shows the average age, weight and body composition of the patients before the start of the KEN treatment. (BCM, body cell mass; FM, fat mass; TBW, total body water).

A 6-fr polyurethane tube was inserted through the nose (Figure 1). The tube was held in place on the patient's cheek and ear by transparent tape.

The patients were given an enteral portable pump and a short course to educate them about its use and about the basics of KEN. The infusion rate was regulated to provide, on a continuous, 24 h daily infusion, 2 l of fluid and a dose of 50 g of protein (K1000®, Table 2) for women and 65 g for men (resulting in an average dose of 0.85 g/kg of ideal body weight in women and 0.89 g/kg in men) and 13–17 mEq of potassium.

Each patient received, in addition, a supplement providing the RDA [29] for all vitamins and essential minerals. They were also given a 50 g dose of polyethylene glycol to be taken on the first, fourth and seventh days of treatment in order to increase intestinal motility and to make up for the absence of fibers in the protein solution.

The KEN cycles were domiciliary and a medical doctor (MD) was available by telephone 24 h/day.

To ensure continuous ketosis during the treatment, the patients had to stop feeding. They were allowed to drink as much as they wanted, however they were only allowed to drink water, tea, coffee and chamomile tea without sweeteners.

During the cycle the patients were given a diary to monitor weight, feeling of hunger (on a visual scale from 1 to 10) and ketonuria (Ketur test, Roche, Italy).

TABLE 2: (g%) Composition of the nutrition powder (K1000®)

Proteins	90.0
Carbohydrates	1.80
Fats	0.80
Calcium	0.40
Potassium	1.00
Phosphorus	0.20
Sodium	0.10
Magnesium	0.05

Table 2 Composition of K1000® (Nutrimed 2000 srl, Italy), the nutrition feed used for the KEN, made of whey proteins enriched with potassium chloride, lecithin and bovine hydrolyzed collagen.

Hypertensive patients were suggested to stop their usual medication to avoid symptomatic hypotension that was described by other authors during PSMF [30,31]. They had to monitor their blood pressure daily and contact the MD in case of increased blood pressure.

As in other PSMF studies [32], diabetic patients were asked to suspend their usual medications to avoid hypoglycemia. They were also asked to monitor glycemia 3 times a day and to contact the MD in case of blood glucose >160 mg%. Stopping or reducing the medications did not cause any trouble, because KEN treatment rapidly reduces hypertension and hyper-glycaemia. Many times we had to discuss this matter with the physicians of our patients.

Patients affected by gout and/or hyperuricemia were supplied with daily doses of allopurinol.

After each KEN cycle, patients returned to the CNS for tube removal, to report all treatment data (including daily evaluation of hunger level on a 1 to 10 visual scale, body weight and ketonuria) and to undergo another impedance test for body composition evaluation.

Each patient was free to choose the number of KEN cycles he or she wanted to undergo. If the patient wanted to undergo another treatment cycle they were first given a rest period of at least 10 days during which they were advised to follow a low–carbohydrate, normocaloric diet.

They were domiciliary patients and it was impossible to schedule from the start of treatment the number of cycles each patient had to undergo. We just told to each patient his ideal body weight and informed him of the risk of been obese or overweight.

All patients during the 5-year period of this study underwent 1 to 21 cycles of KEN treatment (an average of 2.5 ± 0.03). The total duration of treatment time from the first 10-day KEN cycle to the last, including variable-length rest periods (some patients came for a new cycle years later) lasted from 9 to 1400 days (mean 68 ± 96).

Long term results data were collected by a telephone survey which were assessed by nurses.

9.3 RESULTS

Table 3 shows the final results. The male patients lost a mean of 11.9 kg of weight which corresponded to 9.96% of initial body weight. Women also lost about 10% of initial body weight.

The body composition analysis performed before and after treatment showed that 57% of weight loss was came from FM and 22% came from BCM.

No technical complications were reported during the introduction of over 50,000 nasogastric tubes in a 5-year period; neither were there any metabolic complications due to ketonemia or electrolyte imbalances.

Ketonuria was observed in most patients by the 2nd day of the KEN treatment and increased within 2–3 days to 100–120 mg%. Commonly the ketonuria was accompanied by moderate halitosis, however this did not prevent the patients from carrying out normal daily activities.

TABLE 3: Body Composition changes after treatment with KEN in male and female patients (*P<0.0001. Student paired t-test)

Weight and body composition changes after KEN treatment (n=19,036)						
	Total	Variation ± SD	M	Variation ± SD	F	Variation ± SD
Body weight (kg)	91.2	−10.2±7.0*	107.0	−11.9±7.9*	85.4	−9.5±6.5*
BMI (kg/m²)	32.8	−3.7±2.5*	34.3	−3.9±2.6*	32.2	−3.6±2.5*
BCM (kg)	29.4	−2.2*±3.3*	39.7	−3.0±4.2*	25.6	−1.8±2.8*
TBW (kg)	40.1	−3.4*±2.8*	52.7	−4.7±3.5*	35.3	−3.0±3.4*
FM (kg)	35.1	−5.8*±5.5*	34.3	−5.7±6.0*	35.9	−5.8±5.2*

By the 5th day of treatment 24% of patients reported a strong sense of asthenia, even if they had normal blood pressure levels. By the end of the treatment, 12% of patients reported a mild sense of hunger.

Nearly one quarter (22%) of the patients were diabetic and receiving treatment for their condition at the start of treatment. As was observed by other authors [32], 92% of the diabetics in our study also had to suspend their medications during the treatment periods because the lack of carbohydrate in the nutritional solution was sufficient to lower their glycaemia on its own. Of these patients who suspended anti-diabetic therapy, 22% reported glucose values as low as 60 mg/dL. However, no cases of clinical hypoglycemia were reported neither was glucose supplementation needed.

Reduced hypertension during PSMF has been reported previously [30,31]. Similarly, in our study only 20% of the hypertensive patients who had suspended their medications during the treatments needed to resume their medications afterwards, and even then they needed a lower dose.

Complications of KEN:

1. Asthenia 24%
2. Mild sense of hunger 12%
3. Constipation (need to increase Macrogol) 5%
4. Problems with the pump 4%
5. Damage of the external part of the tube (e.g. shaving) 2%
6. Gastric hypersecretion 2%

7.   Nausea and vomiting 1%
8.   Intolerance to the nasal tube 0.03%
9.   Ulcerations or bleeding due to the tube not observed
10. Breakage of the tube in esophagus or in the stomach not observed
11. Perforation or bleeding of the stomach not observed

9.3.1 LONG TERM RESULTS

After the last KEN cycle (after 31–1882 days, average 408 ± 309 days) 15,444 patients could be reached by telephone. We found that 55 patients had undergone bariatric surgery, which is not surprising since many patients had been referred to us for preparation prior to bariatric surgery because a preoperative loss of weight causes an improvement of cardiovascular and thromboembolic risk factors [33]. Regardless these individuals were excluded from the survey. All the other patients had regained an average of 1.57 ± 7.15 kg of body weight (15.4% of the mean weight loss). 38.9% of patients presented a variation of $\pm 3\%$ and we can consider that they maintained their weight loss, 36.9% gained weight (sometimes to a value higher than the weight they had before the KEN treatment) while 24.1% lost more weight because they were able to return to their sporting activities.

9.4 DISCUSSION

It is insightful to compare the results of this study with other PSMF studies in which protein was given by mouth. In one study [15], weight loss after 17 weeks of treatment was 21 kg versus 10.2 kg in 3.5 weeks in the present study. Another smaller study [34] found results are closer to ours: 15 patients lost 14.4 kg after 6 weeks of PSMF with lactalbumin-derived protein dosed at 60 g/day. In a third study [35], patients lost around 8 kg in 4 weeks on either a lean meat, fish, and fowl diet of 450 kcal or an isocaloric high-protein liquid diet. None of the studies reported any significant clinical complications. The last study [35] found that the liquid formula diet was less palatable than the whole food diet. In contrast we found that our patients were able to lose more weight in less time, likely due to the fact that using a 24 h infusion we could further reduce protein (caloric) intake while sparing lean mass.

The KEN diet is a well tolerated treatment that produces very rapid weight loss and gives the patient a psychological boost because he/she sees immediate results. This enthusiasm gives the patient the resolve to continue with the treatment. Remember the thousands of patients that came to us to undergo treatment were not responding to any advertisements, rather they had heard of us by word of mouth.

Another benefit of the KEN treatment is that it is a low-cost treatment. Investments in the procedure include a 3-h course covering the principles of the treatment to new patients, scales, stadiometers, impedance apparati and pumps are relatively inexpensive. Therefore, as all patients stop eating for 10 days, we can say to them that the treatment will cost about the same amount as eating their normal diet for 10 days.

A 6-fr nasogastric tube is very well tolerated; patients get used to sensation within 10 minutes after insertion and no longer feel its presence. Only a very small percentage of patients (0.03%) decided to stop treatment when the tube was placed through the nose. In no cases did the tube cause ulceration or bleeding, nor was there any breakage in the esophagus or stomach. However, in some cases the external part of the tube was damaged by the patients themselves when trying to shave or when trying to replace the tape using scissors. All these problems were solved by replacing the tube itself.

We have assumed that the nasal intubation and the pump are essential to the success of our treatment for controlling the intake of proteins during both day and night and for reducing the catabolism of lean mass. While this assumption should be tested in a double blind study, our results still show that the KEN diet is more effective in promoting weight loss than the PSMF diet and reducing the length of treatment to 10 days prevents the risk of cardiac complications [19-23].

Prof. Jay Mirtallo, President of the American Society for Parenteral and Enteral Nutrition, recently wrote a letter to the New York Times [36] about the nasogastric tube for KEN treatment saying that "to report on someone using this medical therapy as a weight loss method detracts from the health benefit achieved by patients with very severe diseases". We agree with him—enteral nutrition therapy is normally used to feed malnourished patients who are unable to eat food by mouth for various reasons (e.g. dysphagia, cancer) and its utilization has a very important therapeutic value. However, in our experience, extending the use of the nasal tube to obese patients did not in any way impair the use of enteral therapy in malnourished patients. To the contrary, in Italy we noticed that, after thousands of patients began asking for the therapy as a treatment for obesity, the number of malnourished patients asking for the tube as a life support doubled. We think this is likely because they were able to observe how a high quality of life can be maintained during the treatment, and that it is not a big deal to have a small tube in your nose. Furthermore we think the application of enteral therapy in the obese opens new possibilities in healthcare, as worldwide there are the millions of obese patients who could benefit from this treatment, vastly outnumbering the thousands of people with cancer or neurologic dysfunction that require a nasal tube.

With regard to the complications of KEN treatment including asthenia and mild lightheadedness, which have also been reported with the PSMF diet [15], the symptoms were easily relieved by increasing salt intake [15].

Gastric hypersecretion was present as acid reflux or pyrosis in 2% of patients during KEN. This effect could be due to the protein infusion [37,38] or it could be connected with the mild metabolic acidosis [39] that occurs in ketonemic diets [40]. Constipation is also commonly reported during ketonemic diets [15,40], probably due to the lack of fibers in the protein solution. This issue can be resolved by increasing polyethylene glycol (PEG) administration.

Nausea and vomiting has been reported also in another study [15], and they are probably in response to the gastric hypersecretion caused by the ketonemia or by rapid intake of PEG. It is a rare complication but concerning because it can lead to expulsion of the nasal tube which then has to be re-inserted.

KEN treatment is not an option for long-term dieting because it contains 0% carbohydrates and 0% lipids. Rather, KEN is suitable as a 10-day controlled period of starvation during which the protein sparing effect of the continuous infusion of protein allows a fast and safe reduction of weight. Although the weight loss is still 22% BCM, this is to be expected given that the obese and overweight patients show elevated BCM before the start of treatment. This has been confirmed by other authors [41] and a minor loss of BCM is not significant. In future studies we will modulate the protein infusion with respect to the impedance analysis in the aim of reducing BCM loss and of increasing FM loss from their current levels.

Losing 4 kg of fat mass means burning 36,000 calories in 10 days. In other words, to lose 1 kg of fat an individual would need to walk for 75 km [4]2. We tell our patients to live an active life, to maintain their normal daily activities in spite of the presence of the nasal tube and to walk at least one hour per day (if they can). This probably is not enough to burn all those calories. But we must take into account other outputs, such as the loss of ketones in the urine, in the breath and in the sweat; that is, during ketosis there is some insensible loss of calories. Furthermore protein infusions are reported to increase energy expenditure by increasing thermogenesis [42-44].

The long term results from our study were very positive. The data were collected by a telephone survey, and while we could not check the patients' weights directly, we feel the self-reported body weights are accurate and other reports on long term results after weight loss treatments are also based on telephone surveys [45]. At the end of a patient's final KEN cycle they were advised to regularly check their body weight and were given advice on how to reduce their weight again if it began to go back up. They were also advised to consult an MD as needed, however it was rare that they asked for help. In our study we observed a 15.4% weight regain after one year, which is an excellent result if we compare it with other reviews in which a 30-35% weight regain after one year is reported [45]. This difference may be because KEN treatment spares free fat mass, and this reduces weight regain [46]. Furthermore the initial weight of our patients was higher than in most weight maintenance studies [47] which may also account for our improved long-term results [48,49].

Weight loss in our diabetic and hypertensive patients also promoted long-term improvement to their conditions, as has been reported in another study [50], and these results will be the subject of a separate report.

Limitations of this study are related to (1) the lack of a control group, which would be impossible to obtain in our settings. (2) We could not plan the treatment of each patient at the start because they were on domiciliary treatment and (3) many patients come back for a new cycle after years of rest making uncertain the evaluation of their overall clinical outcome."

9.5 CONCLUSIONS

During the course of 5 years nearly 50,000 small 6-French nasogastric tubes were inserted without complications and they were well tolerated by our patients. This study demonstrates that 10-day KEN cycles can induce rapid weight loss; in a very large number of patients we easily obtained a 10% weight loss, 57% of which was FM. No significant adverse effects were found. On a 1-month/5-year follow up, mean weight regain was 15.4%. The KEN cycles are suitable for normal living and the cost is minimal, indeed some patients spend less on the treatment than they would spend on 10 days worth of food. Ultimately we conclude that KEN treatment is safe, fast, inexpensive and has good one-year results for weight maintenance. We propose that KEN is a new approach to obesity treatment which is faster and more effective than hypocaloric diets [47], without the complications of bariatric surgery.

REFERENCES

1. Mayer J: Regulation of energy intake and the body weight: the glucostatic theory and the lipostatic hypothesis. Ann NY Acad Sci 1955, 63:15-43.
2. Schutz Y: Protein turnover, ureagenesis and gluconeogenesis. Int J Vitam Nutr Res 2011, 81:101-107.
3. Drenick EJ, Alvarez LC: Neutropenia in prolonged fasting. Am J Clin Nutr 1971, 24:859-863.
4. Edgren B, Wester PO: Impairment of glomerular filtration in fasting for obesity. Acta Med Scand 1971, 190:389-393.
5. Barrett PV: Hyperbilirubinemia of fasting. JAMA 1971, 217:1349-1353.
6. Owen OE, Felig P, Morgan AP, Wahren J, Cahill GF Jr: Liver and kidney metabolism during prolonged starvation. J Clin Invest 1969, 48:574-583.
7. Elia M: Hunger disease. Clin Nutr. 2000, 19:379-386.
8. Fisch HP, Reutter FW: Late results after zero calorie diet therapy in adiposity. Schweiz Med Wochenschr 1976, 106:339.

9. Blackburn GL, Flatt JP, Clowes GH Jr, O'Donnell TF: Peripheral intravenous feeding with isotonic amino acid solutions. Am J Surg 1973, 125:447.

10. Blackburn GL, Flatt JP, Clowes GH Jr, O'Donnell TF, Hensle TE: Protein sparing therapy during periods of starvation with sepsis or trauma. Ann Surg 1973, 177:588.

11. Madison L, Mebane D, Unger RH, Locher A: The hypoglycemic action of ketones. II. Evidence for stimulatory feedback of ketones on the pancreatic beta cells. J Clin Invest 1964, 43:408.

12. Wieland O: Ketogenesis and its regulation. Advances Metab Dis 1968, 3:1.

13. Atkins RC: Dr Atkin's Diet Revolution. New York: McKay; 1972.

14. Johnstone AM, Lobley GE, Horgan GW, et al.: Effects of a high-protein, low-carbohydrate v. high-protein, moderate-carbohydrate weight-loss diet on antioxidant status, endothelial markers and plasma indices of the cardiometabolic profile. Br J Nutr 2011, 27:1.

15. Palgi A, Read JL, Greenberg I, Hoefer MA, Bistrian BR, Blackburn GL: Multidisciplinary treatment of obesity with a protein-sparing modified fast: results in 668 outpatients. Am J Public Health 1985, 75:1190-1194.

16. Wahren J, Ekberg K: Splanchnic regulation of glucose production. (leggere) Ann Rev Nutr 2007, 27:329.

17. Moore MC, Coate KC, Winnick JJ, An Z, Cherrington : Regulation of hepatic glucose uptake and storage in vivo. Adv Nutr 2012, 1:286.

18. Pagliassotti MJ, Cherrington AD: Regulation of net hepatic glucose uptake in vivo. Annu Rev Physiol 1992, 54:847.

19. Linn R, Stuart SL: The Last Chance Diet. Secaucus: Lyle Stuart Inc; 1976.

20. Gregg MB: Deaths associated with liquid protein diets. Morbidity Mortality Weekly Rep 1977, 26:383.

21. Singh BN, Gaarder TD, Kanegae T, Goldstein M, Montgomerie JZ, Mills H: Liquid protein diets and torsade de pointes. JAMA 1978, 240:115.

22. Brown JM, Yetter JF, Spicer MJ, Jones JD: Cardiac complications of protein-sparing modified fasting. JAMA 1978, 240:120.

23. Michiel RR, Sneider JS, Dickstein RA, Hagman HH, Eich RH: Sudden death in a patient on a liquid protein diet. N Engl J Med 1978, 298:1005.

24. Isner JM, Sours HE, Paris AL, Ferrans VJ, Roberts WC: Sudden, unexpected death in avid dieters using the liquid-protein-modified-fast diet. Observations in 17 patients and the role of the prolonged QT interval. Circulation 1979, 60:6.

25. Wadden TA, Stunkard AJ, Brownell KD: Very low calorie diets: their efficacy, safety, and future. Ann Intern Med 1983, 99:675.

26. Blackburn GL: Protein requirements with very low calorie diets. Postgraduate Med J 1984, 60:59.

27. Li SK, Zhou YB, Zhou CF, et al.: Influence of obesity on short-term surgical outcome in patients with gastric cancer. Zhonghua Wei Chang Wai Ke Za Zhi 2010, 13:133.

28. Sun SS, Chumlea WC, Heymsfield SB, et al.: Development of bioelectrical impedance analysis prediction equations for body composition with the use of a multicomponent model for use in epidemiologic surveys. Am J Clin Nutr 2003, 77:331.

29. RDAhttp://www.salute.gov.it/imgs/C_17_pagineAree_1463_listaFile_item Name_0_file.pdf
30. Cohen N, Flamenbaum W: Obesity and hypertension. Demonstration of a "floor effect". Am J Med 1986, 80:177.
31. Dornfeld LP, Maxwell MH, Waks AU, Schroth P, Tuck ML: Obesity and hypertension: long-term effects of weight reduction on blood pressure. Int J Obes 1985, 9:381.
32. Bistrian BR, Blackburn GL, Flatt JP, Sizer J, Scrimshaw NS, Sherman M: Nitrogen metabolism and insulin requirements in obese diabetic adults on a protein-sparing modified fast. Diabetes 1976, 25:494.
33. Tarnoff M, Kaplan L, Shikora S: An evidence-based assessment of preoperative weight loss in bariatric surgery. Obes Surg 2008, 18:1059-1061.
34. Van Gaal LF, Snyders D, De Leeuw IH, Bekaert JL: Anthropometric and calorimetric evidence for the protein sparing effects of a new protein supplemented low calorie preparation. Am J Clin Nutr 1985, 41:540-544.
35. Wadden TA, Stunkard AJ, Brownell KD, Day SC: A comparison of two very-low-calorie diets: protein-sparing-modified fast versus protein-formula-liquid diet. Am J Clin Nutr 1985, 41:533.
36. Letter to the Editor http:/ / www.nutritioncare.org/ Press_Room/ Press_Releases/ NYTimes_Letter_to_Editor
37. Schubert ML: Gastric secretion. Curr Opin Gastroenterol 2010, 26:598.
38. Ashby DB, Himal HS: Comparison of the effect of different forms of a protein test meal on gastric acid and gastrin secretion. Am J Gastroenterol 1975, 63:321.
39. Malov IS, Kulikov AN, Ivashkina TG: Relations of acid–base balance and gastric secretion of hydrogen carbonate ions in patients with peptic ulcer. Ter Arkh 2001, 73:6.
40. Kang HC, Chung DE, Kim DW, Kim HD: Early- and late-onset complications of the ketogenic diet for intractable epilepsy. Epilepsia 2004, 45:1116.
41. De Lorenzo A, Andreoli A, Serrano P, D'Orazio N, Cervelli V, Volpe SL: Body cell mass measured by total body potassium in normal-weight and obese men and women. J Am Coll Nutr 2003, 22:546-549.
42. Mun EC, Blackburn GL, Matthews JB: Current status of medical and surgical therapy for obesity. Gastroenterology 2011, 120:669.
43. Raben A, Agerholm-Larsen L, Flint A, Holst JJ, Astrup A: Meals with similar energy densities but rich in protein, fat, carbohydrate, or alcohol have different effects on energy expenditure and substrate metabolism but not on appetite and energy intake. Am J Clin Nutr 2003, 77:91.
44. Tappy L: Thermic effect of food and sympathetic nervous system activity in humans. Reprod Nutr Dev 1996, 36:391.
45. Turk MW, Yang K, Hravnak M, Sereika SM, Ewing LJ, Burke LE: Randomized clinical trials of weight loss maintenance: a review. J Cardiovasc Nurs 2009, 24:58.
46. Wadden TA, Butryn ML, Byrne KJ: Efficacy of lifestyle modification for long-term weight control. Obes Res 2004, Suppl 12:151S-162S.
47. Vogels N, Westerterp-Plantenga MS: Categorical strategies based on subject characteristics of dietary restraint and physical activity, for weight maintenance. Int J Obes (Lond) 2005, 29:849.

48. Vogels N, Westerterp-Plantenga MS: Successful long-term weight maintenance: a 2-year follow-up. Obesity (Silver Spring) 2007, 15:1258.
49. Vogels N, Diepvens K, Westerterp-Plantenga MS: Predictors of long-term weight maintenance. Obes Res 2005, 13:2162.
50. Souza GT, Lira FS, Rosa Neto JC, et al.: Dietary whey protein lessens several risk factors for metabolic diseases: a review. Lipids Health Dis 2012, 11:67.

This chapter was originally published under the Creative Commons Attribution License. Cappello, G., Franceschelli, A., Cappello, A., and De Luca, P. Ketogenic Enteral Nutrition as a Treatment for Obesity : Short Term and Long Term Results from 19,000 Patients. Nutrition & Metabolism 2012: 9(96). doi :10.1186/1743-7075-9-96 .

NUTRITION SUPPORT TO PATIENTS UNDERGOING GASTROINTESTINAL SURGERY

NICOLA WARD

10.1 INTRODUCTION

Protein-energy malnutrition is a common problem in hospital patients. Studies have reported 40% of surgical and medical patients to be malnourished on admission to hospital. The majority of patients experienced nutritional depletion during the course of their hospital admission, which was more severe in those patients who were already depleted at the time of their admission [1]. The consequences of pre-operative malnutrition were first recognised in the 1930's. Studley observed a direct relationship between preoperative weight loss and operative mortality rate, independent of factors such as age, impaired cardiorespiratory function and type of surgery [2]. The importance of nutritional depletion as a major determinant of the development of postoperative complications has subsequently been confirmed by Giner et al [3]. The absence of a standardised definition of nutritional depletion has led to surrogate markers of nutritional status being utilised. Albumin, muscle function tests, immunological status and weight loss are used as these show correlation with postoperative morbidity and mortality.

Nutritional depletion is associated with changes in body composition, tissue wasting and impaired organ function which leads to impaired immune and muscle function. Thus, depleted patients are at risk from infectious complications and cardiorespiratory impairment [4,5]. Patients who undergo gastrointestinal surgery are at risk of nutritional depletion from inadequate nutritional intake; both preoperatively and postoperatively, the stress of surgery and the subsequent increase in metabolic rate.

More recently, ensuring adequate nutritional intake has been a major focus of perioperative care and research has focused on the methods of delivering nutritional support, their comparative clinical benefits and minimising the metabolic changes associated with surgical trauma.

10.2 METABOLIC CHANGES IN SURGICAL PATIENTS

The physiological stress of surgical trauma causes a surge of sympathetic activity and an associated rise in catecholamine secretion. These changes are transient. A more prolonged hypermetabolic state associated with a pronounced negative nitrogen balance then follows. Metabolic rate is typically increased by about 10% postoperatively [6]. If adequate nutritional support is not provided at this stage then excessive skeletal muscle proteolysis occurs with further depression of metabolism. Increased energy expenditure is associated with a range of hormonal responses that occur as a result of surgical trauma. Cytokines, including Tumour Necrosis Factor (TNF) and interleukins (IL-1 and IL-6) have an important role in determining longer-term metabolic changes [7]. These changes may not be clinically relevant unless postoperative sepsis or trauma follows surgery but in conjunction with preoperative starvation often results in a significant negative nitrogen balance.

10.3 PHYSIOLOGICAL CHANGES IN SURGICAL PATIENTS

It has been proved that intestinal permeability is increased two to fourfold in the immediate postoperative period, although this normalises within five days [8]. In addition, nutritional depletion is associated with increased intestinal permeability and a decrease in villous height [9]. These findings have lead to the investigation of treatments aimed at maintaining an intact mucosal barrier. Increased intestinal permeability indicates a failure of the gut barrier function to exclude endogenous bacteria and toxins. These have been proposed as causative agents in the systemic inflammatory response syndrome, sepsis and multi-organ failure. However, there has been a failure thus far to prove a correlation between failure of gut barrier function and septic complications after major upper gastrointestinal failure [10].

10.4 CLINICAL BENEFITS TO SURGICAL PATIENTS

Nutritional support leads to improved nutritional status and clinical outcome in severely depleted patients [11]. Studies of postoperative nutritional support have demonstrated reduced morbidity and reduced length of hospital stay [12]. There is also evidence that artificial nutritional support in malnourished patients is cost effective by reducing the costs associated with length of stay and morbidity and improved quality of life [13]. It is important, however, to consider the most clinically appropriate and beneficial means of delivering nutritional support to surgical patients.

10.5 ENTERAL NUTRITION

Conventional treatment after bowel resection has typically entailed starvation with administration of intravenous fluids until passage of flatus, principally due to concerns over post-operative ileus. This was based on the assumption that oral feeding may not be tolerated in the presence of ileus and the integrity of the newly constructed anastomosis may be compromised. However, small intestinal motility recovers 6–8 hours after surgical trauma and moderate absorptive capacity exists even in the absence of normal peristalsis [14]. It has since been shown that postoperative enteral feeding in patients undergoing gastrointestinal resection is safe and well tolerated even when started within 12 hours of surgery [15,16]. The commonest observed adverse effects were gastrointestinal, such as abdominal cramps and bloating [16].

An appropriate delivery method should be selected, depending on the anticipated duration of enteral feeding, aspiration risk and gastrointestinal anatomy. No specific clinical or nutritional advantages have been shown for jejunostomy feeding and this route should be reserved for patients in whom naso-gastric or naso-jejunal feeding is not feasible or safe [17].

Enteral feeding has been shown to result in some specific clinical benefits, including reducing the incidence of post-operative infectious complications [11] and an improved wound healing response [18]. Enteral nutrition may have other beneficial effects including altering antigen exposure and influencing oxygenation of the gut mucosa. More research is required in this area to elucidate whether enteral nutrition truly modulates gut function or whether tolerance of enteral nutrition is predominantly indicative of a patient with healthy organ function [19].

10.6 PARENTERAL NUTRITION

A large multi-centre clinical trial has shown no significant reduction in morbidity or mortality when Total Parenteral Nutrition (TPN) was administered perioperatively to a heterogeneous group of surgical patients. Stratification of patients in this trial according to nutritional status showed that patients with mild malnutrition did not benefit from TPN but had more infectious complications. This led the authors to conclude that perioperative TPN should be limited to severely malnourished patients in the absence of other specific indications [20]. Subsequent studies have principally focussed on severely malnourished patients with gastrointestinal malignancy. These patients have been shown to experience clinically significant reductions in both infectious and non-infectious complications when fed parenterally for a minimum of ten days pre-operatively [21]. A recent meta-analysis of 27 randomised controlled trials concluded that TPN has no statistically significant effects overall on mortality or morbidity in surgical patients. The most recent studies analysed were of better methodological quality and showed fewer benefits than earlier studies. Studies which included only malnourished patients demonstrated a trend to a reduction in complication rates [22].

10.7 ENTERAL VERSUS PARENTERAL NUTRITION

Each route of delivery of nutritional support is associated with different complications. Generally, the complications associated with parenteral nutrition are associated with greater morbidity than those associated with enteral nutrition due to the invasive nature of administration. The route of administration also has effects on organ function, particularly the intestinal tract. Substrates delivered by the enteral route are better utilised by the gut than those administered parenterally. In addition, enteral feeding when compared with TPN solutions may prevent gastrointestinal mucosal atrophy, attenuate the trauma stress response, maintain immunocompetence and preserve normal gut flora [23].

A meta-analysis comparing the nutritional efficacy of early enteral and parenteral nutrition in high-risk surgical patients found that early postoperative enteral nutrition was effective and associated with reduced septic morbidity rates compared with those administered TPN even when catheter sepsis was excluded from the analysis [23]. Enteral nutrition is also an effective option in severely malnourished patients with gastrointestinal cancer and is associated with fewer complications, a shorter post-operative hospital stay [25] and reduced costs compared with TPN [26]. The principal conclusions from these studies was that the enteral route should be used whenever possible, but if the enteral route will not be available for more than one week early administration of TPN should be considered.

10.8 PREOPERATIVE VERSUS POST OPERATIVE

Evidence to support preoperative nutrition support is limited but suggests that if malnourished individuals are adequately fed for at least 7–10 days preoperatively then surgical outcome can be improved [20]. The obvious disadvantage of this is the increased length of hospital stay resulting from admission for nutritional support and the delay in surgical intervention. There is also some evidence to support preoperative nutrition support in patients with inflammatory bowel disease [27]. Studies have also been carried out which cast doubt on the benefits of the standard preoperative fast and have shown reductions in the postoperative catabolic response and improved well-being [28]. As discussed earlier, there is substantially more evidence to support early post-operative nutritional intervention by an appropriate route.

10.9 IMMUNONUTRITION

In addition to ongoing research ascertaining the specific benefits of the routes of delivery for nutrition support, more recent research has also focussed on the composition of nutritional regimens. In particular, much attention has been paid to the potential for specific nutrients to influence the metabolic response to disease.

Glutamine is the most abundant free amino acid in the extra and intracellular compartments. It plays a vital role in nitrogen transport and acid base homeostasis and is a fuel for rapidly dividing cells such as enterocytes, lymphocytes and fibroblasts. It is also involved in antioxidant defence mechanisms by influencing glutathione synthesis. In situations of severe stress or nutritional depletion the demand for glutamine may exceed the body's capacity to synthesise it. Studies have explored the benefits of glutamine-enriched parenteral nutrition regimens, particularly on the gut and immune system. It has been demonstrated that the addition of glutamine to parenteral nutrition regimens given to patients after elective abdominal surgery results in a reduced length of hospital stay [29] and reduced costs [30]. This was accompanied by an improved nitrogen balance and quicker lymphocyte recovery [29]. Glutamine has also been shown to maintain intestinal permeability in postoperative patients [31].

Studies regarding the role of two other potential immunonutrients, arginine and n-3 fatty acids, in gastrointestinal surgery patients have not yet been published.

10.10 CONCLUSIONS

Randomised controlled trials provide evidence to support the use of enteral feeding in surgical patients and indicate no increased morbidity or mortality. However, no meta-analyses have been carried out to pool the data from a plethora of mainly small trials. To date, these show no reductions in mortality have been shown from enterally fed surgical patients. Some useful meta-analyses have been published for parenterally feeding surgical patients, although many studies were small and of flawed methodological quality as they did not take into account the many surgical and anaesthetic variables that can influence post-operative outcomes. Comparative studies show that, compared with parenteral nutrition, enteral nutrition is well tolerated and is associated with reduced septic morbidity, costs and length of stay. These studies form the basis of the current practice of the enteral feeding route being used wherever possible. Further research is needed to elucidate whether, alongside improvements in surgical technique and peri-operative care, enteral nutrition will be associated with overall reductions in morbidity and mortality.

Further research is required to clearly identify which surgical patients will significantly benefit from specific nutritional intervention. This is problematic as assessment of nutritional status is not straightforward and there is also an absence of a standardised definition of nutritional depletion. A standardised, validated definition of nutritional depletion would enable nutrition support to be targeted to those surgical patients most likely to derive significant clinical benefit in terms of improved postoperative outcome. This would also facilitate direct comparison of trial data for large meta-analyses involving "malnourished" patients to provide robust, evidence based guidelines for nutritional support of surgical patients.

REFERENCES

1. McWhirter JP, Pennington CR: The incidence and recognition of malnutrition in hospital. BMJ 1994, 308:945-8.
2. Studley HO: Percentage weight loss, a basic indicator of surgical risk in patients with chronic peptic ulcer. JAMA 1936, 106:458-460.
3. Giner M, Laviano A, Meguid MM, Gleason JR: In 1995 a correlation between malnutrition and poor outcome in critically ill patients still exists. Nutrition 1996, 12:23-9.
4. Windsor JA, Hill GL: Risk factors for post operative pneumonia: the importance of protein depletion. Ann Surg 1988, 17:181-5.

5. Arora NS, Rochester DF: Respiratory muscle strength and maximal voluntary ventilation in undernourished patients. Am Rev Respir Dis 1982, 126:5-8.
6. Kinney JM, Duke JH Jr, Long CL, Gump FE: Tissue fuel and weight loss after injury. J Clin Path 1970, Suppl 4:65-72.
7. Douglas RG, Shaw JHF: Metabolic response to sepsis and trauma. Br J Surg 1989, 76:115-122.
8. Beattie AH, Prach AT, Baxter AT, Pennington CR: A randomised controlled trial evaluating the use of enteral nutritional supplements postoperatively in malnourished surgical patients. Gut 2000, 46:813-818.
9. van der Hulst RR, von Meyenfeldt MF, van Freel BK, Thunnissen FB, Brummer RJ, Arends JW, Soeters PB: Gut permeability, intestinal morphology, and nutritional depletion. Nutrition 1998, 14:1-6.
10. Kanwar S, Windsor AC, Welsh F, Barclay GR, Guillou PJ, Reynolds JV: Lack of correlation between failure of gut barrier function and septic complications after major upper gastrointestinal surgery. Ann Surg 2000, 231:88-95.
11. Beier-Holgersen SR, Boesby S: Influence of postoperative enteral nutrition on post surgical infections. Gut 1996, 39:833-5.
12. Askanazi J, Starker PN, Olsson C, Hensle TW, Lockhart SH, Kinney JM, Lasala PA: Effect of immediate post-operative nutritional support on the length of hospitalisation. Ann Surg 1986, 203:236-9.
13. Robinson G, Goldstein M, Levine G: Impact of nutritional status on DRG length of stay. JPEN 1987, 11:49-51.
14. Woods JH, Erickson LW, Condon RE: Post-operative ileus: a colonic problem. Surgery 1978, 84:527-533.
15. Reissman P, Teoh TA, Cohen SM, Weiss EG, Nogueras JJ, Wexner SD: Is early oral feeding safe after elective colorectal surgery? A prospective randomized trial. Ann Surg 1995, 222:73-77.
16. Braga M, Gianotti L, Gentilini S, Liotta S, Di Carlo V: Feeding the gut early after digestive surgery: results of a nine-year experience. Clinical Nutrition 2002, 21:59-65.
17. Smith RC, Hartemink RJ, Hollinshead JW, Gillett DJ: Fine bore jejunostomy feeding following major abdominal surgery: a controlled randomised clinical trial. Br J Surg 1985, 72:458-61.
18. Schroeder D, Gillanders L, Mahr K, Hill GL: Effects of immediate postoperative enteral nutrition on body composition, muscle function and wound healing. JPEN 1991, 15:376-383.
19. Reynolds JV: Gut barrier function in the surgical patient. Br J Surg 1996, 83:1668-1669.
20. Veterans Affairs Total Parenteral Nutrition Cooperative Study Group: Periperative Total Parenteral Nutrition in surgical patients. NEJM 1991, 325:525-32.
21. Bozzetti F, Gavazzi C, Miceli R, Rossi N: Perioperative total parenteral nutrition in malnourished, gastrointestinal cancer patients: a randomised, clinical trial. JPEN 2000, 24:7-14.
22. Heyland DK, Montalvo M, MacDonald S, Keefe L, Xiang YS, Drover JW: Total Parenteral Nutrition in the surgical patient: a meta-analysis. Can J Surg 2001, 44:102-11.

23. Saito H, Trocki O, Alexander JW: The effect of route of nutrient administration on the nutritional state, catabolic hormone secretion, and gut mucosal integrity after burn injury. JPEN 1987, 11:1-7.

24. Moore FA, Feliciano DV, Andrassy RJ, McArdle AH, Booth FV, Morgenstein-Wagner TB, Kellum JM, Welling RE, Moore EE: Early enteral feeding, compared with parenteral, reduced postoperative septic complications. The results of a meta-analysis. Ann Surg 1992, 216:172-183.

25. Bozzetti F, Braga M, Gianotti L, Gavazzi C, Mariani L: Postoperative enteral versus parenteral nutrition in malnourished patients with gastrointestinal cancer: a randomised multicentre trial. Lancet 2001, 358:1487-92.

26. Braga M, Gianotti L, Gentilini O, Parisi V, Salis C, Di Carlo V: Early postoperative enteral nutrition improves gut oxygenation and reduces costs compared with total parenteral nutrition. Crit Care Med 2001, 29:242-248.

27. Rombeau JL, Barot LR, Williamson CE, Mullen JL: Preoperative total parenteral nutrition and surgical outcome in patients with inflammatory bowel disease. Am J Surg 1982, 143:139-43.

28. Ljungqvist O, Soreide E: Preoperative fasting. Br J Surg 2003, 90:400-6.

29. Morlion BJ, Stehle P, Wachtler P, Siedhoff HP, Koller M, Konig W, Furst P, Puchstein C: Total parenteral nutrition with glutamine dipeptide after major abdominal surgery. Ann Surg 1998, 227:302-8.

30. Mertes N, Schulzki C, Goeters C, Winde G, Benzing S, Kuhn KS, van Aken H, Stehle P, Furst P: Cost containment through L-alanyl-L-glutamine supplemented total parenteral nutrition after major abdominal surgery: a prospective randomised double-blind controlled study. Clin Nutrition 2000, 19:395-401.

31. Jiang ZM, Cao JD, Zhu XG, Zhao WX, Yu JC, Ma EL, Wang XR, Zhu MW, Shu H, Liu YW: The impact of alanyl-glutamine on clinical safety, nitrogen balance, intestinal permeability, and clinical outcome in postoperative patients: a randomised, double-blind, controlled study of 120 patients. JPEN 1999, 23:S62-66.

CHAPTER 11

MICRONUTRIENT DEFICIENCY IN OBESE SUBJECTS UNDERGOING LOW CALORIE DIET

NTJE DAMMS-MACHADO, GESINE WESER,
and STEPHAN C. BISCHOFF

11.1 BACKGROUND

In general, occurrence of malnutrition is thought to be disease-related and/ or associated with undernourishment. During the past few years, evidence has been raised that obesity can also be associated with substantial nutrient deficiencies [1-5]. In fact, the prevalence of micronutrient deficiencies in obese individuals is higher compared to normal weight controls of the same age and sex [6,7], and affects several micronutrients such as zinc [4,8], selenium [4,6,8,9], folate [4,6,8,10], vitamin B1[11], vitamin B12[4,6,8,10,12], vitamin A [6,8], vitamin E [4,6], and 25-hydroxyvitamin D [25(OH)D] [4,6,8,11]. Imbalances or deficiencies of essential micronutrients significantly influence day-to-day performance, behavior and emotional state, as well as intellectual and physical activity [13-15]. It has been hypothesized that toxic by-products of incomplete biochemical reactions resulting from excessive intake of kilocalories and states of micronutrient deficiencies could lead to further weight gain or development of associated metabolic diseases [13,16]. Considering the worldwide prevalence of obesity, a significant part of the population could be afflicted by this type of micronutrient deficiency, even in wealthy Western countries.

The dietary reference intakes (DRI) for daily supply of vitamins and mineral nutrients apply to healthy, normal weight individuals. They account for individual variations and distinguish between age groups and sex [17,18], but they do not apply to patients with metabolic alterations or other disease, or individuals using pharmaceuticals on a regular basis. Hence, DRI do not necessarily meet the metabolic needs of obese individuals. Especially in physiologic stress situations like significant weight loss or periods of weight cycling, obese patients potentially need different amounts of micronutrients.

The first aim of this pilot study was to investigate the micronutrient intake in obese subjects compared to a reference population and DRI recommendations. Second aim was to determine both serum and intracellular micronutrient status after a standardized DRI-covering low-calorie formula diet over three months in order to analyze if DRI for micronutrients apply to obese patients in a period of major weight loss. This setting was chosen, because it offers a unique possibility to study this issue using an entirely standardized diet consumed by high-grade obese individuals over a longer-term period.

11.2 METHODS

11.2.1 INTERVENTION AND STUDY POPULATION

This pilot study included obese individuals participating in a multidisciplinary weight loss program (OPTIFAST®52) causing an average weight loss of 26.0 kg in men and 19.6 kg in women within one year [19]. Briefly, the program consists of a five-phase lifestyle modification program designed for 52 weeks, including (i) a 1-week introduction during which a detailed nutrition analysis is performed; (ii) a 12 week period of low-calorie diet (LCD) (800 kcal/day) during which participants consume a formula diet exclusively (daily consumption of 5 sachets at 160 kcal each,

Optifast 800® formula, Nestlé Inc.); (iii) a 6 weeks refeeding phase, (iv) a 7 weeks stabilization phase and (v) a 26 weeks maintenance phase. We previously reported more detailed information about the program [19]. The five daily consumed formula meals in the second phase contain vitamins, minerals and trace elements according to DRI for healthy adults (Table 1), except for the flavor potato/leek, which contains less amounts of vitamin C, vitamin B12, folate and calcium. However, flavor selection was documented, recording that the latter one was only consumed occasionally.

Table 1. Content of selected micronutrients in the formula diet and comparison with DRI (D-A-CH reference values)

Micronutrient	Unit	Per sachet flavor A (42 g)	% of DRI per 5 sachets	Per sachet flavor B (42 g)	% of DRI per 5 sachets
Vitamin A	mg	0.3	♀188; ♂150	0.2	♀125; ♂100
Vitamin D	µg	1.0	101	1.2	118
Vitamin E	mg	4.0	♀142; ♂166	3.4	♀122; ♂143
Vitamin C	mg	20.0	100	10.8	54
Vitamin B12	µg	0.6	98	0.4	60
Folate	µg	80.2	100	48.0	60
Calcium	mg	290.6	145	168.1	84
Iron	mg	4.0	♂133; ♀199	3.8	♂127; ♀191
Zinc	mg	3.0	♂149; ♀213	2.3	♂114; ♀163
Selenium	µg	20.2	144-336	13.6	97-227

Flavor A: vanilla, chocolate, strawberry, coffee, and tomato; flavor B: potato/leek.

To determine micronutrient intake in obese individuals we analyzed dietary record data obtained during the introduction week from all participants enrolled from 02/2006 to 02/2010 (n=104). A randomly assigned subgroup of subjects (n=32) participated in a pilot study, and was followed up for micronutrient measurement before and after the three-month formula diet period (LCD intervention group). Patients with a history of bariatric surgery were excluded from study participation. The measurements were performed by intracellular micronutrient analysis in buccal mucosa cells (BMC) and by additional serum micronutrient analysis in 14 of the subjects. The latter subjects did not differ in initial body weight and weight loss to the whole LCD intervention group. For 9 subjects, long-term data on intracellular vitamin concentrations were also obtained at the end of the program year, 9 months after completion of the LCD phase. The nutrients evaluated in this study were vitamin C (BMC, serum, leukocytes), vitamin E (BMC, serum), lycopene (BMC), β-carotene (BMC), vitamin A, 25(OH)D, vitamin B12, folate, selenium, iron, zinc and calcium (all serum). Deficiency was defined as a concentration below the reference interval: vitamin A 0.2-1.2 mg/ml, vitamin E 5–16 mg/ml (serum)/9.5-20.3 pmol/μg DNA (BMC), 25(OH)D, 20–70 ng/ml, vitamin C 28.3-85.1 μg/ml (serum)/57–114 nmol/108 cells (leukocytes)/3.9-11.1 pmol/μg DNA (BMC), vitamin B12 191–663 pg/ml, folate 4.6-18.7 ng/ml, selenium 74–139 μg/ml, iron 40–170 μg/dl, zinc 70–150 μg/dl, calcium 2.2-2.6 mmol/l, β-carotene 0.1-05 pmol/μg DNA, and lycopene 0.1-05 pmol/μg DNA. Moreover, C-reactive protein (CRP) concentrations were analyzed in serum samples. Drug use was monitored and documented on standardized forms. We calculated body mass index (BMI) and relative weight loss in percent (RWL; = 100xΔweight loss in kg/initial body weight in kg). Body composition was analyzed using bioelectrical impedance analysis at all study visits (Data Input Nutriguard M, Darmstadt, Germany). The study protocol was part of a multicenter clinical trial, research project "Obesity and the gastrointestinal tract" (ClinicalTrials.gov identifier: NCT01344525), approved by the ethics committee of the University Hospital of Tübingen, Germany. Informed consent was obtained from every subject prior to participation.

11.2.2 DIETARY RECORDS

Food intake was recorded using a predesigned daily journal. Subjects had to document time, amount (in gram) and situation, in which a food or beverage was consumed. They were instructed to: (1) document all consumed foods and beverages in as much detail as possible, (2) to weigh foods (or to estimate doses, if weighing was not possible in some situations), (3) to document food or beverage intake immediately after consumption and

(4) not to change usual eating habits. Data analysis was performed using the nutrition software EBISpro, version 8.0 for Windows. In analyzing the eating records, nutrients were studied in relation to the DRI (D-A-CH reference values) [18]. The DRI utilized corresponds to the age group and sex. Furthermore, data were compared with the Second National Nutrition Survey (NNSII), which is representative for the German population. The dietary assessment in this survey was performed using controlled interviews according to the diet history method, which were reinforced by dietary record collection and 24 hour-recalls in a representative sub-sample.

11.2.3 INTRACELLULAR MICRONUTRIENT CONCENTRATIONS IN BUCCAL MUCOSA CELLS (BMC)

BMC were collected using a kit from Day-med-concept GmbH, Berlin, Germany. Subjects first had to rinse their mouths with water thoroughly to remove food particles and then brush the inner lining of their cheeks with a soft toothbrush twenty times, twice on each side. The toothbrush was washed in 25 ml NaCl solution (0.9%) gently after each brushing. The samples were then centrifuged at 1,600 rpm for 3 minutes. The supernatant was discarded; the cells were completely resuspended in rinsing solution (phosphor float 0.15% w/v) and centrifuged again at 1,800 rpm for 3 minutes. After removal of the supernatant fraction, the stabilizing solution (heat-sensitive reducing agent 0.09% w/v) was added; and the cells were resuspended and stored. The micronutrients in BMC (pmol/μg DNA) of the samples were measured by BioTeSys GmbH (Esslingen, Germany) using an accredited RP-HPLC method according to DIN EN ISO/IEC 17025. The reference values are based on a statistical distribution reflecting the 25th and 75th percentile of a data set covering analysed BMC samples over one year.

Micronutrient concentrations were expressed in pmol/μg DNA. Micronutrient detection was possible when the amount of DNA in BMC was at least sufficient (>1 μg). If the amount of DNA extracted was < 1 μg, the data was excluded from analysis. Micronutrients below detection limit were defined as suboptimal cellular concentrations according to the analysis laboratory and therefore were included.

11.2.4 SERUM CONCENTRATIONS OF MICRONUTRIENTS

For serum micronutrient analysis, blood was collected by venipuncture between 8.00 a.m. and 10.00 a.m. after an overnight fast. Serum was separated by centrifugation at 2,000 x g for 15 min at 4°C. Aliquots were immediately stored at −80°C and sent to an external laboratory on the same day. HPLC was used to assay vitamin A and α-tocopherol. Measurement of vitamin C, calcium and iron was performed by photometry. Furthermore, serum was analyzed for 25(OH)D (radioimmunoassay), zinc and selenium (atomic absorption spectrometry) and vitamin B12 and folate (luminescence immunoassay).

11.2.5 VITAMIN C CONCENTRATIONS IN LEUKOCYTES

Isolation of leucocytes for vitamin C analysis was performed immediately after blood withdrawal. Briefly, sedimentation of erythrocytes was performed in a hermetic tube in dark environment using 6% Dextran according to the method of Denson et al.[20]. Supernatant was centrifuged for 10 min at 320 x g. After resuspension with HA buffer lysis of remaining erythrocytes was performed by 5 min incubation with 10 ml ammonium chloride. After centrifugation (10 min, 600 x g), leukocytes were manually counted and pellets frozen at −80 °C until analysis. Determination of total ascorbic acid concentrations in leukocytes was performed by HPLC. In summary, after thawing, leukocyte pellets reducing agent (20 µl 20% TCEP solution [tris (2- carboxyethyl) phosphine hydrochlorid]) was added, thoroughly mixed and incubated on ice for 5 min. For cell lysis 80 µl 10% meta-phosphoric acid was added, mixed and centrifuged (10 min, 13,000 x g, 4°C). Ascorbic acid concentrations in the supernatant were determined by UV/VIS detector at 245 nm.

All samples for vitamin C analysis were rapidly processed and shielded from light exposure.

11.2.6 STATISTICAL ANALYSIS

Values are expressed as means $\pm$ SD if not indicated otherwise. For the comparison of dietary record parameters with the reference population, Gaussian distribution was assumed due to sample size (n = 15,371). Differences between the obese study population and the NNSII data were analyzed using unpaired t-tests. The paired t-test was applied to compare repeated measures of micronutrients. If Gaussian distribution could not be assumed Wilcoxon signed-rank test was used instead of t-tests. Frequencies were analyzed with cross tables according to the method of McNemar. Analysis of covariance (ANCOVA) was performed to control for the effect of sex, age, energy, and medication use on micronutrient concentrations. Relations between continuous variables were analyzed by calculating the Spearman's rank correlation coefficient or, in case of normal distribution of the data, the Pearson's correlation coefficient. P values <0.001 were interpreted as statistically highly significant, p-values between 0.001 and <0.01 as very significant and p-values between 0.01 and <0.05 as significant differences. All analyses were carried out by using the statistics software SPSS, version 19.0 (IBM®SPSS®, Chicago, IL), and Graph Pad Prism, version 5.0 (GraphPad Software, Inc., La Jolla, CA).

11.3 RESULTS

11.3.1 BASELINE CHARACTERISTICS, WEIGHT LOSS AND DRUG INTAKE

Prior to intervention all subjects had at least grade I obesity (BMI $\geq$ 30 kg/m²), about 50% even obesity grade III (BMI $\geq$ 40 kg/m²). The obese study group (dietary records) and the reference population were well matched in respect to age, but the obese group comprised more females (Table 2).

BMI of the reference population was significantly lower compared to the obese study group (26.5 kg/m² versus 40.9 kg/m², p < 0.001). 32 out of 104 obese individuals (31%) underwent the LCD intervention. On average, these subjects lost 16.2% of initial body weight during the three-month LCD period. The LCD intervention subgroup (n=9), which was followed up until program end (12 months after start of intervention), did not differ in weight loss during the LCD period compared with the whole LCD intervention group (Table 3).

TABLE 2: Subjects characteristics of the obese study population (dietary record analysis) and a subgroup undergoing low-calorie diet

	Reference population (NNSII)	Obese study population (n=104)	LCD intervention group (n=32)	LCD intervention subgroup (follow-up until program end) (n=9)
Sex (%)				
male	46.2	26.9	12.5	33.3
female	53.8	73.1	87.5	66.7
Age	45.8	45.8±11.0	47.0±10.23	48.9±8.94
Weight [kg]	76.7	117.8±29.85	118.4±19.93	125.5±22.54
BMI [kg/m²]	26.5	40.9±7.20	41.8±7.21	43.0±6.42

Data are presented as mean ± SD.

TABLE 3: Weight loss during low-calorie diet (n=32) and further follow-up until program end (n=9)

	WL after LCD [kg]	RWL after LCD [%]	WL 12 at program end [kg]	RWL at program end [%]
LCD intervention group (n=32)	19.5±5.65	16.2±3.24		
LCD intervention subgroup[a] (n=9)	21.8±8.41	17.0±4.12	19.9±15.0	15.5±10.6

[a]follow-up until program end.
Abbreviations: WL Weight loss, RWL Relative weight loss.

86% of the subjects undergoing LCD took medication on a regular basis, which may have resulted in drug-nutrient interaction effects, thus influencing micronutrient bioavailability: ACE inhibitor (21%), proton pump inhibitor (8%), antidepressants (14%), L-thyroxine (14%), biguanide (7%), insulin (7%), loop diuretics (8%), NSAID (7%) and xanthine oxidase inhibitor (14%). Frequencies and dosage of medication decreased slightly in 36% of the cases during the LCD period. Controlling for sex, age, energy intake, and medication use, did not reveal significant effects on micronutrient concentrations.

11.3.2 MICRONUTRIENT INTAKE

Micronutrient intakes in obese subjects are shown in Table 4. Micronutrient intake in female subjects was significantly lower for five micronutrients compared to the reference population, in male subjects for six micronutrients, respectively. Women consumed nine micronutrients in amounts below DRI whereas with men this applied to seven micronutrients. Lowest micronutrient intakes compared to DRI were observed for retinol, ß-carotene, vitamin D, folate, iron and iodine (>75% of the obese study population below DRI) and vitamin E, C and calcium (>50% respectively).

Micronutrient intake did not differ between the whole study group (n = 104) and the subset of obese individuals undergoing LCD, which were further subjected to intracellular and serum micronutrient analysis.

11.3.3 MICRONUTRIENT DEFICIENCIES IN SERUM BEFORE AND AFTER LCD

Baseline deficiencies in serum micronutrient concentrations were observed for 25(OH)D, vitamin C, selenium and iron (Table 5). Except for 25(OH)D, the number of cases with deficiencies either remained (selenium, iron, both n.s.) or tended to further increase, which was the case for vitamin C (+15% of subjects with deficiency, n.s.). After the formula period, additional deficiency in zinc (7.7%) and calcium (53.8%) occurred. Figure 1 shows serum concentrations that decreased (calcium ($p < 0.01$)

and iron (p<0.05)) or increased (25(OH)D (p<0.01), folate (p<0.05) and zinc (p<0.01)), or remained unchanged (vitamin C (n.s.)) in the course of intervention using formula diet.

TABLE 4: Micronutrient intake of the obese study population compared to DRI and the reference population

Micronutrients		Female subjects (n = 76)					Male subjects (n = 28)				
		DRIa	Obese study population	Reference population (NNS II)	Pb	Obese subjects [%] below DRI	DRIa	Obese study population	Reference population (NNS II)	Pb	Obese subjects [%] below DRI
Retinol	[µg]	800	629.0±76.57	600.0±0.01	ns	86	1000	594.2±55.92	1000.0±0.01	<.001	89
β-Carotene	[mg]	4.8	3.0±0.24	5.4±0.04	<.001	86	6	2.7±0.31	5.1±0.04	<.001	93
Vitamin D	[µg]	5	2.5±0.32	2.9±0.03	<.05	87	5	2.4±0.31	3.8±0.04	<.001	93
Vitamin E	[mg]	12	11.7±0.56	13.4±0.08	<.05	55	14	11.4±0.80	16.0±0.12	<.05	75
Vitamin B1	[mg]	1	1.2±0.04	1.3±0.01	ns	25	1.2	1.4±0.10	1.8±0.01	<.05	39
Vitamin B2	[mg]	1.2	1.4±0.04	1.7±0.01	<.05	33	1.4	1.5±0.09	2.2±0.02	<.01	39
Niacin-equivalent	[mg]	13	31.2±0.98	28.6±0.13	ns	0	16	34.9±1.67	39.8±0.22	ns	0
Vitamin B6	[mg]	1.2	1.5±0.04	2.0±0.01	<.001	24	1.5	1.7±0.09	2.6±0.02	<.01	43
Folate-equivalent	[µg]	400	215.2±8.07	290.0±1.94	<.001	99	400	213.4±11.07	338.0±3.09	<.001	100
Vitamin B12	[µg]	3	4.9±0.31	4.3±0.02	ns	30	3	5.7±0.36	6.5±0.04	ns	4
Vitamin C	[mg]	100	92.1±5.30	152.0±0.95	<.001	66	100	86.2±8.50	152.0±1.14	<.001	71

TABLE 4: *Cont.*

Micronutrients		DRIa	Female subjects (n = 76) Obese study population	Reference population (NNS II)	Pb	Obese subjects [%] below DRI	DRIa	Male subjects (n = 28) Obese study population	Reference population (NNS II)	Pb	Obese subjects [%] below DRI
Sodium	[g]	550	3321.7±119.01	2494.0±9.41	<.001	0	550	3981.6±246.13	3458.0±15.72	<.05	0
Potassium	[mg]	2000	2649.1±72.92	3243.0±11.29	<.001	14	2000	2757.2±146.67	3789.0±15.06	<.001	11
Calcium	[mg]	1000	979.9±46.72	1019.0±4.33	ns	63	1000	1020.4±75.47	1143.0±5.93	ns	61
Magnesium	[mg]	300	365.2±12.23	376.0±1.23	ns	29	350	380.9±23.01	452.0±1.74	<.05	46
Iron	[mg]	15	12.9±0.36	12.3±0.04	ns	78	10	14.7±0.79	15.2±0.06	ns	7
Zinc	[mg]	7	12.0±0.36	9.5±0.03	<.001	3	10	14.2±0.71	12.3±0.05	<.05	4
Iodine	[µg]	200	83.9±4.08	98.0±0.45	ns	99	200	92.8±6.67	107.0±0.5	ns	100

Abbreviations: DRI = Dietary Reference Intake, NNS II = National Nutrition Survey II.

Data are presented as mean±SE.

ᵃ Recommendations for nutrient intake in Germany, Austria and Switzerland (D-A-CH reference values)[18].

[b] *Obese study population compared to German reference population (NNS II).*

TABLE 5: Serum micronutrient levels and deficiencies in obese subjects before and after low-calorie diet (n = 14)

		Before formula diet		After formula diet		
		Mean ± SD	Deficiency [%]	Mean ± SD	Deficiency [%]	p[a]
Vitamin A	[mg/l]	0.67 ± 0.19	0	0.78 ± 0.22	0	n.s.
Vitamin E	[mg/l]	11.57 ± 4.31	0	12.54 ± 2.66	0	n.s.
25(OH)D	[ng/ml]	17.22 ± 4.02	57.1	24.32 ± 7.25	30.8	<.01
Vitamin C	[mg/l]	52.01 ± 10.65	10.0	43.86 ± 15.96	25.0	n.s.
Vitamin B12	[pg/ml]	474.1 ± 155.3	0	528.3 ± 165.3	0	n.s.
Folate	[ng/ml]	10.51 ± 4.7	0	15.42 ± 4.9	0	<.05
Selenium	[µg/l]	87.71 ± 11.74	14.3	95.42 ± 18.67	16.7	<.05
Iron	[µg/dl]	81.50 ± 35.05	14.3	61.62 ± 26.17)	15.4	<.05
Zinc	[µg/dl]	82.14 ± 10.64	0	94.85 ± 13.80	7.7	<.01
Calcium	[mmol/l]	2.44 ± 0.10	0	2.18 ± 0.28	53.8	<.01

[a] *p-values were calculated in relation to absolute values using paired t-tests.*

11.3.4 MICRONUTRIENT DEFICIENCIES IN BMC BEFORE AND AFTER LCD

Intracellular antioxidant status in BMC is displayed in Figure 2. Before intervention, deficiencies were observed for vitamin C (63.3%), ß-carotene (20.0%) and lycopene (10.0%). After the LCD period BMC concentrations of vitamin C (p<0.05) and lycopene (p<0.05) decreased, resulting in a higher percentage of subjects with deficiencies (vitamin C +30.2%, p<0.01 and lycopene +6.1%, n.s.). At the end of the weight loss program (9 months after termination of the formula diet) antioxidative status was optimal or even above reference range, except for vitamin C (deficiencies in 77.8% of subjects), which also tended to improve (n.s.).

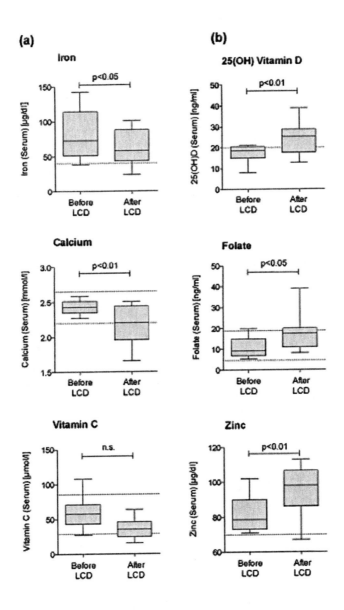

FIGURE 1: Serum micronutrients levels that decreased (a) or increased (b) in the course of intervention using a DRI- covering low-calorie formula diet (n = 14). The dotted lines indicate the reference limits for adequate serum levels. Data are presented as median +/− quartiles (boxes) and 1.5 interquartile ranges (whiskers).

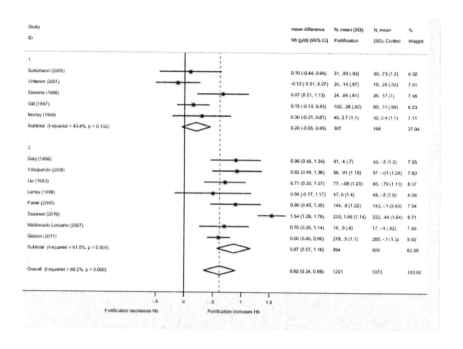

Study ID	mean difference Hb (g/dl) (95% CI)	N, mean (SD); Fortification	N, mean (SD), Control	% Weight
1				
Schümann (2005)	0.10 (-0.44, 0.64)	31, .83 (.93)	30, .73 (1.2)	6.92
Virtanen (2001)	-0.12 (-0.51, 0.27)	20, .14 (.57)	16, .26 (.52)	7.91
Stevens (1998)	0.67 (0.21, 1.13)	24, .84 (.61)	26, .17 (1)	7.45
Gill (1997)	0.15 (-0.13, 0.43)	192, .26 (.92)	60, .11 (.99)	8.53
Morley (1999)	0.30 (-0.21, 0.81)	40, 2.7 (1.1)	32, 2.4 (1.1)	7.11
Subtotal (I-squared = 43.4%, p = 0.132)	0.20 (-0.05, 0.45)	307	164	37.94
3				
Daly (1996)	0.90 (0.46, 1.34)	41, .4 (.7)	43, -.5 (1.3)	7.55
Villalpando (2006)	0.92 (0.48, 1.36)	58, .91 (1.18)	57, -.01 (1.24)	7.60
Liu (1993)	0.71 (0.35, 1.07)	77, -.08 (1.23)	85, -.79 (1.11)	8.07
Laney (1999)	0.50 (-0.17, 1.17)	47, 0 (1.4)	48, -.5 (1.9)	6.06
Faber (2005)	0.90 (0.45, 1.35)	144, .8 (1.22)	142, -.1 (2.43)	7.54
Sazzawal (2010)	1.54 (1.29, 1.79)	233, 1.98 (1.14)	232, .44 (1.54)	8.71
Maldonado Lonzano (2007)	0.70 (0.26, 1.14)	16, .3 (.4)	17, -.4 (.82)	7.60
Gibson (2011)	0.60 (0.40, 0.80)	278, .5 (1.1)	285, -.1 (1.3)	8.92
Subtotal (I-squared = 81.6%, p = 0.000)	0.87 (0.57, 1.16)	894	909	62.06
Overall (I-squared = 86.2%, p = 0.000)	0.62 (0.34, 0.89)	1201	1073	100.00

-.5   0   .5   1   1.5
Fortification decreases Hb   Fortification increases Hb

FIGURE 2: Intraepithelial micronutrient levels before and after obesity therapy using a low-calorie formula diet (n=32) and during further follow-up (n=9). Samples with no detectable micronutrient levels were excluded in this analysis. Data are presented as median +/− quartiles (boxes) and 1.5 interquartile ranges (whiskers). The dotted lines indicate the reference ranges. Statistical analysis: paired t-test.

11.3.5 VITAMIN C IN SERUM, BMC AND LEUKOCYTES BEFORE AND AFTER LCD

No correlation between vitamin C serum, BMC and leukocyte concentrations was observed. Serum and BMC vitamin C levels tended to decrease during the formula period (serum 59.44±22.73 µmol/l before intervention, 37.29±13.48 µmol/l after formula diet (n.s.), BMC 6.62±1.52 pmol/µg DNA and 2.95±1.10 pmol/µg DNA (p<0.001), respectively), whereas leukocyte vitamin C concentrations increased (81.64±16.30 ng/108 cells to 111.2±36.32 ng/108 cells, p<0.05) (Figure 3).

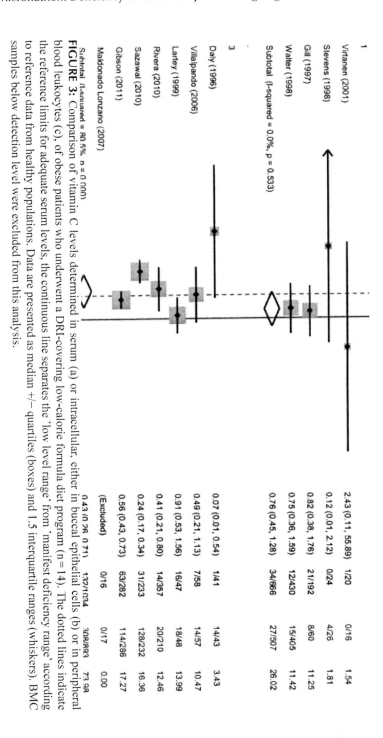

FIGURE 3: Comparison of vitamin C levels determined in serum (a) or intracellular, either in buccal epithelial cells (b) or in peripheral blood leukocytes (c), of obese patients who underwent a DRI-covering low-calorie formula diet program (n=14). The dotted lines indicate the reference limits for adequate serum levels, the continuous line separates the 'low level range' from 'manifest deficiency range' according to reference data from healthy populations. Data are presented as median +/- quartiles (boxes) and 1.5 interquartile ranges (whiskers). BMC samples below detection level were excluded from this analysis.

11.3.6 CORRELATIONS WITH C-REACTIVE PROTEIN (CRP), BODY WEIGHT AND BODY FAT

CRP concentrations positively correlated with body weight ($r=0.6558$, $p<0.0001$). There was a negative correlation between iron and CRP ($r=-0.456$, $p<0.05$). Lipophilic vitamins were negatively associated with body fat in percent of total body weight (25(OH)D: $r=-0,6369$, $p<0.0001$, vitamin A: $r=-0,4663$, $p<0.05$, vitamin E (serum): $r=-0,4378$, $p<0.05$).

11.4 DISCUSSION

The present study clearly confirms previous observations stating that obese individuals are characterized by micronutrient deficiencies [4,6-8,10-13]. The deficiencies are suggested by both low intake and low serum and intracellular levels as shown by our data.

The study demonstrates an insufficient dietary micronutrient supply of retinol, ß-carotene, vitamin D, vitamin E, vitamin C, folate, iron, and calcium in obese individuals. A highly significant difference compared to the reference population, both in men and women, was observed for ß-carotene, folate, vitamin C, and fiber - nutrients which are essentially found in fruits, vegetables and whole-grain products, thus pointing to an unbalanced diet leading to micronutrient deficiencies.

Evaluation of nutritional intake has some methodological weakness such as underreporting that limits the interpretation of dietary record data. The resulting error is possibly even more distinct in obese subjects [21-24]. However, underreporting especially applies to carbohydrate-rich snacks [25], which are low in micronutrient content by nature, and not to 'healthy' food. Therefore we assume that this error is negligible regarding micronutrient intake.

Before intervention, obese subjects showed deficiencies of several micronutrients in serum or BMC, namely 25(OH) vitamin D, vitamin C, selenium, iron, ß-carotene and lycopene. We did not find any statistically significant correlation between micronutrient intake and serum or BMC concentrations, which could be due to the limited subject number. However, the reported intakes of ß-carotene, vitamin D, vitamin C, and iron were clearly below DRI and point to a relation between micronutrient intake and body micronutrient status.

Based on our data, we conclude that a DRI-covering low-calorie formula diet does not meet the demands of obese individuals. The reasons can be manifold and could cover metabolic alterations during a period of major weight loss, unbalanced dispersal of lipophilic compounds and fat-tissue specific oxidative stress. Indeed, we observed even more subjects with deficiencies in some micronutrients after a three-month period of formula diet compared to the baseline status before intervention. In particular, vitamin C, selenium, iron, zinc, and lycopene deficiencies increased or could not be corrected by protein-rich formula diet containing vitamins and minerals according to DRI. The formula meal replacement products contained micronutrients in amounts often even higher than those recommended for the general population. We also observed an increase in subjects with calcium deficiency. However, serum calcium concentration is not an adequate measure for dietary calcium intake, but indicates an electrolyte imbalance induced by weight loss and accompanying fluid changes in the body.

Possible interaction effects between pharmaceuticals and micronutrients have to be considered, which may account for increased demands. Within this study, frequency and dosage of drug use did not change during the LCD period in most of the cases and thus most likely did not confound the results. In 36% of the subjects the dosage of at least one drug was slightly reduced, which would, if anything, have improved micronutrient bioavailability.

We did not find statistically significant correlations between vitamin E in serum and BMC, but the decrease in BMC concentrations could point to the fact that intracellular levels respond more sensitively to altered oxidative stress, which particularly occurs in a period of major weight loss [26]. This is explained by an upregulation of the renin-angiotensin system and a reduction of glutathione and glutathione peroxidase in erythrocytes, resulting in higher concentrations of reactive oxygen species which again promote the metabolic syndrome [6]. All three lipophilic vitamins negatively correlated with total body fat, assessed by bioelectric impedance analysis. This is most likely due to the storage capacity for lipophilic compounds, which is so far only suggested for 25(OH)D [27,28]. It is tempting to speculate that this also applies to other lipophilic compounds. Thus, a higher amount of fat tissue could lead to an increase in accumulation of lipophilic vitamins, which in turn are lacking in the serum pool. The positive association between adipose tissue mass and systemic 25(OH)D concentrations, the almost 2fold reduction of 25(OH)D deficiency following LCD, and the significant increase in 25(OH)D serum concentrations observed in our study all suggest storage in adipose tissue and release during weight loss, also described elsewhere [29,30].

McClung et al.[31] hypothesized that obesity influences iron absorption by inflammatory mediated mechanisms. Proinflammatory cytokines promote hepcidin release in liver and fat tissue, which is involved in iron homeostasis, inhibiting absorption in enterocytes [31]. This hypothesis is supported by a significantly negative correlation of iron concentration with CRP levels observed in our obese subjects.

Measurement of vitamins in blood samples might not reflect the amount of vitamins absorbed or the concentration in tissues [32,33]. To gain information on body distribution we monitored both serum and intracellular levels of vitamins. BMC are easily available and serve as a model system for assessment of the nutritional and antioxidative status, as well as to control for the success of supplementation and effect of medicamentous therapies [33-35]. With a cellular turnover of 5 to 25 days, BMC are supposed to reflect the current cellular supply [36].

We evaluated the level of vitamin C, lycopene, α-tocopherol, and ß-carotene and thus the antioxidative capacity directly in BMC. These dietary-derived antioxidants are an important component to support the exogenous antioxidative system [33]. Except for ß-carotene and α-tocopherol, which were only slightly reduced, we observed a significant decrease in vitamin C and lycopene during the three-month formula diet suggesting again an enhanced oxidative stress in obese individuals and thus a higher demand of antioxidative vitamins compared to healthy, normal weight subjects, especially in a period of major weight loss.

The current choices for functional markers of vitamin C status are vitamin C concentrations in plasma and leukocytes. Plasma or serum vitamin C levels are highly sensitive to recent dietary intakes, but may not reflect tissue content as well as leukocyte levels [37,38]. Serum vitamin C concentrations remained unchanged during the vitamin C enriched formula diet, whereas leukocyte levels improved. Leukocyte concentrations more reliably display long-term supply and deficiencies [37,38]. Bioavailability of vitamin C is a complex issue involving distribution to the tissues and utilization by the tissues [35]. Before intervention, leukocyte levels were depleted and might replete preferentially due to their high metabolic priority [37]. Contrary to our expectations intracellular vitamin C concentrations in BMC significantly decreased. To obtain a state of complete saturation, the repletion dynamics of vitamin C in certain tissues may be more specific than others when the vitamin intake during repletion is limited [37]. However, the results should be interpreted carefully because of the small sample size, the variation of vitamin C content throughout cell types and the reliability of sampling and analysis procedure due to the unstable nature of vitamin C. In contrast to the fat-soluble antioxidants α-tocopherol, lycopene and ß-carotene, which were demonstrated to be reliable markers in BMC [32,33,35,39,40], the capacity of BMC vitamin C concentrations and its reliability as a biomarker for vitamin C status has not been described so far.

Interestingly, we observed a significant increase in all antioxidants measured in BMC at the end of the program year. This subgroup only included nine subjects, but suggests a change in dietary habits following intensive weight reduction and diet counseling. These subjects were successful in losing weight and were able to maintain this weight after the formula diet, therefore most likely putting their nutritional knowledge into practice. However, this finding needs to be confirmed by other studies.

A potential limitation of the study is that the dietary assessment strategies differed in the two study populations. In the NNSII a comprehensive dietary history method including cross-check features was used. The dietary record approach in this study was chosen to provide quantitatively accurate information on food consumption as well as influence of food processing, but may be biased due to the estimation of the weight of food consumed in some cases instead of weighing, and also by affecting eating behavior. Moreover, for several micronutrients simple blood concentrations were measured, which might not always reflect a complete picture of the nutritional status. At this stage we only included a small sample size, which limits the explanatory power of the study results.

11.5 CONCLUSIONS

To the best of our knowledge, this is the first report analyzing if DRI of micronutrients meet the demands of obese individuals consuming a standardized LCD diet. Our pilot study provides evidence that a poor micronutrient status in obesity is not only caused by intakes that are below the DRI. A formula diet providing 100% of micronutrients according to DRI did not cover the demands of some micronutrients in obese subjects. This can be explained by metabolic alterations during a period of major weight loss, unbalanced dispersal of lipophilic compounds and fat-tissue specific oxidative stress. The underlying mechanisms should be further addressed, as well as whether obese individuals receiving an energy-balanced DRI-covering diet also manifest micronutrient deficiencies.

REFERENCES

1. Schneider A: Malnutrition with Obesity. Aktuelle Ernährungsmedizin. 2008, 33:280-283.
2. Grzybek A, Klosiewicz-Latoszek L, Targosz U: Changes in the intake of vitamins and minerals by men and women with hyperlipidemia and overweight during dietetic treatment. Eur J Clin Nutr 2002, 56:1162-1168.
3. Aasheim ET, Hofso D, Hjelmesaeth J, Birkeland KI, Bohmer T: Vitamin status in morbidly obese patients: a cross-sectional study. Am J Clin Nutr 2008, 87:362-369.
4. Ernst B, Thurnheer M, Schmid SM, Schultes B: Evidence for the necessity to systematically assess micronutrient status prior to bariatric surgery. Obes Surg 2009, 19:66-73.
5. Xanthakos SA: Nutritional deficiencies in obesity and after bariatric surgery. Pediatr Clin North Am 2009, 56:1105-1121.
6. Kimmons JE, Blanck HM, Tohill BC, Zhang J, Khan LK: Associations between body mass index and the prevalence of low micronutrient levels among US adults. MedGenMed 2006, 8:59.
7. Kaidar-Person O, Person B, Szomstein S, Rosenthal RJ: Nutritional deficiencies in morbidly obese patients: a new form of malnutrition? Part B: minerals. Obes Surg 2008, 18:1028-1034.
8. Madan AK, Orth WS, Tichansky DS, Ternovits CA: Vitamin and trace mineral levels after laparoscopic gastric bypass. Obes Surg 2006, 16:603-606.

9. Sanchez C, Lopez-Jurado M, Aranda P, Llopis J: Plasma levels of copper, manganese and selenium in an adult population in southern Spain: influence of age, obesity and lifestyle factors. Sci Total Environ 2010, 408:1014-1020.

10. Brolin RE, Gorman JH, Gorman RC, Petschenik AJ, Bradley LJ, Kenler HA, Cody RP: Are vitamin B12 and folate deficiency clinically important after roux-en-Y gastric bypass? J Gastrointest Surg 1998, 2:436-442.

11. Flancbaum L, Belsley S, Drake V, Colarusso T, Tayler E: Preoperative nutritional status of patients undergoing Roux-en-Y gastric bypass for morbid obesity. J Gastrointest Surg 2006, 10:1033-1037.

12. Skroubis G, Sakellaropoulos G, Pouggouras K, Mead N, Nikiforidis G, Kalfarentzos F: Comparison of nutritional deficiencies after Roux-en-Y gastric bypass and after biliopancreatic diversion with Roux-en-Y gastric bypass. Obes Surg 2002, 12:551-558.

13. Kaidar-Person O, Person B, Szomstein S, Rosenthal RJ: Nutritional deficiencies in morbidly obese patients: a new form of malnutrition? Part A: vitamins. Obes Surg 2008, 18:870-876.

14. Bourre JM: Effects of nutrients (in food) on the structure and function of the nervous system: update on dietary requirements for brain. Part 1: micronutrients. J Nutr Health Aging 2006, 10:377-385.

15. Reynolds E: Vitamin B12, folic acid, and the nervous system. Lancet Neurol 2006, 5:949-960.

16. Muscogiuri G, Sorice GP, Prioletta A, Policola C, Della Casa S, Pontecorvi A, Giaccari A: 25-Hydroxyvitamin D concentration correlates with insulin-sensitivity and BMI in obesity. Obesity (Silver Spring) 2010, 18:1906-1910.

17. Institute of Medicine, Food and Nutrition Board: Dietary Reference Intakes: RDA and AI for Vitamins and Elements. [http://fnic.nal.usda.gov/]

18. Wolfram G: New reference values for nutrient intake in Germany, Austria and Switzerland (DACH-Reference Values). Forum Nutr 2003, 56:95-97.

19. Bischoff SC, Damms-Machado A, Betz C, Herpertz S, Legenbauer T, Low T, Wechsler JG, Bischoff G, Austel A, Ellrott T: Multicenter evaluation of an interdisciplinary 52-week weight loss program for obesity with regard to body weight, comorbidities and quality of life-a prospective study. Int J Obes (Lond) 2012, 36:614-624.

20. Denson KW, Bowers EF: The determination of ascorbic acid in white blood cells. A comparison of W.B.C. ascorbic acid and phenolic acid excretion in elderly patients. Clin Sci 1961, 21:157-162.

21. Bandini LG, Schoeller DA, Cyr HN, Dietz WH: Validity of reported energy intake in obese and nonobese adolescents. Am J Clin Nutr 1990, 52:421-425.

22. Goris AH, Westerterp-Plantenga MS, Westerterp KR: Undereating and underrecording of habitual food intake in obese men: selective underreporting of fat intake. Am J Clin Nutr 2000, 71:130-134.

23. Lichtman SW, Pisarska K, Berman ER, Pestone M, Dowling H, Offenbacher E, Weisel H, Heshka S, Matthews DE, Heymsfield SB: Discrepancy between self-reported and actual caloric intake and exercise in obese subjects. N Engl J Med 1992, 327:1893-1898.

24. Pryer JA, Vrijheid M, Nichols R, Kiggins M, Elliott P: Who are the 'low energy reporters' in the dietary and nutritional survey of British adults? Int J Epidemiol 1997, 26:146-154.
25. Poppitt SD, Swann D, Black AE, Prentice AM: Assessment of selective under-reporting of food intake by both obese and non-obese women in a metabolic facility. Int J Obes Relat Metab Disord 1998, 22:303-311.
26. Yanagawa Y, Morimura T, Tsunekawa K, Seki K, Ogiwara T, Kotajima N, Machida T, Matsumoto S, Adachi T, Murakami M: Oxidative stress associated with rapid weight reduction decreases circulating adiponectin concentrations. Endocr J 2010, 57:339-345.
27. Wortsman J, Matsuoka LY, Chen TC, Lu Z, Holick MF: Decreased bioavailability of vitamin D in obesity. Am J Clin Nutr 2000, 72:690-693.
28. Earthman CP, Beckman LM, Masodkar K, Sibley SD: The link between obesity and low circulating 25-hydroxyvitamin D concentrations: considerations and implications. Int J Obes (Lond) 2012, 36:387-396.
29. Lin E, Armstrong-Moore D, Liang Z, Sweeney JF, Torres WE, Ziegler TR, Tangpricha V, Gletsu-Miller N: Contribution of adipose tissue to plasma 25-hydroxyvitamin D concentrations during weight loss following gastric bypass surgery. Obesity (Silver Spring) 2011, 19:588-594.
30. Damms-Machado A, Friedrich A, Kramer K, Stingel K, Meile T, Küper M, Königsrainer A, Bischoff SC: Pre- and postoperative nutritional deficiencies in obese patients undergoing laparoscopic sleeve gastrectomy. Obes Surg 2012, 22:881-889.
31. McClung JP, Karl JP: Iron deficiency and obesity: the contribution of inflammation and diminished iron absorption. Nutr Rev 2009, 67:100-104.
32. Peng YM, Peng YS, Lin Y, Moon T, Roe DJ, Ritenbaugh C: Concentrations and plasma-tissue-diet relationships of carotenoids, retinoids, and tocopherols in humans. Nutr Cancer 1995, 23:233-246.
33. Erhardt JG, Mack H, Sobeck U, Biesalski HK: beta-Carotene and alpha-tocopherol concentration and antioxidant status in buccal mucosal cells and plasma after oral supplementation. Br J Nutr 2002, 87:471-475.
34. Sobeck U, Fischer A, Biesalski HK: Uptake of vitamin A in buccal mucosal cells after topical application of retinyl palmitate: a randomised, placebo-controlled and double-blind trial. Br J Nutr 2003, 90:69-74.
35. Paetau I, Rao D, Wiley ER, Brown ED, Clevidence BA: Carotenoids in human buccal mucosa cells after 4 wk of supplementation with tomato juice or lycopene supplements. Am J Clin Nutr 1999, 70:490-494.
36. Gillespie GM: Renewal of buccal epithelium. Oral Surg Oral Med Oral Pathol 1969, 27:83-89.
37. Jacob RA: Assessment of human vitamin C status. J Nutr 1990, 120(Suppl 11):1480-1485.
38. Yamada H, Yamada K, Waki M, Umegaki K: Lymphocyte and plasma vitamin C levels in type 2 diabetic patients with and without diabetes complications. Diabetes Care 2004, 27:2491-2492.
39. Gabriel HE, Liu Z, Crott JW, Choi SW, Song BC, Mason JB, Johnson EJ: A comparison of carotenoids, retinoids, and tocopherols in the serum and buccal mucosa of

chronic cigarette smokers versus nonsmokers. Cancer Epidemiol Biomarkers Prev 2006, 15:993-999.
40. Reifen R, Haftel L, Faulks R, Southon S, Kaplan I, Schwarz B: Plasma and buccal mucosal cell response to short-term supplementation with all trans-beta-carotene and lycopene in human volunteers. Int J Mol Med 2003, 12:989-993.

This chapter was originally published under the Creative Commons Attribution License. Damms-Machado, A., Weser, G., and Bischoff, S. C. Micronutrient Deficiency in Obese Subjects Undergoing Low Calorie Diet. Nutrition Journal 2012: 11(34). doi:10.1186/1475-2891-11-34.

DIABETES-SPECIFIC NUTRITION ALGORITHM: A TRANSCULTURAL PROGRAM TO OPTIMIZE DIABETES AND PREDIABETES CARE

JEFFREY I. MECHANICK, ALBERT E. MARCHETTI,
CAROLINE APOVIAN, ALEXANDER KOGLIN BENCHIMOL,
PETER H. BISSCHOP, ALEXIS BOLIO-GALVIS, REFAAT A. HEGAZI,
DAVID JENKINS, ENRIQUE MENDOZA, MIGUEL LEON SANZ,
WAYNE HUEY-HERNG SHEU, PATRIZIO TATTI,
MAN-WO TSANG, and OSAMA HAMDY

12.1 INTRODUCTION

Type 2 diabetes (T2D) and prediabetes impose a huge burden of illness on developed and developing nations through high disease prevalence (6.6% overall, >10% in many countries), direct and indirect multisystem pathophysiologic effects, and financial liabilities (US$376 billion annually worldwide) [1]. This enormous disease burden can be reduced by deliberate application of interventions with proven effectiveness [2–14]. Ideally, diagnostic and therapeutic interventions should be accessible, facile, affordable, cost-effective, and culturally sensitive [1]. To improve efficiency, they can be combined in coordinated disease management programs. Lifestyle management, including physical activity and diabetes-specific nutrition therapy, is an essential and necessary component of any comprehensive care plan for diabetes [15••, 16, 17]. Care plan implementation is facilitated by clinical practice guidelines (CPGs) intended to inform clinical decisions, standardize and optimize patient care, improve outcomes, and control costs [18, 19]. Recommendations within CPGs should be evidence-based, precise, clear, relevant, authoritative, and compatible with existing norms [20, 21••]. The purpose of this report is to describe pertinent background material and the development process of a transcultural diabetes-specific nutrition algorithm (tDNA) that can facilitate portability of evidence-based recommendations to better enable their implementation and validation across a broad geographic and cultural spectrum.

12.2 BENEFITS AND PROBLEMS ASSOCIATED WITH CPGS

Although CPGs may have distinct flaws or problems intrinsic to their development, interpretation, and implementation, they are useful tools to aid clinical decision making and improve patient care [21••, 22–26]. Benefits are derived from the characteristics and attributes of the CPGs. For example, authoritative guidelines are developed by expert panels from specialized areas of medicine and reflect group consensus on specific aspects of patient care. These CPGs are evidence-based, transparently incorporating relevant research findings, and contain recommendations with the greatest potential for superior clinical outcomes. Depending on the methodology used, CPGs may consider subjective factors such as risk-benefit perceptions and cost-effectiveness. They may also engage such principles as middle-range question-oriented literature searching, patient-oriented evidence, cascades of recommendations for a particular clinical question based on variations in clinical settings, multiple levels of review, and diligent screening of writers and reviewers with respect to credentialing and conflicts of interest [21••]. Through these exacting methodologies and resultant credible content, CPGs empower practitioners, patients, and the larger universe of other health care stakeholders to make better decisions regarding the applicability of care.

CPGs also have limitations [1, 19, 27]. Even if their recommendations are appropriate, their implementation and performance can be impeded by untimeliness, complexity, and/or incompatibility with other recommendations. Their adoption and adherence may be further hindered by idiosyncratic physician and patient attitudes as well as the unique characteristics of a practice setting [28]. Guidelines may not accommodate disruptions in the continuity of care that arise among health care providers, facilities, and time frames [29]. Moreover, selected recommendations may reflect only a professional perspective, which may discount patient predilections or values and compromise clinical adherence and outcomes [19, 28]. Finally, CPGs may not be able to be generalized for all patients or populations. Patient age, gender, and genomics, as well as culture, customs, and environment, must be factored into any decision to apply a particular recommendation to a particular patient in a particular setting [29]. In effect, CPGs are simply not portable across divergent clinical settings. In light of the globalization and impact of the diabetes epidemic, this significant problem must be resolved.

12.3 ADDRESSING THE PORTABILITY PROBLEM

Whenever possible, either de novo or the most recent up-to-date CPGs on a particular topic should be used as a resource for specific patient management issues [30]. For ease of implementation, the CPGs should be straightforward and readily understood [20]. Derivative products (i.e., decision trees, flow charts, or algorithms) can be used to reduce the complexity of comprehensive CPGs, aid comprehension, and facilitate successful implementation and validation [31–33]. Such tools not only improve the standardization of care, but also help to coordinate the activities of all members of a treatment team for patients with diabetes. A diabetes flow sheet was shown to increase CPG adherence in a recent outcomes study based on medical audits [34].

12.4 TRANSCULTURAL FACTORS

To address the problem of generalizability and the effect of cultural differences among patients on a global scale, CPG development must begin with a robust decision-tree template amenable to strategic modification that does not sacrifice performance. Thus, the tDNA template was designed for the optimization of nutritional care for patients with T2D and prediabetes on a global scale (Fig. 1, Tables 1, ,2,2, ,3,3, ,4,4, ,5,5, ,66 and and7)7) [15••, 35–40, 41••, 42]. This instrument extends evidence-based nutritional recommendations from the American Association of Clinical Endocrinologists (AACE) [15••, 43] and the American Diabetes Association (ADA) [41••] and provides nodes that can be populated with information based on geographic and ethnocultural factors for individualization and implementation at regional and local levels worldwide. The tDNA is intended to 1) increase awareness of the benefits of nutritional interventions for patients with T2D and prediabetes; 2) encourage healthy dietary patterns that accommodate regional differences in genetic factors, lifestyles, foods, and cultures; 3) enhance the implementation of existing CPGs for T2D and prediabetes management; and 4) simplify nutritional therapy for ease of application and portability.

TABLE 1: Classification of body composition by BMI, WC, and disease risk for Caucasians

	BMI, kg/m²	Obesity class	Disease risk	
			WC: M ≤ 40 in F ≤ 35 in	WC: M > 40 in F > 35 in
Underweight	<18.5			
Normal	18.5–24.9			
Overweight	25.0–29.9		Increased	High
Obese	30.0–34.9	I	High	Very high
	35.0–39.9	II	Very high	Very high
Extremely obese	≥40	III	Extremely high	Extremely high

BMI body mass index; F female; M male; WC waist circumference
(Adapted from: Bantle JP, Wylie-Rosett J, Albright AL, et al. Nutrition recommendations and interventions for diabetes: a position statement of the American Diabetes Association. Diabetes Care. 2008;31 Suppl 1:S61–78) [41••]

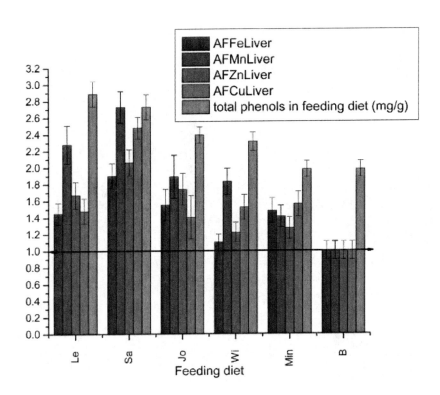

FIGURE 1: Transcultural medical nutrition algorithm for prediabetes and type 2 diabetes. AACE—American Association of Clinical Endocrinologists; ADA—American Diabetes Association; BMI—body mass index; DASH—Dietary Approaches to Stop Hypertension; FPG—fasting plasma glucose; HbA1c—glycosylated hemoglobin A1c; IFG—impaired fasting glucose; IGT—impaired glucose tolerance; MNT—medical nutrition therapy; OGTT—oral glucose tolerance test; PG—plasma glucose; WC—waist circumference; WHR—waist-to-hip ratio

TABLE 2: Classification of body composition by BMI, WC, and disease risk for Southeast Asians and Asian Americans

	BMI, kg/m²	Obesity class	Disease risk	
			WC: M ≤ 90 cm F ≤ 80 cm	WC: M > 90 cm F > 80 cm
Underweight	<18.5			
Normal	18.5–22.9		Average	Average
Overweight	23–24.9	I	Increased	High
Obese	25.0–29.9	II	High	Very high
			Very high	Very high
Extremely obese	≥30	III	Severe	Severe

BMI body mass index; F female; M male; WC waist circumference
(Adapted from: Wildman RP, Gu D, Reynolds K, et al. Appropriate body mass index and waist circumference cutoffs for categorization of overweight and central adiposity among Chinese adults. Am J Clin Nutr. 2004;80:1129–36) [36]
(Adapted from: Appropriate body-mass index for Asian populations and its implications for policy and intervention strategies. WHO Expert Consultation. Lancet. 2004;363:157–63) [37]

TABLE 3: Physical activity guidelines for the management of diabetes

Intensity level	Physical activity
Low	Patients should be encouraged to achieve an active lifestyle and to avoid sedentary living, because physical activity and exercise provide many health benefits and facilitate glycemic control. Participation in any physical activity provides some health benefits
	For substantial benefits:
	≥150 min/week of moderate-intensity activity, or
	≥75 min/week of vigorous-intensity aerobic activity, or
	some combination of equivalent moderate/vigorous activity
Medium	Aerobic activity should be performed in episodes of ≥10 min and preferably spread throughout the week
	For additional, more extensive benefits:
	≥300 min/week of moderate-intensity activity, or
	≥150 min/week of vigorous-intensity aerobic activity, or
	some combination of equivalent moderate/vigorous activity
	additional health benefits are gained beyond this amount

TABLE 3: *Cont.*

Intensity level	Physical activity
High	Moderate- or high-intensity resistance exercise training for all major muscle groups, as a separate modality from aerobic exercise, has been shown to increase muscle mass and strength, alter body composition, and improve glycemic control; therefore, it should be combined with aerobic activity in each individual ≥2 days per week

Exercise should be undertaken only after cardiac clearance has been obtained
(Adapted from: US Department of Health and Human Services. 2008 Physical activity
guidelines for Americans. 2008.http://www.health.gov/paguidelines/guidelines/summary.
aspx. Accessed June 22, 2011) [35]

TABLE 4: AACE/ADA nutritional guidelines for the management of diabetes

Hypocaloric (weight loss) diet: 250–1000 kcal/d deficit
Target: decrease weight by 5% to 10% for overweight/obese, 15% for class 3 obesity
Target: decrease BMI by 2 to 3 units
Carbohydrates (preferably low-glycemic index): 45% to 65% daily energy intake and not less than 130 g/d in patients on low calorie diet
Protein: 15% to 20% daily energy intake
Dietary fat: <30% daily energy intake
Saturated fat: <7% daily energy intake
Cholesterol: <200 mg/d
Fiber: 25–50 g/d
Trans fats: minimize or eliminate

AACE American Association of Clinical Endocrinologists; ADA American Diabetes
Association; BMI body mass index
(Adapted from: National Guideline Clearinghouse. Guideline synthesis: Nutritional
management of diabetes mellitus. 2009.http://www.guideline.gov.syntheses/synthesis.
aspx?id+16430. Accessed June 22, 2011.) [40]

TABLE 5: Diabetes-specific (glycemia targeted specialized) nutrition formulas for the management of prediabetes and diabetes

Overweight/obese	Use 2 to 3 diabetes-specific nutrition formulasa as part of a reduced calorie meal plan, as a calorie replacement for meal, partial meal, or snack (grade C; LOE 3)	
	Calorie goals:	
	<250 lb = 1200 to 1500 calories	
	>250 lb = 1500 to 1800 calories	
	Calories from diabetes-specific nutrition formulas	
	Calories from other healthy dietary source	
Normal weight	Uncontrolled diabetes	1 to 2 diabetes-specific nutrition formulas per day to be incorporated into a meal plan, as a calorie replacement for meal, partial meal, or snack (grade D; LOE 4)
	$HbA_{1c} > 7\%$	
	Controlled diabetes	Use of diabetes-specific nutrition formulas should be based on clinical judgment and individual assessmentb(grade D; LOE 4)
	$HbA_{1c} \leq 7\%$	
Underweight	Use diabetes-specific nutrition supplementsc 1 to 3 units/d per clinical judgment based on desired rate of weight gain and clinical tolerance (grade D; LOE 4)	

LOE 1: data defined as conclusive results from prospective, randomized controlled trials that have large subject populations representative of the target population and results that are easily generalized to the target population. Data also include results from meta-analyses of randomized controlled trials, results from multicenter trials, and "all or none" evidence; LOE 2: data include conclusive results from individual randomized controlled trials that have limited subject numbers or target population representation; LOE 3: data include all other conclusive clinical findings from nonrandomized studies, studies without controls, and nonexperimental or observational studies. These data may require interpretation and, by themselves, are not compelling; LOE 4: data are defined as information based solely on experience or expert opinion and are not necessarily substantiated by any conclusive scientific data. Frequently, only LOE 4 data are available
aDiabetes-specific nutrition formulas are nutritional products used as replacement for meals, partial meals, or snacks to replace calories in the diet
bIndividuals who may have muscle mass and/or function loss and/or micronutrient deficiency may benefit from diabetes-specific nutrition supplements. Individuals who need support with weight maintenance and/or a healthy meal plan could benefit from diabetes-specific nutrition
cDiabetes-specific nutrition supplements are complete and balanced nutritional products used in addition to a typical meal plan, to help promote increased nutritional intake
HbA1c glycosylated hemoglobin A1c; LOE level of evidence

TABLE 6: Criteria for bariatric surgery for the management of diabetes

BMI ≥ 40 kg/m² (about 100 lb overweight for men and 80 lb for women) or
BMI 35–39.9 kg/m² and an obesity-related comorbidity, such as T2D, coronary heart disease, or severe sleep apnea
BMI 30–34.9 kg/m² under special circumstances
According to the International Diabetes Federation, bariatric surgery should be considered an alternative treatment option in patients with a BMI of 30–35 kg/m² when diabetes is not adequately controlled by a medical regimen and especially when there are cardiovascular disease risk factors
Consideration may be given to laparoscopic-assisted gastric banding in patients with T2D who have a BMI > 30 kg/m² or Roux-en-Y gastric bypass for patients with a BMI > 35 kg/m² to achieve at least short-term weight reduction
And for each of the above:
Failure to achieve and sustain weight loss after attempts at lifestyle modification
Tolerable operative risks
Understanding of operation
Commitment to treatment and long-term follow-up
Acceptance of required lifestyle changes

BMI body mass index; T2D type 2 diabetes
(Adapted from: Weight-control Information Network—an information service of the National Institute of Diabetes and Digestive and Kidney Diseases (NIDDK). Bariatric surgery for severe obesity. 2009.http://win.niddk.nih.gov/publications/gastric.htm. Accessed November 14, 2011) [38]
(Adapted from: International Diabetes Federation. Bariatric surgical procedures and interventions in the treatment of obese patients with type 2 diabetes: a position statement from the International Diabetes Federation Taskforce on Epidemiology and Prevention. http://www.idf.org/webdata/docs/IDF-Position-Statement-Bariatric-Surgery.pdf. Accessed June 27, 2011) [39]
(Adapted from: Handelsman Y, Mechanick JI, Blonde L, et al. American Association of Clinical Endocrinologists Medical Guidelines for Clinical Practice for developing a diabetes mellitus comprehensive care plan. Endocr Pract. 2011;17 Suppl 2:1–53) [15••]

12.5 METHODOLOGY TO DEVELOP THE TDNA

The methods and procedures used to develop the tDNA are widely recognized as state-of-the-art within medical organizations and were rigorously applied throughout this endeavor. The task force chair initiated the project via live meetings and telephone or digital communications. Internationally respected health care experts in diabetes and nutrition from Brazil, Canada, China, Mexico, The Netherlands, Panama, Spain, Taiwan, and the

United States were identified through literature searches and peer recommendations. Each expert was contacted, briefed on the project, and questioned about his or her current activities and interest in participating in the program. Based on responses, invitations were extended until a complement of specialists, sufficient for advisory activities, accepted the request to be included in the task force.

TABLE 7: Antihypertensive diet: daily nutrient goals used in the DASH studies

Carbohydrate	55% of calories
Total fat	27% of calories
Protein	18% of calories
Saturated fat	6% of calories
Cholesterol	150 mg
Fiber	30 g
Sodium	1500 mg
Potassium	4700 mg
Calcium	1250 mg
Magnesium	500 mg

DASH Dietary Approaches to Stop Hypertension
Based on a 2100-calorie eating plan
(Adapted from: US Department of Health and Human Services. Your guide to lowering your blood pressure with DASH. NIH publication no. 06-408. 2006. http://www.nhlbi.nih.gov/health/public/heart/hbp/dash/new_dash.pdf. Accessed June 22, 2011) [42]

Members of the task force provided data, culturally meaningful information, and expert opinion to guide algorithm development. During a meeting in New York City on November 12 to 13, 2010, members discussed clinical evidence and the influence of various diabetes risk factors and comorbidities (cardiovascular events, obesity, hypertension, and dyslipidemia) in the construction of the tDNA template. Task force members also deliberated over the relative merits of specific metrics (body weight, waist-to-hip ratio [WHR], fasting blood glucose, and glycosylated hemoglobin [HbA1c]) and nutritional therapies (foods, diets, and calorie supplementation and replacement with prepared diabetes-specific formulas) that would be cited in the template. Diabetes-specific formulas (glycemia-targeted specialized nutrition formulas) may be used for calorie replacement or supplementation as part of medical nutrition therapy (MNT). Transcultural factors influencing dietary practices, food choices, and diabetes health care interventions were also considered. For example, energy-dense fast foods are ubiquitous but may take different forms throughout the world. Likewise, healthy foods take different forms based on geography and seasonality. Table 8 lists common international foods and their glycemic indices [44]. Such information becomes essential at the local level to make nutritional therapy meaningful.

TABLE 8: Common international foods and glycemic indices

Carbohydrate foods	Glycemic index		Glycemic index
Common foods		Fruits	
White wheat bread	75	Apple	36
Whole wheat bread	74	Banana	51
Multigrain bread	53	Dates	42
Wheat roti	62	Mango	51
Chapati	52	Orange	43
Corn tortilla	46	Peaches	43
White rice	73	Pineapple	59
Brown rice	68	Watermelon	76
Barley	28	Vegetables	
Corn	52	Potato, boiled	78
Spaghetti	49	Potato, instant mash	87
Rice noodles	53	Potato, fried	63
Udon noodles	55	Sweet potato	63
Couscous	65	Carrots, boiled	39
Dairy products		Pumpkin, boiled	64
Whole milk	39	Plantain	55
Skim milk	37	Taro, boiled	53
Soy milk	37	Vegetable soup	48
Rice milk	86	Legumes	
Ice cream	51	Chickpeas	28
Yogurt	41	Kidney beans	24
Cereals		Lentils	32
Cornflakes	81	Soy beans	16

TABLE 8: *Cont.*

Carbohydrate foods	Glycemic index		Glycemic index
Rolled oat meal	55	Snacks	
Instant oat meal	79	Chocolate	40
Rice congee	78	Popcorn	65
Muesli	57	Potato chips	56
Millet porridge	67	Soda	59
Biscuits	69	Rice crackers	87

Glycemic index (GI) ranks carbohydrates according to their effect on blood glucose levels. High GI = ≥70; medium GI = 56–69; low GI = ≤55
(Adapted from: Atkinson FS, Foster-Powell K, Brand-Miller JC. International tables of glycemic index and glycemic load values: 2008. Diabetes Care. 2008;31:2281–3. 45. Baker R, Feder G. Clinical guidelines: where next? Int J Qual Health Care. 1997;9:399–404) [44]

The evidence supporting task force recommendations was rated and assigned a numerical descriptor according to levels of scientific substantiation provided by the 2010 AACE protocol for the development of CPGs (Table 9) [21••]. The cumulative information was then codified using an alphabetic descriptor (grade A, B, C, D), reflecting the respective strength of the recommendation [21••]. The data and information used to construct the algorithm, as well as the included recommendations, closely reflect similar information and grading found in the diabetes nutrition sections of the AACE [15••, 43] and ADA [41••] CPGs.

Following the initial task force meeting, a subcommittee reviewed a meeting transcript to adopt points of agreement and resolve points of disagreement to achieve consensus on all major topics of discussion. Subsequently, all task force members received abstract summaries of the proceedings for their review and subsequent modification or approval. Consensus recommendations were discussed at a second task force meeting held on June 17 to 18, 2011 in New York City. At that time, recommendations were critiqued, refined, and prepared for transcultural adaptation by an expanded task force team that included additional experts from Canada, India, and Spain.

TABLE 9: Levels of substantiation and their respective numerical and semantic descriptors

Level of evidence	Study design or information type
1	RCTs
1	Meta-analyses of RCTs
2	Nonrandomized RCTs
2	Meta-analyses of nonrandomized RCTs
2	Prospective cohort studies
2	Retrospective case–control studies
3	Cross-sectional study
3	Surveillance study
3	Consecutive case series
3	Single case report
4	Expert consensus
4	Expert opinion based on experience
4	Theory-driven conclusions
4	Experience-based information
4	Review

RCT randomized controlled trial
(Adapted from: Mechanick JI, Camacho PM, Cobin RH, et al. American Association of Clinical Endocrinologists Protocol for Standardized Production of Clinical Practice Guidelines—2010 update. Endocr Pract. 2010;16:270–83) [21••]

12.6 TRANSCULTURALIZATION STANDARDS

The transculturalization of CPGs addresses problems that arise when recommendations are considered for implementation in an environment beyond that of the sponsoring individuals or organization [45]. In regard to nutrition therapy, transcultural factors relate to genetic differences within a given population, food preferences, religious practices, socioeconomic status, and others. Attributes of the transculturalization process should include evidence-based methodology, scientific rigor, transparency, relevance, and authority commensurate with the original CPGs [30, 46–50]. To obtain the cooperation and acceptance of key regional stakeholders in the implementation of the CPGs, their participation in the transculturalization process is essential. Likewise, a mechanism to have regional experts train local stakeholders and then continue the iterative process is vital, along with a validation and evaluation process to further modify the CPGs, if needed [50, 51]. To accommodate patient opinion and choice, subjective patient preferences for health care interventions that are locally available should be considered [52–54], as well as cascades of alternative strategies for a specific action [55, 56] and patient aids to inform their decisions [53].

12.7 TRANSCULTURALIZATION OF THE DIABETES-SPECIFIC NUTRITION ALGORITHM

On July 8, 2011, clinical experts from the Philippines, Hong Kong, Indonesia, Malaysia, Taiwan, Singapore, and Thailand met in Taipei, Taiwan to learn about the tDNA and begin the process of adapting the algorithm to their territories. This transcultural group was composed of endocrinologists, dietitians, and primary care practitioners who represented the health care specialties serving the patient populations that were targeted for the adaptive process. During the meeting, participants received information on diabetes and lifestyle modification, nutrition therapy and related clinical outcomes, and tDNA program goals and objectives. A point-by-point review of the algorithm was undertaken to explore pathways, content, and supportive evidence and to elicit information for the cultural adaptation of the algorithm and related recommendations for Southeast Asian patients. Subcommittee meetings were subsequently held in Taiwan (July 18, 2011) and India (September 23, 2011) to explicitly populate the nodes of the algorithm and the cells of the calorie supplement/replacement matrix (Table 5) with specific transcultural information and recommendations for their respective regions. Companion articles in this issue of Current Diabetes Reports describe the adaptive process and related output [57, 58].

12.8 RESULTS

An amalgam of the deliberations and conclusions of the expanded international task force is presented here, displaying the consensus composite template of the tDNA, which is being used in the transculturalization process. Adaptations will be considered in ongoing regional meetings until provincial versions of the algorithm are available for local implementation and validation throughout the world.

12.8.1 R1

Diets, meals, and foods influence glycemic status and the risk of diabetic complications (grade A) [16, 59–61].

12.8.2 R2

MNT is important and should be implemented as an essential component of comprehensive management programs for all patients with T2D and prediabetes (grade A) [41••, 43, 62–67].

12.8.3 R3

Diets should be based on individual risk factors for impaired glucose tolerance, obesity, hypertension, and dyslipidemia (grade A) [64, 65, 67, 68].

12.8.4 R4

Cultural factors should guide the selection of local foods and meals to adhere with general nutrition recommendations from the AACE and ADA (grade D) [1, 41••, 43].

12.8.5 R5

Diabetes-specific formulas may be used for calorie replacement or supplementation as part of MNT (grade A) [41••, 43, 69•, 70, 71]. Prepared and packaged diabetes-specific formulas contain nutrients that are designed to facilitate glycemic control [69•]. Such nutrients include modified malto-dextrin, fructose, fiber, soy protein, monounsaturated fatty acids, and antioxidants. Clinical studies have demonstrated improvements in glycemic profiles and reductions in disease complications among patients who consume prepared formula products as part of MNT. For patients with low body mass index (BMI) and/or insufficiency states, such as the elderly, caloric supplementation is helpful for weight gain, amelioration of nutritional deficiencies, and prevention of diabetic complications [69•, 72–75]. For patients with normal or elevated BMI, caloric replacement is helpful to achieve weight loss, greater metabolic control, and avoidance of subtle deficits of vitamins or other nutrients that can accompany simple calorie restriction [69•]. Intensification or reduction in the number of replacements and supplements is a stepped process based on clinical appraisals and modification of regimens to meet individual patient goals [73].

12.8.6 R6

Geographic location and ethnocultural classifications should be used to tailor the algorithm for specific patient populations. Risk factors are the leading determinants of patient pathways and related recommendations; one or more risk factors identify patients who are more likely to experience disease progression and/or complications (grade A) [75–77]. Dietary modification can mitigate the following risk factors: T2D or prediabetes, excessive weight or obesity, hypertension, and dyslipidemia (grade A) [64, 65, 67].

12.8.7 R7

Anthropometric measures—BMI, waist circumference (WC), or WHR—should be used to assess body composition and risk of progression [41••]. Although each of these measures has merit in clinical practice, differences in values and interpretations arising from phenotypic and cultural differences among populations have confounded global standardization.

Likewise, difficulty using some methods (eg, WHR) has created regional preferences in medical practice and influenced general recommendations. Consequently, BMI and WC were chosen as the preferred prioritized measures of body composition in the algorithm. Values for normal and abnormal composition can be adjusted via ethnocultural inputs for local applicability (grade B) [78, 79].

12.8.8 R8

Irrespective of patient risk factors, lifestyle intervention mandates professional counseling, physical activity, and healthy eating patterns consistent with current CPGs or evidence (grade A) [41••, 43]. Professional counseling may be impeded by local attitudes and costs as well as the lack of perceived value by patients who may be economically disadvantaged. Although both low-risk and high-risk patients should comply with these basic recommendations, high-risk patients should intensify their efforts according to their specific needs and conditions.

12.8.9 R9

A registered dietitian (RD) who is familiar with the components of MNT should be involved in patient management (grade B) [41••]. Long-term changes in behavior are difficult to achieve for many patients. To assist implementation, physicians should encourage and support patients through the behavior modification process. However, physicians are limited by time and experience in behavior modification techniques. Therefore, the use of other health care professionals with expertise in patient self-management may be necessary. Research has shown that lifestyle case management by RDs can improve health outcomes among patients with T2D [80, 81•, 82]. In cultures and regions (e.g., Hong Kong) where patients may oppose or decline nutrition consultation by health care providers who are not physicians, we encourage physicians to develop skills in nutrition medicine by participating in appropriate continuing medical education.

12.8.10 R10

Patients should be encouraged to lead an active lifestyle and avoid seden-tary living, as physical activity and exercise independently confer health benefits and facilitate glycemic control (grade A) [35, 83–85]. Substantial benefit is achieved with ≥150 min per week of moderate activity or ≥75 min per week of vigorous aerobic activity [83–86]. Resistance exercise training, as a separate modality from aerobic exercise, can increase muscle mass and improve glycemic control and should be combined with aerobic activity (grade D) [87]. Additional time spent on any physical activity can augment benefit and represents an intensification strategy for patients with higher risk stratification or those who do not achieve their goals with less intense activity.

12.8.11 R11

MNT was introduced in 1994 by the American Dietetic Association to better express the concept of therapeutic nutrition [65, 88]. It consists of specific nutritional interventions that include assessment, counseling, and dietary modification, with and without specialized nutritional formulas for calorie supplementation or replacement [65]. Diabetes-specific MNT has been considered a cornerstone of diabetes treatment because it can im-prove glycemic profiles and reduce the risk of disease complications [65, 67, 89]. Formalized recommendations for T2D in the medical literature include the following: carbohydrates, preferentially from low-glycemic index foods, for 45% to 65% of daily energy intake and not less than 130 g/day in patients on low-calorie diets (grade D) [41••, 43, 90, 91]; fats for less than 30% of daily energy intake (grade D) [41••, 43, 90]; saturated fat for less than 7% of daily energy intake (grade A) [41••, 43, 90, 92]; pro-tein for 15% to 20% of energy intake and not less than 1 g/kg in patients with normal kidney function (grade D) [41••, 43]; cholesterol restricted to less than 200 mg daily (grade A) [41, 43, 90, 92]; trans fats eliminated or reduced to minimal intake (grade D) [41••, 43, 90, 92]; and fiber for 25 to 50 g daily (grade A) [41••, 43, 90].

12.8.12 R12

Overweight or obese patients should adhere to these guidelines and try to achieve a gradual weight loss of 5% to 10% by reducing caloric intake, for a total daily deficit of 250 to 1000 kcal (grade A) [15••, 16, 17, 41••, 43, 70, 93, 94]. Patients with class 3 obesity should shed 15% of body weight (grade D) [15••, 16, 17, 41••, 43, 70, 93, 94]. BMI should be decreased by 2 to 3 units (grade D) [41••, 43, 70, 93, 94]. Any amount of weight loss is associated with metabolic benefits, even if clinical targets are not met.

12.8.13 R13

Bariatric surgery may be considered for patients with T2D and obesity who 1) fail to respond to lifestyle and pharmacologic interventions; 2) meet established criteria related to body composition, comorbidities, and surgical risk; and 3) commit to durable lifestyle changes and follow-up evaluations [95–98]. The recent statement by the International Diabetes Federation on criteria for bariatric surgery should be considered when making treatment decisions [39].

12.8.14 R14

Patients with T2D or prediabetes complicated by hypertension require further nutritional management. Sodium intake should already be limited to 1,500 mg/day per recent recommendations provided by the Dietary Guidelines for Americans, 2010 (grade A) [99–102, 103•, 104]. The principles of the Dietary Approaches to Stop Hypertension (DASH) diet, particularly increasing the consumption of fresh fruits and vegetables, should also be incorporated into the patient's diet.

12.8.15 R15

Patients with lipid abnormalities must pay closer attention to fat intake based on their dyslipidemic profiles and may benefit from viscous fibers and plant sterols (grade A) [91, 92, 105–111]. The reduction of simple sugars and alcohol is important for patients with hypertriglyceridemia.

12.8.16 R16

When multiple comorbidities exist in a patient with T2D or prediabetes, recommended interventions are applied simultaneously and at a higher level of intensity, but individual patient factors, such as potential for adherence, adverse effects, and dietary customs and practices, are also taken into account (grade D).

12.8.17 R17

Follow-up evaluations for all patients should occur at appropriate intervals depending on need (grade D). Assessments should include a history and physical examination (anthropometrics, blood pressure); blood chemistries (glucose, HbA1c, lipids, renal function, and liver enzymes depending on clinical status); and urinary microalbumin determination. Improvements in disease states based on follow-up assessments create an opportunity to diminish the intensity of interventions and to spare resources. Although deterioration of clinical status creates a need to increase the intensity of interventions, it also creates an opportunity to search for ways to improve care and possibly adherence.

12.9 DISCUSSION

Within North America, the national prevalence of diabetes and prediabetes ranges from 10.1% in Mexico to 11.6% in Canada and 12.3% in the United States [1]. The global prevalence is significantly lower, at 6.6%, but rates in the Arab countries are much higher at 13.4% (Oman) to 18.7% (United Arab Emirates) [1]. These figures reflect accurate estimates of the size of affected populations, but do not convey the complexities that underlie the epidemiology of the disease. Hidden behind these numbers are the details that illuminate the nature of the problem. Today, societies are heterogeneous not only in North America, but in many other places around the world. Continents, countries, states, municipalities, and even neighborhoods can be characterized by ethnicity, customs, mores, habits, and beliefs. All of these demographics influence personal choices that contribute to health or illness and the prevention or development and perpetuation of diabetes.

Health care providers must understand the culture of diabetes to effectively manage their patients with diabetes. Although general cultural sensitivity training is offered in medical school and through postgraduate activities, most practitioners are woefully deficient in the knowledge and skill to maneuver medically through the intricacies of a diverse patient population [112–115]. Clinical guidance rarely cites the cultural differences that truly matter in the delivery of health care. This may be especially true—and particularly important—with respect to diabetes, a disease that is intimately associated with lifestyles and foods. For these reasons, the international task force sought to identify and incorporate regional differences in genetic factors, diet, exercise, and culture into CPGs for nutrition therapy in T2D and prediabetes.

For example, based on clinical evidence, it was abundantly clear to the task force members that a principal cause of obesity and diabetes was the consumption of energy-rich or fast foods. Such foods are characterized by high concentrations of fats and refined carbohydrates with high glycemic indices. Describing foods in terms of composition, however, may limit comprehension and corrective action. Instead, citing examples that are culturally meaningful (e.g., fried white rice with pork drippings or quarter-pound cheeseburgers with french fries and soda) may be more relevant.

Assessing an individual for diabetes risk seems relatively straightforward until one realizes that Southeast Asians tend to develop the disease at a younger age and lower BMI. Disease management in Southeast Asian patients is also complicated by a greater prominence of postprandial hyperglycemia and renal complications.

Economics and education affect the likelihood that a health care intervention, regardless of its benefit, will be adopted and faithfully used by a particular segment of society. Task force members noted that the acceptance of dietitians or nutrition counselors, for instance, is low in Southeast Asia because the importance of such individuals is probably undervalued or misunderstood, not only by patients but occasionally by physicians, too. The cost and relative inaccessibility of these allied professionals may impede their participation in health care, especially when community resources are not available for targeted education. Moreover, broader education in the form of CPGs for comprehensive care of patients with diabetes as well as specific lifestyle interventions are needed worldwide, but guidance comes mostly from developed countries, especially Europe and North America, where interpretation of sophisticated recommendations is easier than in developing non-English-speaking nations. Couple this problem to a lack of familiarity with nutrition therapy in general and prepared liquid formulas in particular, and the likelihood of effective nutrition management is greatly reduced

In response to these problems, we developed the tDNA. It has four major strengths: 1) simplicity that fosters not only an understanding of diabetes-specific nutrition therapy but also the cultural adaptation necessary for worldwide implementation; 2) incorporation of advice from national and international associations and respected publications; 3) inclusion of important clinical evidence and experience from multinational health care stakeholders who contributed to the developmental process; 4) openness to scientific and cultural adaptation.

Dietary and culinary habits within many diverse global communities must still be identified, and guidance must be further tailored along ethnic and cultural lines. To reach this end point within the tDNA program, diabetes and nutrition experts from around the world continue to be organized, familiarized with program goals, and invited to contribute to the transculturalization process. Adapted versions of the algorithm have already emerged for Southeast Asian and Asian Indian populations [57, 58]. Implementation will require education initiatives and follow-up assessments to determine if clinical benefit is truly achieved. These activities are currently being planned within the tDNA program. If found to be successful in optimizing comprehensive diabetes care, the tDNA and related educational resources will be made available for widespread dissemination and worldwide implementation.

12.10 CONCLUSIONS

The algorithm presented here incorporates established standards used for CPG development, adaptation, and implementation. It is comprehensive and authoritative, yet brief and easy to use. Importantly, it is designed for simplicity and global cultural adaptation, or transculturalization. In large part, it conveys established clinical guidance from highly respected organizations for nutrition therapy and lifestyle management. It also references calorie augmentation or replacement with diabetes-specific liquid meals, a relatively novel addition to traditional nutrition therapy. It remains open to modification of content and context.

REFERENCES

Papers of particular interest, published recently, have been highlighted as: • Of importance •• Of major importance

1. IDF diabetes atlas. 4. Brussels: International Diabetes Federation; 2009.
2. The effect of intensive treatment of diabetes on the development and progression of long-term complications in insulin-dependent diabetes mellitus. The Diabetes Control and Complications Trial Research Group. N Engl J Med. 1993;329:977–86.
3. Intensive blood-glucose control with sulphonylureas or insulin compared with conventional treatment and risk of complications in patients with type 2 diabetes (UKPDS 33). UK Prospective Diabetes Study (UKPDS) Group. Lancet. 1998;352:837–53.

4. Effect of intensive therapy on the microvascular complications of type 1 diabetes mellitus. JAMA. 2002;287:2563–9.

5. Charlton-Menys V, Betteridge DJ, Colhoun H, et al. Targets of statin therapy: LDL cholesterol, non-HDL cholesterol, and apolipoprotein B in type 2 diabetes in the Collaborative Atorvastatin Diabetes Study (CARDS) Clin Chem. 2009;55:473–80. doi: 10.1373/clinchem.2008.111401.

6. Daly CA, Fox KM, Remme WJ, et al. The effect of perindopril on cardiovascular morbidity and mortality in patients with diabetes in the EUROPA study: results from the PERSUADE substudy. Eur Heart J. 2005;26:1369–78. doi: 10.1093/eurheartj/ehi225.

7. Esposito K, Giugliano D, Nappo F, Marfella R. Regression of carotid atherosclerosis by control of postprandial hyperglycemia in type 2 diabetes mellitus. Circulation. 2004;110:214–9. doi: 10.1161/01.CIR.0000134501.57864.66.

8. Hansson L, Zanchetti A, Carruthers SG, et al. Effects of intensive blood-pressure lowering and low-dose aspirin in patients with hypertension: principal results of the Hypertension Optimal Treatment (HOT) randomised trial. HOT study group. Lancet. 1998;351:1755–62. doi: 10.1016/S0140-6736(98)04311-6.

9. Nathan DM, Cleary PA, Backlund JY, et al. Intensive diabetes treatment and cardiovascular disease in patients with type 1 diabetes. N Engl J Med. 2005;353:2643–53. doi: 10.1056/NEJMoa052187.

10. Neil HA, DeMicco DA, Luo D, et al. Analysis of efficacy and safety in patients aged 65–75 years at randomization: Collaborative Atorvastatin Diabetes Study (CARDS) Diabetes Care. 2006;29:2378–84. doi: 10.2337/dc06-0872.

11. Newman CB, Szarek M, Colhoun HM, et al. The safety and tolerability of atorvastatin 10 mg in the Collaborative Atorvastatin Diabetes Study (CARDS) Diabetes Vasc Dis Res. 2008;5:177–83. doi: 10.3132/dvdr.2008.029.

12. Ohkubo Y, Kishikawa H, Araki E, et al. Intensive insulin therapy prevents the progression of diabetic microvascular complications in Japanese patients with non-insulin-dependent diabetes mellitus: a randomized prospective 6-year study. Diabetes Res Clin Pract. 1995;28:103–17. doi: 10.1016/0168-8227(95)01064-K.

13. Stratton IM, Adler AI, Neil HA, et al. Association of glycaemia with macrovascular and microvascular complications of type 2 diabetes (UKPDS 35): prospective observational study. BMJ. 2000;321:405–12. doi: 10.1136/bmj.321.7258.405.

14. Turnbull F, Neal B, Ninomiya T, et al. Effects of different regimens to lower blood pressure on major cardiovascular events in older and younger adults: meta-analysis of randomised trials. BMJ. 2008;336:1121–3. doi: 10.1136/bmj.39548.738368.BE.

15. Handelsman Y, Mechanick JI, Blonde L, et al. American Association of Clinical Endocrinologists Medical Guidelines for Clinical Practice for developing a diabetes mellitus comprehensive care plan. Endocr Pract. 2011;17(Suppl 2):1–53.

16. Knowler WC, Barrett-Connor E, Fowler SE, et al. Reduction in the incidence of type 2 diabetes with lifestyle intervention or metformin. N Engl J Med. 2002;346:393–403. doi: 10.1056/NEJMoa012512.

17. Tuomilehto J, Lindstrom J, Eriksson JG, et al. Prevention of type 2 diabetes mellitus by changes in lifestyle among subjects with impaired glucose tolerance. N Engl J Med. 2001;344:1343–50. doi: 10.1056/NEJM200105033441801.

18. Scalzitti DA. Evidence-based guidelines: application to clinical practice. Phys Ther. 2001;81:1622–8.

19. Woolf SH, Grol R, Hutchinson A, et al. Clinical guidelines: potential benefits, limitations, and harms of clinical guidelines. BMJ. 1999;318:527–30. doi: 10.1136/bmj.318.7182.527.

20. Grol R, Dalhuijsen J, Thomas S, et al. Attributes of clinical guidelines that influence use of guidelines in general practice: observational study. BMJ. 1998;317:858–61. doi: 10.1136/bmj.317.7162.858.

21. Mechanick JI, Camacho PM, Cobin RH, et al. American Association of Clinical Endocrinologists protocol for standardized production of clinical practice guidelines–2010 update. Endocr Pract. 2010;16:270–83.

22. Burgers JS, Cluzeau FA, Hanna SE, et al. Characteristics of high-quality guidelines: evaluation of 86 clinical guidelines developed in ten European countries and Canada. Int J Technol Assess Health Care. 2003;19:148–57. doi: 10.1017/S026646230300014X.

23. Field MJ, Lohr KN. Guidelines for clinical practice: from development to use. Washington, D.C: Institute of Medicine, National Academy Press; 1992.

24. Shapiro DW, Lasker RD, Bindman AB, Lee PR. Containing costs while improving quality of care: the role of profiling and practice guidelines. Annu Rev Public Health. 1993;14:219–41. doi: 10.1146/annurev.pu.14.050193.001251.

25. Thomson R, Lavender M, Madhok R. How to ensure that guidelines are effective. BMJ. 1995;311:237–42. doi: 10.1136/bmj.311.6999.237.

26. Wollersheim H, Burgers J, Grol R. Clinical guidelines to improve patient care. Neth J Med. 2005;63:188–92.

27. Feder G, Eccles M, Grol R, et al. Clinical guidelines: using clinical guidelines. BMJ. 1999;318:728–30. doi: 10.1136/bmj.318.7185.728.

28. Davis DA, Taylor-Vaisey A. Translating guidelines into practice. A systematic review of theoretic concepts, practical experience and research evidence in the adoption of clinical practice guidelines. CMAJ. 1997;157:408–16.

29. Beller SE, Monatesti SJ. Problems with current practice guidelines and quality improvement (QI) programs and how to solve them. http://wellness.wikispaces.com/Problems+with+Current+Practice+Guidelines+and+Quality+Improvement+%28QI%29+Programs+and+How+to+Solve+Them. Accessed November 14 2011.

30. Fervers B, Burgers JS, Haugh MC, et al. Adaptation of clinical guidelines: literature review and proposition for a framework and procedure. Int J Qual Health Care. 2006;18:167–76. doi: 10.1093/intqhc/mzi108.

31. Cook R. Clinical algorithms and flow charts as representations of guideline knowledge. 2005. http://www.hinz.org.nz/journal/2005/09/Clinical-Algorithms-and-Flow-Charts-as-Representations-of-Guideline-Knowledge/923. Accessed October 17 2011.

32. Shiffman RN. Representation of clinical practice guidelines in conventional and augmented decision tables. J Am Med Inform Assoc. 1997;4:382–93. doi: 10.1136/jamia.1997.0040382.

33. Shiffman RN, Michel G, Essaihi A, Thornquist E. Bridging the guideline implementation gap: a systematic, document-centered approach to guideline implementation. J Am Med Inform Assoc. 2004;11:418–26. doi: 10.1197/jamia.M1444.

34. Hahn KA, Ferrante JM, Crosson JC, et al. Diabetes flow sheet use associated with guideline adherence. Ann Fam Med. 2008;6:235–8. doi: 10.1370/afm.812.

35. US Department of Health and Human Services. 2008 physical activity guidelines for Americans. 2008. http://www.health.gov/paguidelines/guidelines/summary.aspx. Accessed June 22, 2011.

36. Wildman RP, Gu D, Reynolds K, et al. Appropriate body mass index and waist circumference cutoffs for categorization of overweight and central adiposity among Chinese adults. Am J Clin Nutr. 2004;80:1129–36.

37. Appropriate body-mass index for Asian populations and its implications for policy and intervention strategies. WHO Expert Consultation. Lancet. 2004;363:157–63.

38. Weight-control Information Network—an information service of the National Institute of Diabetes and Digestive and Kidney Diseases (NIDDK). Bariatric surgery for severe obesity. 2009. http://win.niddk.nih.gov/publications/gastric.htm. Accessed November 14, 2011.

39. International Diabetes Federation. Bariatric surgical procedures and interventions in the treatment of obese patients with type 2 diabetes: a position statement from the International Diabetes Federation Taskforce on Epidemiology and Prevention. http://www.idf.org/webdata/docs/IDF-Position-Statement-Bariatric-Surgery.pdf. Accessed June 27, 2011.

40. National Guideline Clearinghouse. Guideline synthesis: nutritional management of diabetes mellitus. 2009. http://www.guideline.gov.syntheses/synthesis.aspx?id+16430. Accessed June 22, 2011.

41. Bantle JP, Wylie-Rosett J, Albright AL, et al. Nutrition recommendations and interventions for diabetes: a position statement of the American Diabetes Association. Diabetes Care. 2008;31(Suppl 1):S61–78.

42. US Department of Health and Human Services. Your guide to lowering your blood pressure with DASH. NIH publication no. 06-408. 2006. http://www.nhlbi.nih.gov/health/public/heart/hbp/dash/new_dash.pdf. Accessed June 22, 2011.

43. Rodbard HW, Blonde L, Braithwaite SS, et al. American Association of Clinical Endocrinologists medical guidelines for clinical practice for the management of diabetes mellitus. Endocr Pract. 2007;13(Suppl 1):1–68.

44. Atkinson FS, Foster-Powell K, Brand-Miller JC. International tables of glycemic index and glycemic load values: 2008. Diabetes Care. 2008;31:2281–3. doi: 10.2337/dc08-1239.

45. Baker R, Feder G. Clinical guidelines: where next? Int J Qual Health Care. 1997;9:399–404.

46. Development and validation of an international appraisal instrument for assessing the quality of clinical practice guidelines: the AGREE project. AGREE Collaboration. Qual Saf Health Care. 2003;12:18–23.

47. Graham ID, Harrison MB, Brouwers M. Evaluating and adapting practice guidelines for local use: a conceptual framework. In: Pickering S, Thompson J, editors. Clinical governance in practice. London: Harcourt; 2003. pp. 213–29.

48. Graham ID, Harrison MB, Brouwers M, et al. Facilitating the use of evidence in practice: evaluating and adapting clinical practice guidelines for local use by health care organizations. J Obstet Gynecol Neonatal Nurs. 2002;31:599–611. doi: 10.1111/j.1552-6909.2002.tb00086.x.

49. Atkins D, Best D, Briss PA, et al. Grading quality of evidence and strength of recommendations. BMJ. 2004;328:1490. doi: 10.1136/bmj.328.7454.1490.

50. Fretheim A, Schunemann HJ, Oxman AD. Improving the use of research evidence in guideline development: 3. Group composition and consultation process. Health Res Pol Syst. 2006;4:15. doi: 10.1186/1478-4505-4-15.

51. Harrison MB, Graham ID, Lorimer K, et al. Nurse clinic versus home delivery of evidence-based community leg ulcer care: a randomized health services trial. BMC Health Serv Res. 2008;8:243. doi: 10.1186/1472-6963-8-243.

52. Chong C, Chen I, Naglie C, Krahn M. Do clinical practice guidelines incorporate evidence on patient preferences? Med Decis Making. 2007;27:E63–4.

53. Weijden T, Legare F, Boivin A, et al. How to integrate individual patient values and preferences in clinical practice guidelines? A research protocol. Implement Sci. 2010;5:10. doi: 10.1186/1748-5908-5-10.

54. Schunemann HJ, Fretheim A, Oxman AD. Improving the use of research evidence in guideline development: 10 Integrating values and consumer involvement. Health Res Pol Syst. 2006;4:22. doi: 10.1186/1478-4505-4-22.

55. Oppenheim PI, Sotiropoulos G, Baraff LJ. Incorporating patient preferences into practice guidelines: management of children with fever without source. Ann Emerg Med. 1994;24:836–41. doi: 10.1016/S0196-0644(94)70201-2.

56. Latoszek-Berendsen A, Talmon J, Clercq P, Hasman A. With good intentions. Int J Med Inform. 2007;76(Suppl 3):S440–6. doi: 10.1016/j.ijmedinf.2007.05.012.

57. Su H-Y, Tsang M-W, Huang S-Y, et al. Transculturalization of a diabetes-specific nutrition algorithm: Asian application. Curr Diab Rep. 2012, in press.

58. Joshi SR, Mohan V, Joshi SS, et al. Transcultural diabetes nutrition therapy algorithm: the Asian Indian application. Curr Diab Rep. 2012, in press.

59. Lindstrom J, Louheranta A, Mannelin M, et al. The Finnish Diabetes Prevention Study (DPS): lifestyle intervention and 3-year results on diet and physical activity. Diabetes Care. 2003;26:3230–6. doi: 10.2337/diacare.26.12.3230.

60. Ratner R, Goldberg R, Haffner S, et al. Impact of intensive lifestyle and metformin therapy on cardiovascular disease risk factors in the diabetes prevention program. Diabetes Care. 2005;28:888–94. doi: 10.2337/diacare.28.4.888.

61. Gillies CL, Abrams KR, Lambert PC, et al. Pharmacological and lifestyle interventions to prevent or delay type 2 diabetes in people with impaired glucose tolerance: systematic review and meta-analysis. BMJ. 2007;334:299. doi: 10.1136/bmj.39063.689375.55.

62. Fung TT, Rimm EB, Spiegelman D, et al. Association between dietary patterns and plasma biomarkers of obesity and cardiovascular disease risk. Am J Clin Nutr. 2001;73:61–7.

63. Liu E, McKeown NM, Newby PK, et al. Cross-sectional association of dietary patterns with insulin-resistant phenotypes among adults without diabetes in the Framingham Offspring Study. Br J Nutr. 2009;102:576–83. doi: 10.1017/S0007114509220836.

64. Yu-Poth S, Zhao G, Etherton T, et al. Effects of the National Cholesterol Education Program's Step I and Step II dietary intervention programs on cardiovascular disease risk factors: a meta-analysis. Am J Clin Nutr. 1999;69:632–46.

65. Pastors JG, Warshaw H, Daly A, et al. The evidence for the effectiveness of medical nutrition therapy in diabetes management. Diabetes Care. 2002;25:608–13. doi: 10.2337/diacare.25.3.608.

66. Imamura F, Lichtenstein AH, Dallal GE, et al. Generalizability of dietary patterns associated with incidence of type 2 diabetes mellitus. Am J Clin Nutr. 2009;90:1075–83. doi: 10.3945/ajcn.2009.28009.

67. Pastors JG, Franz MJ, Warshaw H, et al. How effective is medical nutrition therapy in diabetes care? J Am Diet Assoc. 2003;103:827–31. doi: 10.1016/S0002-8223(03)00466-8.

68. Turner RC, Millns H, Neil HA, et al. Risk factors for coronary artery disease in non-insulin dependent diabetes mellitus: United Kingdom Prospective Diabetes Study (UKPDS: 23) BMJ. 1998;316:823–8. doi: 10.1136/bmj.316.7134.823.

69. • Tatti P, di Mauro P, Neri M, et al. Effect of a low-calorie high-nutrition value formula on weight loss in type 2 diabetes mellitus. Mediterr J Nutr Metab. 2009; doi:10.1007/s12349-009-0050-7. This discusses evidence of the value of calorie replacement in the nutritional management of diabetes.

70. Elia M, Ceriello A, Laube H, et al. Enteral nutritional support and use of diabetes-specific formulas for patients with diabetes: a systematic review and meta-analysis. Diabetes Care. 2005;28:2267–79. doi: 10.2337/diacare.28.9.2267.

71. Livesey G, Taylor R, Hulshof T, Howlett J. Glycemic response and health–a systematic review and meta-analysis: relations between dietary glycemic properties and health outcomes. Am J Clin Nutr. 2008;87:258S–68S.

72. Clinical guidelines on the identification, evaluation, and treatment of overweight and obesity in adults—the evidence report. National Institutes of Health. Obes Res. 1998;6 Suppl 2:51S-209S.

73. Turnbull PJ, Sinclair AJ. Evaluation of nutritional status and its relationship with functional status in older citizens with diabetes mellitus using the mini nutritional assessment (MNA) tool–a preliminary investigation. J Nutr Health Aging. 2002;6:185–9.

74. Benbow SJ, Hoyte R, Gill GV. Institutional dietary provision for diabetic patients. QJM. 2001;94:27–30. doi: 10.1093/qjmed/94.1.27.

75. Bonadonna RC, Cucinotta D, Fedele D, et al. The metabolic syndrome is a risk indicator of microvascular and macrovascular complications in diabetes: results from Metascreen, a multicenter diabetes clinic-based survey. Diabetes Care. 2006;29:2701–7. doi: 10.2337/dc06-0942.

76. Goldberg IJ. Clinical review 124: Diabetic dyslipidemia: causes and consequences. J Clin Endocrinol Metab. 2001;86:965–71. doi: 10.1210/jc.86.3.965.

77. Grossman E, Meserli F. Hypertension and diabetes. In: Fisman EZ, Tenenbaum A, editors. Cardiovascular diabetology: clinical, metabolic and inflammatory facets. Basel: Karger; 2008. pp. 82–106.

78. Janiszewski PM, Janssen I, Ross R. Does waist circumference predict diabetes and cardiovascular disease beyond commonly evaluated cardiometabolic risk factors? Diabetes Care. 2007;30:3105–9. doi: 10.2337/dc07-0945.

79. Lukaski HC. Methods for the assessment of human body composition: traditional and new. Am J Clin Nutr. 1987;46:537–56.

80. Franz MJ, Monk A, Barry B, et al. Effectiveness of medical nutrition therapy provided by dietitians in the management of non-insulin-dependent diabetes mellitus: a randomized, controlled clinical trial. J Am Diet Assoc. 1995;95:1009–17. doi: 10.1016/S0002-8223(95)00276-6.

81. Huang MC, Hsu CC, Wang HS, Shin SJ. Prospective randomized controlled trial to evaluate effectiveness of registered dietitian-led diabetes management on glycemic and diet control in a primary care setting in Taiwan. Diabetes Care. 2010;33:233–9. doi: 10.2337/dc09-1092.

82. Wolf AM, Conaway MR, Crowther JQ, et al. Translating lifestyle intervention to practice in obese patients with type 2 diabetes: Improving Control with Activity and Nutrition (ICAN) study. Diabetes Care. 2004;27:1570–6. doi: 10.2337/diacare.27.7.1570.

83. Pan XR, Li GW, Hu YH, et al. Effects of diet and exercise in preventing NIDDM in people with impaired glucose tolerance. The Da Qing IGT and Diabetes Study. Diabetes Care. 1997;20:537–44. doi: 10.2337/diacare.20.4.537.

84. Boule NG, Haddad E, Kenny GP, et al. Effects of exercise on glycemic control and body mass in type 2 diabetes mellitus: a meta-analysis of controlled clinical trials. JAMA. 2001;286:1218–27. doi: 10.1001/jama.286.10.1218.

85. Nelson ME, Rejeski WJ, Blair SN, et al. Physical activity and public health in older adults: recommendation from the American College of Sports Medicine and the American Heart Association. Med Sci Sports Exerc. 2007;39:1435–45. doi: 10.1249/mss.0b013e3180616aa2.

86. Albright A, Franz M, Hornsby G, et al. American College of Sports Medicine position stand. Exercise and type 2 diabetes. Med Sci Sports Exerc. 2000;32:1345–60. doi: 10.1097/00005768-200007000-00024.

87. Villareal DT, Apovian CM, Kushner RF, Klein S. Obesity in older adults: technical review and position statement of the American Society for Nutrition and NAASO, The Obesity Society. Am J Clin Nutr. 2005;82:923–34.

88. Identifying patients at risk: ADA's definitions for nutrition screening and nutrition assessment. Council on Practice (COP) Quality Management Committee. J Am Diet Assoc. 1994;94:838–9.

89. Mann JI, Leeuw I, Hermansen K, et al. Evidence-based nutritional approaches to the treatment and prevention of diabetes mellitus. Nutr Metab Cardiovasc Dis. 2004;14:373–94. doi: 10.1016/S0939-4753(04)80028-0.

90. Anderson JW, Randles KM, Kendall CW, Jenkins DJ. Carbohydrate and fiber recommendations for individuals with diabetes: a quantitative assessment and meta-analysis of the evidence. J Am Coll Nutr. 2004;23:5–17.

91. Jenkins DJ, Kendall CW, McKeown-Eyssen G, et al. Effect of a low-glycemic index or a high-cereal fiber diet on type 2 diabetes: a randomized trial. JAMA. 2008;300:2742–53. doi: 10.1001/jama.2008.808.

92. Third Report of the National Cholesterol Education Program (NCEP) expert panel on detection, evaluation, and treatment of high blood cholesterol in adults (Adult Treatment Panel III) final report. Circulation. 2002;106:3143–421.

93. Caterson ID. Medical management of obesity and its complications. Ann Acad Med Singapore. 2009;38:22–7.

94. Klein S, Sheard NF, Pi-Sunyer X, et al. Weight management through lifestyle modification for the prevention and management of type 2 diabetes: rationale and strategies: a statement of the American Diabetes Association, the North American Association for the Study of Obesity, and the American Society for Clinical Nutrition. Diabetes Care. 2004;27:2067–73. doi: 10.2337/diacare.27.8.2067.

95. Dixon JB, O'Brien PE, Playfair J, et al. Adjustable gastric banding and conventional therapy for type 2 diabetes: a randomized controlled trial. JAMA. 2008;299:316–23. doi: 10.1001/jama.299.3.316.

96. Mechanick JI, Kushner RF, Sugerman HJ, et al. American Association of Clinical Endocrinologists, The Obesity Society, and American Society for Metabolic & Bariatric Surgery Medical guidelines for clinical practice for the perioperative nutritional, metabolic, and nonsurgical support of the bariatric surgery patient. Endocr Pract. 2008;14(Suppl 1):1–83.

97. Brolin RE. Bariatric surgery and long-term control of morbid obesity. JAMA. 2002;288:2793–6. doi: 10.1001/jama.288.22.2793.

98. Pinkney J, Kerrigan D. Current status of bariatric surgery in the treatment of type 2 diabetes. Obes Rev. 2004;5:69–78. doi: 10.1111/j.1467-789X.2004.00119.x.

99. Appel LJ, Moore TJ, Obarzanek E, et al. A clinical trial of the effects of dietary patterns on blood pressure. DASH Collaborative Research Group. N Engl J Med. 1997;336:1117–24. doi: 10.1056/NEJM199704173361601.

100. Appel LJ, Brands MW, Daniels SR, et al. Dietary approaches to prevent and treat hypertension: a scientific statement from the American Heart Association. Hypertension. 2006;47:296–308. doi: 10.1161/01.HYP.0000202568.01167.B6.

101. Dietary guidelines for Americans, 2010. 7. Washington, DC: US Government Printing Office; 2010.

102. Appel LJ, Sacks FM, Carey VJ, et al. Effects of protein, monounsaturated fat, and carbohydrate intake on blood pressure and serum lipids: results of the OmniHeart randomized trial. JAMA. 2005;294:2455–64. doi: 10.1001/jama.294.19.2455.

103. Blumenthal JA, Babyak MA, Sherwood A, et al. Effects of the dietary approaches to stop hypertension diet alone and in combination with exercise and caloric restriction on insulin sensitivity and lipids. Hypertension. 2010;55:1199–205. doi: 10.1161/HYPERTENSIONAHA.109.149153.

104. Sacks FM, Svetkey LP, Vollmer WM, et al. Effects on blood pressure of reduced dietary sodium and the Dietary Approaches to Stop Hypertension (DASH) diet. DASH-Sodium Collaborative Research Group. N Engl J Med. 2001;344:3–10. doi: 10.1056/NEJM200101043440101.

105. Levine GN, Keaney JF, Jr, Vita JA. Cholesterol reduction in cardiovascular disease. Clinical benefits and possible mechanisms. N Engl J Med. 1995;332:512–21. doi: 10.1056/NEJM199502233320807.

106. Superko HR, Krauss RM. Coronary artery disease regression. Convincing evidence for the benefit of aggressive lipoprotein management. Circulation. 1994;90:1056–69.

107. Jenkins DJ, Jones PJ, Lamarche B, et al. Effect of a dietary portfolio of cholesterol-lowering foods given at 2 levels of intensity of dietary advice on serum lipids in hyperlipidemia: a randomized controlled trial. JAMA. 2011;306:831–9. doi: 10.1001/jama.2011.1202.

108. Grundy SM, Cleeman JI, Merz CN, et al. Implications of recent clinical trials for the National Cholesterol Education Program Adult Treatment Panel III guidelines. Circulation. 2004;110:227–39. doi: 10.1161/01.CIR.0000133317.49796.0E.
109. Shepherd J, Cobbe SM, Ford I, et al. Prevention of coronary heart disease with pravastatin in men with hypercholesterolemia. West of Scotland Coronary Prevention Study Group. N Engl J Med. 1995;333:1301–7. doi: 10.1056/NEJM199511163332001.
110. Buse JB, Ginsberg HN, Bakris GL, et al. Primary prevention of cardiovascular diseases in people with diabetes mellitus: a scientific statement from the American Heart Association and the American Diabetes Association. Circulation. 2007;115:114–26. doi: 10.1161/CIRCULATIONAHA.106.179294.
111. Randomised trial of cholesterol lowering in 4444 patients with coronary heart disease: the Scandinavian Simvastatin Survival Study (4S). Lancet. 1994;344:1383–9.
112. Carrillo JE, Green AR, Betancourt JR. Cross-cultural primary care: a patient-based approach. Ann Intern Med. 1999;130:829–34.
113. Culhane-Pera KA, Reif C, Egli E, et al. A curriculum for multicultural education in family medicine. Fam Med. 1997;29:719–23.
114. Green AR, Betancourt JR, Carrillo JE. Integrating social factors into cross-cultural medical education. Acad Med. 2002;77:193–7. doi: 10.1097/00001888-200203000-00003.
115. Like RC, Steiner RP, Rubel AJ. STFM core curriculum guidelines. Recommended core curriculum guidelines on culturally sensitive and competent health care. Fam Med. 1996;28:291–7.

This chapter was originally published under the Creative Commons Attribution License. Mechanick, J. I., Marchetti, A. E., Apovian, C., Benchimol, A. K., Bisschop, P. H., Bollo-Galvis, A., Hegazi, R. A., Jenkins, D., Mendoza, E., Sanz, M. L., Sheu, WH-H, Tatti, P., Tsang, M-W, and Hamdy, O. Diabetes-Specific Nutrition Algorithim: A Transcultural Program to Optimize Diabetes and Prediabetes Care. Current Diabetes Reports 2012. 12(2). doi:10.1007/s11892-012-0253-z.

EFFECT OF FRUIT RESTRICTION ON GLYCEMIC CONTROL IN PATIENTS WITH TYPE 2 DIABETES: A RANDOMIZED TRIAL

ALLAN S. CHRISTENSEN, LONE VIGGERS, KJELD HASSELSTRÖM, and SØREN GREGERSEN

13.1 BACKGROUND

The prevalence of type 2 diabetes (T2DM) is still rising and has reached epidemic proportions in most countries [1]. It is estimated that around 350 million people worldwide have T2DM [1]. Individuals with T2DM have increased morbidity and mortality and represent a huge economic burden for society. The importance of medical nutrition therapy (MNT) is recognized as one of the cornerstones in the treatment of T2DM [2-4]. Several evidence-based nutrition guidelines have been published and show that both diet quality and quantity have a huge impact on T2DM [3-5]. A variety of fibre-rich food like fruit and vegetables are generally recommended [4,5].

Fruit contain a wide range of specific bioactive substances which can act through multiple pathways in the human body e.g. as antioxidants, reduce inflammation and improve endothelial function [6-8]. High fruit intake has been shown to reduce the risk of e.g. cardiovascular disease [9,10] and some cancer types [11].

Health professionals often have concerns about the sugar content of fruit and therefore advice individuals with T2DM to restrict their intake to a maximum of two pieces a day. Few studies have addressed whether high fruit intake is associated with glycemic control and these have shown either no association [12-15] or an inverse association [16] between fruit intake and either HbA1c or blood glucose. However, these are all observational studies and none are performed in subjects with T2DM. Therefore sparse data exist to answer the question whether or not fruit has a negative impact on blood glucose levels in subjects with T2DM. We carried out this study to test the hypothesis that an advice to restrict fruit intake to a maximum of two pieces a day compared to at least two pieces a day results in an improved glycemic control in adults with type 2 diabetes.

13.2 METHODS

13.2.1 SUBJECTS

Volunteers were selected from patients referred to MNT by their GP to the Outpatient Clinic at Department of Nutrition, Regional Hospital West Jutland. Eligible patients were adults with T2DM (duration of T2DM < 12 months), HbA1c values 12.0% or less and who accepted to adhere to the protocol. Exclusion criteria were clinically significant cardiovascular, renal or endocrine disease. A total of 136 subjects were invited and 63 subjects were randomized. Each subject gave informed, written consent and the study was approved by The Regional Committee on Biomedical Research Ethics.

13.2.2 STUDY DESIGN

This study was a 12 week open randomized parallel diet intervention trial. Sequentially numbered, sealed envelopes containing a computer-generated allocation were used. The intervention consisted of standard MNT and an advice to either: 1) Eat at least two pieces of fruit each day (high-fruit) or 2) eat no more than two pieces of fruit each day (low-fruit). Both groups had two consultations with an experienced registered dietitian at the Outpatient Clinic. One consultation in the beginning and one at the end of the study period. Shortly before consultations in the Outpatient Clinic the subjects had a blood sample drawn at their GP. During the intervention subjects were treated at the GP's discretion. The primary outcome was change in HbA1c. Secondary outcomes were changes in fruit intake, body weight and waist circumference.

13.2.3 NUTRITIONAL INTERVENTION

The MNT was given on an individual basis and focused on the individual needs and personal preferences [3]. All overweight subjects were advised to restrict the energy intake. The only difference in the MNT between the groups was the advice concerning fruit intake. The patients were recommended to eat fresh and whole fruit only and to exclude fruit juice, canned and dried fruit from their diet or keep it as low as possible. One piece of fruit was standardized to the amount of a fruit that contained approximately 10 grams of carbohydrate e.g. 100 grams apple, 50 grams banana or 125 grams orange. The patients were given written information and pictures about the amount of the most common fruit that corresponded to one piece.

13.2.4 ANTHROPOMETRY MEASUREMENTS

Height was measured at the first visit only. Body weight and waist circumference were measured at both visits. Subjects were weighed barefooted and in light clothing on a calibrated scale. Height was measured using a wall measuring stick scale. Waist circumference was measured horizontally at the level of the umbilicus in a relaxed standing position.

13.2.5 BIOCHEMICAL ANALYSIS

Blood samples were taken at the subjects GP using standard procedures. The blood samples were analyzed at Department of Clinical Biochemistry, Regional Hospital West Jutland using standard laboratory procedures. HbA1c was analyzed using HPLC.

13.2.6 FRUIT INTAKE

The subjects filled in a weighed 3-day fruit record before and after the intervention. At each visit the fruit intake was estimated using dietary recalls. Portion sizes were estimated and translated to grams using pictures and table values of mean weight for a given standard portion [17,18]. This was compared with the fruit record to avoid errors. Fruit intake was calculated at each visit as mean intake using the 3-day fruit record.

13.2.7 PHYSICAL ACTIVITY

A self-reported questionnaire was used at each visit to estimate physical activity level [19].

13.2.8 STATISTICAL ANALYSIS

Statistical analysis was performed using Stata statistical software package 11.1 (Stata, College Station, TX, USA). All analyses were performed on an intention-to-treat basis, with a two-sided 0.05 significance level ($\alpha=0.05$). We used paired t-test to analyze if a variable changed significantly from before to after the intervention. For each outcome we compared mean difference (after - before) between the two groups using an unpaired t-test. For the primary outcome we also used multiple regression analysis controlling for potential confounders. Results are given as mean ± standard error unless otherwise stated.

A sample of 38 subjects in each arm was estimated to detect a difference of 0.7% in HbA1c. The sample size was based on achieving an 80% power with $\alpha = 0.05$, SD = 1.0 and dropout = 10%. The inclusion rate was slower than anticipated. The study was terminated prematurely due to limited time and research funding. Fortunately, the variation in HbA1c was smaller than estimated in the power calculation and there were no dropouts. Therefore the actual power in the study was around 90% to detect a difference of 0.7% in HbA1c between the groups.

TABLE 1: Baseline characteristics of study participants*

	High-fruit (n = 32)	Low-fruit (n = 31)
Age (years)	59 ± 12	57 ± 12
Sex (female)	14 (44)	18 (58)
Height (cm)	170 ± 8	169 ± 10
Body weight (kg)	92 ± 17	91 ± 17
BMI (kg/m²)	32 ± 5	32 ± 6
Waist circumference (cm)	104 ± 11	107 ± 9
HbA1c (%)	6.7 ± 1.2	6.5 ± 1.1
Physical activity level (PAL)	1.7 ± 0,1	1.6 ± 0,1
Fruit intake (g)	194 ± 87	186 ± 82
Duration of diabetes (days)	22 (12–107)	33 (14–54)
Start on OAD prior to intervention†		
1-30 days	10 (45)	7 (58)
31-60 days	6 (27)	3 (25)
> 60 days	6 (27)	2 (17)

*Baseline values are presented as mean ± SD, median (25th-75th centile), and number (%). † OAD = oral antidiabetic drugs.

13.3 RESULTS

13.3.1 BASELINE CHARACTERISTICS

Recruitment took place from November 2009 to March 2011 with the last visit in June 2011. In total 63 T2DM subjects were included. Baseline characteristics are shown in Table 1. At baseline significantly more subjects were taking oral antidiabetic drugs (OADs) on the high-fruit diet than on the low-fruit diet (22 vs 12; p=0.02). There were no significant differences between the groups for any of the other baseline variables.

13.3.2 COMPLIANCE TO INTERVENTION

Based on the fruit records and recalls, the reported fruit intake was altered as expected (Table 2). One subject on the high-fruit diet kept the fruit intake steady just below two pieces a day. The outcomes were unaffected by exclusion of this non-compliant subject.

TABLE 2: Body weight, waist circumference and fruit intake before and after intervention

	High-fruit		Low-fruit		Differences between groups	
	Before	After	Before	After	Means (CI 95%)	p-value
Body weight (kg) †	92.4 ± 2.9	89.9 ± 3.0*	91.2 ± 3.0	89.6 ± 2.9*	−0.9 (−2.2 to 0.4)	0.18
Waist circumference (cm)	103 ± 2	99 ± 2*	107 ± 2	103 ± 2*	−1.2 (−3.0 to 0.5)	0.17
Fruit intake (grams)	194 ± 15	319 ± 24*	186 ± 15	135 ± 7*	175 (119 to 232)	< 0.0001

* Significant difference between before and after.
† Body weight: high-fruit (n = 32), low-fruit (n = 31), waist circumference: high-fruit (n = 27), low-fruit (n = 22), fruit intake: high-fruit (n = 32), low-fruit (n = 31).

13.3.3 HBA1C

As expected, there was a significant reduction in HbA1c in both groups. The high-fruit group had a change from 6.74 ± 0.2 to $6.26 \pm 0.1\%$ and the low-fruit group a change from 6.53 ± 0.2 to $6.24 \pm 0.1\%$. The reductions were 0.49 ± 0.2 and $0.29 \pm 0.1\%$ in the high-fruit and low-fruit diet respectively. There was no significant difference between the groups (Table 3). Adjusting for use of OAD at baseline did not significantly change the result (Table 3). Five subjects (high-fruit = 2; low-fruit = 3) increased OAD dosage during the study period. They had a significantly higher HbA1c at baseline and reduced their HbA1c significantly more during the study (Figure 1).

TABLE 3: Mean difference between the groups in HbA1c (%)

	Difference*	CI 95%	p-value
Unadjusted	0.19	−0.23 to 0.62	0.37
Adjusted for baseline OAD†	0.06	−0.38 to 0.49	0.80

* Difference between the diets (high-fruit (n = 32) – low-fruit (n = 31)) analyzed by multiple regression. † OAD = oral antidiabetic drugs.

13.3.4 WEIGHT AND WAIST CIRCUMFERENCE

Both groups had a significant reduction in body weight and waist circumference with no differences between groups (Table 2). The reductions in body weight were 2.5 ± 0.5 and 1.7 ± 0.5 kg in the high-fruit and low-fruit diet respectively. In waist circumference the reductions were 4.3 ± 0.6 and 3.0 ± 0.6 cm in the high-fruit and low-fruit group, respectively. Neither change in body weight ($r=-0.07$, $p=0.61$; $r=0.17$, $p=0.19$) nor in waist circumference ($r=-0.15$, $p=0.31$; $r=0.13$, $p=0.36$) was associated with change in fruit intake or change in HbA1c respectively.

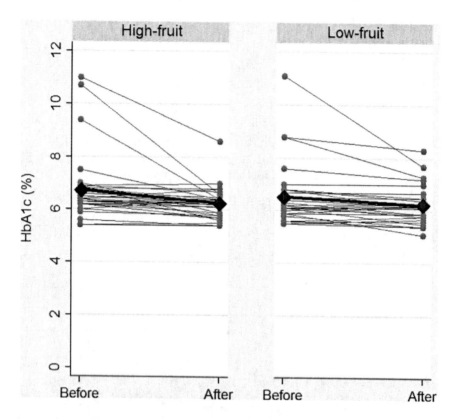

FIGURE 1: HbA1c values before and after intervention by groups. Each thin line represents one subject. Thick line represents mean change.

13.3.5 PHYSICAL ACTIVITY

A significant change in physical activity was seen in the high-fruit group (0.07 ± 0.02 PAL; p=0.005) but not in the low-fruit group (0.04 ± 0.03 PAL; p=0.19). However, there was no difference between the groups (0.04 PAL; p=0.31).

13.3.6 SIDE EFFECTS

One subject on the high-fruit diet, who increased fruit intake from 145 to 310 grams, reported mild gastrointestinal side effects, but the subject remained compliant throughout the study.

13.4 DISCUSSION

Our pragmatic trial demonstrated that, in adults with newly diagnosed T2DM, MNT with an advice to restrict fruit intake resulted in a decreased fruit intake while MNT with an advice to eat more fruit resulted in an increased fruit intake. However this difference in fruit intake did not significantly affect glycemic control, body weight or waist circumference.

To our knowledge, this is the first randomized intervention study examining the effects of dietary advice to restrict fruit intake on glycemic control in T2DM. Most intervention studies with fruit have investigated fruit as a part of a whole diet, fruit mixed with vegetables or only one type of fruit and often as a single meal study e.g. glycemic index studies. Very few intervention studies have tested a variety of fruit over several weeks and none have investigated long-term glycemic control in T2DM subjects.

In our study we found that restriction of fruit intake does not significantly affect HbA1c. In a study by Rodriguez et al. 15 obese women randomized to either a low-fruit or a high-fruit diet for 8 weeks a difference between the groups of 550 kJ from fructose was obtained [20]. This is around twice the difference obtained in the present study. The study reported no differences in HOMA, glucose or insulin levels between the groups. In another study by Madero et al. 131 obese subjects were randomized to a low-fructose diet or a moderate-natural- fructose diet for 6 weeks [21]. The groups' intake of fruit corresponded to approximately 250 and 2200 kJ, respectively in low-fructose and moderate-natural-fructose which corresponds to a difference between the groups about three times as large as in the present study. Significant reductions in HOMA and glucose values were seen within the moderate-natural-fructose group, but no difference between the groups was seen. Cross-sectional studies have shown that fruit intake is not associated [12-15] or inversely associated [16] with HbA1c or other parameters reflecting glycemic control. Further, cohort studies addressing the impact of fruit intake on the incidence of T2DM have shown either no association or an inverse association [22,23]. The evidence, including our present study, therefore suggests that a high fruit intake does not have a negative impact on glycemic control.

We found a tendency towards reduced body weight and waist circumference in the group that ingested most fruit 0.9 (CI 95%; −0.4 to 2.2) kg and 1.2 (CI 95%; −0.5 to 3.0) cm respectively. This corroborates with a few intervention studies. The study by Rodriguez et al. in which the high-fruit group had a significant reduction in waist circumference compared to low-fruit group (5.5 vs. 2.4 cm; p=0.048) [20]. Weight loss was similar in the two groups (6.1 vs. 6.4 kg; p=0.78). In another intervention study 49 obese women were randomized to add either three apples, three pears or three oat cookies to their usual diet for 10 weeks [24]. The total energy and fiber content of the supplements were matched. The two groups with fruit supplements lost significantly more body weight than the group with oat cookies (−0.9 vs −0.8 vs 0.2 kg). In a third study by Madero et al. the moderate-natural-fructose group reduced body weight more than the low-fructose group (4.1 vs 2.9 kg; p=0.02) [21]. A recent review study concluded that in most studies a higher fruit intake has a beneficial effect on body weight and that no studies have found a negative effect [25].

In spite of a difference in fruit intake of about two pieces daily between the groups we did not find any effect on HbA1c, body weight or waist circumference. The most likely explanation is that fruit is eaten as a part of a daily diet and therefore when changing the fruit intake it will lead to other changes in the diet. We did not measure total energy intake, but weight and physical activity were similar between the groups and therefore energy intake must have been more or less the same in both groups too. When changing the fruit intake other changes in the diet most likely occur and this would explain that there was no difference in HbA1c, body weight and waist circumference despite the significant difference in fruit intake.

Our study has several strengths. It is the first randomized controlled study investigating the relevant scientific question: does fruit intake matter in relation to glycemic control in T2DM subjects? We chose to do this in a "real life" setting. Thus, almost all subjects were fully compliant and there were no drop-outs.

However, our study also has some weaknesses. First, it can be argued that a greater difference in fruit intake between the high and low fruit groups would have resulted in a significant effect, positive or negative. However, we consider a difference of about two pieces of fruit as clinically relevant and we think it reflects a "real life" situation. We admit that testing whether an even higher fruit intake may impact significantly the glycemic control would be interesting, but this was not the intention in this pragmatic trial. Secondly, we did not control (and had no pre-trial intention to do so) the intake of medication. A difference in baseline use of OADs could bias the results. However, adjustments did not significantly change the results (Table 3). Therefore we do not believe it has biased the results. Thirdly, fruit intake and physical activity were self-reported and therefore could have been subject to under or over-reporting. Measurement of biomarkers of fruit intake, e.g. plasma vitamin C and plasma carotenoids would have strengthened the study.

13.5 CONCLUSIONS

We conclude that an advice to restrict fruit intake as part of standard MNT in overweight adults with newly diagnosed TDM2 does not improve glycemic control, body weight or waist circumference. Considering the many possible beneficial effects of fruit, we recommend that fruit intake should not be restricted in T2DM subjects.

REFERENCES

1. Danaei G, Finucane MM, Lu Y, Singh GM, Cowan MJ, Paciorek CJ, Lin JK, Farzadfar F, Khang YH, Stevens GA, Rao M, Ali MK, Riley LM, Robinson CA, Ezzati M: National, regional, and global trends in fasting plasma glucose and diabetes prevalence since 1980: systematic analysis of health examination surveys and epidemiological studies with 370 country-years and 2.7 million participants. Lancet 2011, 378:31-40.
2. Morris SF, Wylie-Rosett J: Medical Nutrition Therapy: A Key to Diabetes Management and Prevention. Clinical diabetes 2010, 28:12-18.

3. Franz MJ, Powers MA, Leontos C, Holzmeister LA, Kulkarni K, Monk A, Wedel N, Gradwell E: The evidence for medical nutrition therapy for type 1 and type 2 diabetes in adults. J Am Diet Assoc 2010, 110:1852-1889.
4. Bantle JP, Wylie-Rosett J, Albright AL, Apovian CM, Clark NG, Franz MJ, Hoogwerf BJ, Lichtenstein AH, Mayer-Davis E, Mooradian AD, Wheeler ML: Nutrition recommendations and interventions for diabetes: a position statement of the American Diabetes Association. Diabetes Care 2008, 31(Suppl 1):S61-78.
5. Mann JI, De Leeuw I, Hermansen K, Karamanos B, Karlstrom B, Katsilambros N, Riccardi G, Rivellese AA, Rizkalla S, Slama G, Toeller M, Uusitupa M, Vessby B: Evidence-based nutritional approaches to the treatment and prevention of diabetes mellitus. Nutr Metab Cardiovasc Dis 2004, 14:373-394.
6. Gonzalez-Gallego J, Garcia-Mediavilla MV, Sanchez-Campos S, Tunon MJ: Fruit polyphenols, immunity and inflammation. Br J Nutr 2010, 104(Suppl 3):S15-27.
7. Chong MF, Macdonald R, Lovegrove JA: Fruit polyphenols and CVD risk: a review of human intervention studies. Br J Nutr 2010, 104(Suppl 3):S28-39.
8. Feeney MJ: Fruits and the prevention of lifestyle-related diseases. Clin Exp Pharmacol Physiol 2004, 31(Suppl 2):S11-13.
9. Dauchet L, Amouyel P, Hercberg S, Dallongeville J: Fruit and vegetable consumption and risk of coronary heart disease: a meta-analysis of cohort studies. J Nutr 2006, 136:2588-2593.
10. Martinez-Gonzalez MA, Lamuela-Raventos RM: The unparalleled benefits of fruit. Br J Nutr 2009, 102:947-948.
11. Aune D, Lau R, Chan DS, Vieira R, Greenwood DC, Kampman E, Norat T: Non-linear reduction in risk for colorectal cancer by fruit and vegetable intake based on meta-analysis of prospective studies. Gastroenterology 2011, 141:106-118.
12. Overby NC, Margeirsdottir HD, Brunborg C, Andersen LF, Dahl-Jorgensen K: The influence of dietary intake and meal pattern on blood glucose control in children and adolescents using intensive insulin treatment. Diabetologia 2007, 50:2044-2051.
13. Gulliford MC, Ukoumunne OC: Determinants of glycated haemoglobin in the general population: associations with diet, alcohol and cigarette smoking. Eur J Clin Nutr 2001, 55:615-623.
14. Buyken AE, Toeller M, Heitkamp G, Irsigler K, Holler C, Santeusanio F, Stehle P, Fuller JH: Carbohydrate sources and glycaemic control in Type 1 diabetes mellitus. EURODIAB IDDM Complications Study Group. Diabet Med 2000, 17:351-359.
15. Panagiotakos DB, Tzima N, Pitsavos C, Chrysohoou C, Papakonstantinou E, Zampelas A, Stefanadis C: The relationship between dietary habits, blood glucose and insulin levels among people without cardiovascular disease and type 2 diabetes; the ATTICA study. Rev Diabet Stud 2005, 2:208-215.
16. Sargeant LA, Khaw KT, Bingham S, Day NE, Luben RN, Oakes S, Welch A, Wareham NJ: Fruit and vegetable intake and population glycosylated haemoglobin levels: the EPIC-Norfolk Study. Eur J Clin Nutr 2001, 55:342-348.
17. Andersen LT, Jensen H, Haraldsdottir J: Typiske vægte for madvarer. Scand J Nutr 1996, 40:S129-152.
18. The Danish Diabetes Association: Sund mad - når du har diabetes. Odense; 2001.

19. Johansson G, Westerterp KR: Assessment of the physical activity level with two questions: validation with doubly labeled water. Int J Obes (Lond) 2008, 32:1031-1033.

20. Rodriguez MC, Parra MD, Marques-Lopes I, De Morentin BE, Gonzalez A, Martinez JA: Effects of two energy-restricted diets containing different fruit amounts on body weight loss and macronutrient oxidation. Plant Foods Hum Nutr 2005, 60:219-224.

21. Madero M, Arriaga JC, Jalal D, Rivard C, McFann K, Perez-Mendez O, Vazquez A, Ruiz A, Lanaspa MA, Jimenez CR, Johnson RJ, Lozada LG: The effect of two energy-restricted diets, a low-fructose diet versus a moderate natural fructose diet, on weight loss and metabolic syndrome parameters: a randomized controlled trial. Metabolism 2011, 60:1551-1559.

22. Carter P, Gray LJ, Troughton J, Khunti K, Davies MJ: Fruit and vegetable intake and incidence of type 2 diabetes mellitus: systematic review and meta-analysis. BMJ 2010, 341:c4229.

23. Hamer M, Chida Y: Intake of fruit, vegetables, and antioxidants and risk of type 2 diabetes: systematic review and meta-analysis. J Hypertens 2007, 25:2361-2369.

24. de Oliveira MC, Sichieri R, Venturim Mozzer R: A low-energy-dense diet adding fruit reduces weight and energy intake in women. Appetite 2008, 51:291-295.

25. Alinia S, Hels O, Tetens I: The potential association between fruit intake and body weight–a review. Obes Rev 2009, 10:639-647.

This chapter was originally published under the Creative Commons Attribution License. Christensen, A. S., Viggers, L., Hasselström , K., and Gregersen, S. Effect of Fruit Restriction on Glycemic Control in Patients with Type 2 Diabetes: A Randomized Trial. Nutrition Journal 2013: 12(29). doi:10.1186/1475-2891-12-29.

IS THERE A ROLE FOR CARBOHYDRATE RESTRICTION IN THE TREATMENT AND PREVENTION OF CANCER?

RAINER J. KLEMENT and ULRIKE KÄMMERER

14.1 INTRODUCTION

When defining the factors of a healthy lifestyle that aims at preventing a disease like cancer, a logical approach is to compare individuals that get the disease with those that don't. Cancer, which might be considered a disease of civilization, has consistently been reported to be very rare among uncivilized hunter-gatherer societies [1-4]. This observation makes sense from an evolutionary perspective from which it is reasonable to assume that the lifestyle factors that protect our genome against tumorigenesis have been selected for early in the history of the genus homo when humans lived as hunter-gatherers [5]. In particular, the time since the neolithic revolution, which meant the transition from foraging and nomadism to agriculture and settlement, spans a fraction less than 1% of human history. Thus, the switch from the "caveman's diet" consisting of fat, meat and only occasionally roots, berries and other sources of carbohydrate (CHO) to a nutrition dominated by easily digestible CHOs derived mainly from grains as staple food would have occurred too recently to induce major adoptions in our genes encoding the metabolic pathways. This is even more the case for the changes that occurred over the past 100 years, in particular the switch from labor in the field to a sedentary lifestyle and an increase in the consumption of easily digestible CHOs with high glycemic indices (GIs), leading to diseases of civilization that are strongly associated with the so-called Western way of life [6]. Despite a large heterogeneity in regional occupation, modern hunter-gatherers share certain lifestyle factors that are not frequently met in Westernized societies, including regular physical activity, sun exposure, sufficient sleep, low chronic stress and the lack of foods that would also not have been available to our pre-neolithic ancestors. While there is already compelling evidence for the beneficial roles of regular physical activity and sufficient vitamin D in the prevention and treatment of cancer, the influence of the altered nutritional patterns in the Western diet is less clearly defined.

14.1.1 MODERN HUNTER-GATHERERS' DIET

Data from 229 hunter-gatherer societies included in the revised Ethnographic Atlas indicate that hunter-gatherer diets differ from typical Western ones in basically two aspects: first, a strong reliance on animal foods (45-65% of energy or E%) and second, the consumption of low-GI plant foods such as vegetables, fruits, seeds and nuts [7]. This is consistent with stable isotope studies of human fossils [8,9]. As a consequence, the amount and type of carbohydrates in the typical western diet differ markedly from the ones that our genes adapted to. In particular, Cordain and colleagues estimated that modern hunter-gatherers derived about 22-40 E% from CHOs and 19-30 E% from protein, which is lower and higher, respectively, than recommended by Western food agencies. Recently, Ströhle & Hahn confirmed that the energy derived from CHOs—despite being dependent upon geographic latitude and ecological environment - in modern hunter-gatherers is markedly lower than in Westernized societies [10]. High CHO intake, in particular in the form of sugar and other high GI foods, has been linked to modern diseases like metabolic syndrome [11], Alzheimer's disease [12,13], cataract and macula degeneration [14-16] and gout [17]. Intriguingly, with the possible exception of Alzheimer's disease [18], the occurrence and prognosis of cancer seems positively associated with both the prevalence of these diseases [19-28] and the GI and glycemic load (GL) of the diet [29-32]; this implies a possible role of high CHO intake in cancer as well.

In this review, we are going to present some arguments that support the hypothesis that lowering the amount of CHOs in the diet can have direct beneficial effects on the prevention and treatment of malignant diseases. The main focus will be on very low CHO, ketogenic diets as an effective supportive therapy option for cancer patients.

14.2 TUMOR CELL METABOLISM—IT'S ALL ABOUT GLUCOSE

That there exists an intimate connection between CHOs and cancer has been known since the seminal studies performed by different physiologists in the 1920s. Treating diabetic patients, A. Braunstein observed in 1921 that in those who developed cancer, glucose secretion in the urine disappeared. Further, culturing tissue of benign and malign origin in glucose-containing solutions, he quantified the much higher consumption by cancer tissue compared to muscle and liver [33]. One year later, R. Bierich described the remarkable accumulation of lactate in the micromilieu of tumor tissues [34] and demonstrated lactate to be essential for invasion of melanoma cells into the surrounding tissue [35]. The most accurate and well known experiments were published by Otto Warburg and colleagues from 1923 on [36-38]. Warburg observed that tumor tissue ex vivo would convert high amounts of glucose to lactate even in the presence of oxygen (aerobic glycolysis), a metabolic phenotype now referred to as the Warburg effect. This meant a sharp contrast to normal tissue which was known to exhibit the Pasteur effect, i.e., a decrease of glucose uptake and inhibition of lactate production under aerobic conditions. Today, the Warburg effect is an established hallmark of cancer, i.e., a pathological capability common to most, if not all, cancer cells [39]. At first sight, the reason why many cancers should run preferentially on glucose to produce energy seems counter-intuitive: basic biochemistry textbooks tell us that glycolysis partially oxidizes the carbon skeleton of one mole of glucose to two moles of pyruvate, yielding two moles of ATP and NADH. In normal cells under normoxic conditions, pyruvate is oxidized in the mitochondria by the enzyme pyruvate dehydrogenase, creating acetyl-CoA which is further utilized in the tricarboxylic acid cycle (TCA or Krebs cycle) to yield a total of 32+ moles of ATP. Thus, the oxidation of pyruvate in the mitochondria supplies 30+ additional moles of ATP compared to its reduction to lactate via lactate dehydrogenase A (LDHA), which happens in case of insufficient oxygen levels or - in case of cancer cells - due to the Warburg effect.

14.2.1 POSSIBLE CAUSES FOR THE "WARBURG EFFECT"

Over the past years, however, it has become increasingly clear that malignant cells compensate for this energy deficit by up-regulating the expression of key glycolytic enzymes as well as the glucose transporters GLUT1 and GLUT3, which have a high affinity for glucose and ensure high glycolytic flux even for low extracellular glucose concentrations. This characteristic is the basis for the wide-spread use of the functional imaging modality positron emission tomography (PET) with the glucose-analogue tracer 18F-fluoro-2-deoxyD-glucose (FDG) (Figure 1). There are mainly four possible drivers discussed in the literature that cause the metabolic switch from oxidative phosphorylation to aerobic glycolysis in cancer cells. The first one is mitochondrial damage or dysfunction [40], which was already proposed by Warburg himself as the cause for tumorigenesis [41]. Somatic mutations in mitochondrial DNA (mtDNA) and certain OX-PHOS genes can lead to increased production of reactive oxygen species (ROS) and accumulation of TCA cycle intermediates (succinate and fumarate) that trigger the stabilization of hypoxia inducible factor (HIF)-1α, inactivation of tumor suppressors including p53 and PTEN and upregulation of several oncogenes of the phosphoinositide 3-kinase (PI3K)/Akt/mammalian target of rapamycin (mTOR) signaling pathway [42]. In tumor cells, Akt plays a major role in resisting apoptosis and promoting proliferation, and it does so by reprogramming tumor cell metabolism [43-45]. Akt suppresses β-oxidation of fatty acids [46], but enhances de novo lipid synthesis in the cytosol [47,48]. Akt also activates mTOR, a key regulator of cell growth and proliferation that integrates signaling from insulin and growth factors, amino acid availability, cellular energy status and oxygen levels [49,50]. In cancer cells, mTOR has been shown to induce aerobic

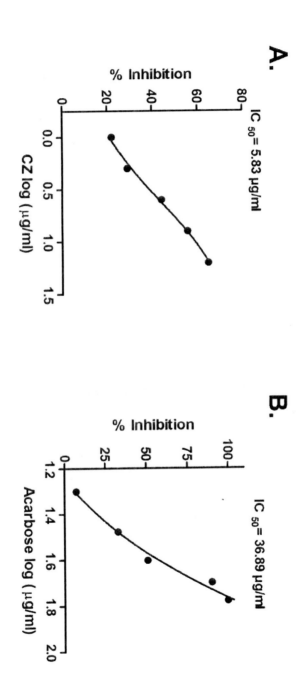

FIGURE 1: PET image of a patient with a left central lung carcinoma (arrows). Note also the high FDG uptake by the kidneys (Fig D), brain and myocard (Figure E). Source: PET/CT Imaging Centre, University Hospital of Würzburg.

glycolysis by up-regulating key glycolytic enzymes, in particular through its downstream effectors c-Myc and HIF-1α. Both of these transcription factors are involved in the expression of pyruvate kinase M2, a crucial glycolytic enzyme for rapidly proliferating cells [51].

HIF-1α is further important for the adaption to hypoxia by increasing the expression of glycolytic enzymes including GLUT1 and hexokinase (HK) II as well as several angiogenic factors [49,52]. The observation that certain malignant cells are able to use both glycolysis and OXPHOS under aerobic conditions has been taken to argue that mitochondrial dysfunction alone is not a sufficient cause for the Warburg effect [53]. Indeed, somatic mutations in most oncogenes and tumor suppressor genes have been shown to directly or indirectly activate glycolysis even in the presence of oxygen. As described above, they do so mainly by hyperactivating major metabolic signaling pathways such as the insulin-like growth facor-1 receptor (IGFR1)-insulin receptor (IR)/PI3K/Akt/mTOR signaling pathway (Figure 2). In principle, hyperactivation of this pathway can occur at several points from alterations in either upstream (receptor) or downstream (transducer) proteins and/or disruption of negative feedback loops via loss-of-function mutations in suppressor genes [44,45,54]. Thus, genetic alterations in oncogenes and tumor suppressor genes are a second possible cause for the Warburg effect.

As a third mechanism, with advanced tumorigenesis, non-mutation induced stabilization of HIF-1α occurs through a lack of oxygen in hypoxic tumor regions and contributes to increased glycolysis. Proliferation of aggressive tumors proceeds too fast for concurrent vascularization, so that hypoxic regions will develop. Because the diffusion coefficients for glucose are larger than for oxygen, these regions rely heavily on glycolysis. Hypoxic cancer cells are particularly radio- and chemoresistant. In PET-studies, tumor areas with high FDG uptake have been consistently linked to poor prognosis [55,56] and are now being considered as important biological target volumes to receive dose escalations in radiation treatment [57].

14.2.2 THE IMPACT OF INSULIN AND IGF1

Finally, chronic activation of the IGFR1-IR/PI3K/Akt survival pathway through high blood glucose, insulin and inflammatory cytokines has been

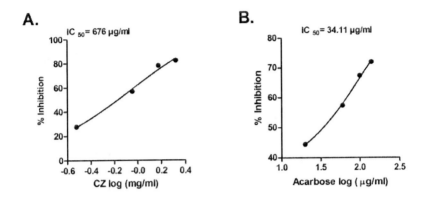

FIGURE 2: The IGF1R-IR/PI3K/Akt/mTOR pathway and its manipulation through diet. Elevations in blood glucose concentrations lead to secretion of insulin with subsequent elevation of free IGF1. Binding of insulin and IGF1 to their receptor tyrosine kinases induces autophosphorylation of the latter which leads to subsequent activation of PI3K by one of at least three different pathways [54]. Further downstream, PI3K signaling causes phosphorylation and activation of the serine/threonine kinase Akt (also known as protein kinase B). Akt activates mammalian target of rapamycin (mTOR), which itself induces aerobic glycolysis by up-regulating key glycolytic enzymes, in particular via its downstream effectors c-Myc and hypoxia inducible factor (HIF)-1α. mTOR is negatively affected through activation of AMPK, which can be achieved by dietary restriction [67]. In addition, a possible negative interaction between insulin and AMPK is discussed in vivo [60].

proposed as a cause of carcinogenesis [30,58,59] and switch towards aerobic glycolysis. In this theory, hyperactivation of the IGFR1-IR signalling
pathway does not occur primarily through somatic gene mutations, but
rather through elevated concentrations of insulin and IGF1, allowing for
more ligands binding to their receptors. Interestingly, gain-of-function
mutations resulting in ligand-independent overactivation of both IGFR1
and IR are uncommon [60]. Furthermore, loss-of-function of the tumor
suppressor PTEN may result in hypersensitivity to insulin/IGF1-mediated
activation of the IGFR1-IR pathway rather than constitutive downstream
activation [60]. Thus, it seems possible that high levels of insulin and
IGF1 in the microenvironment favor cell survival and evolution towards
malignancy instead of apoptosis in DNA-damaged cells. Indeed, both hyperglycemia and hyperinsulinemia are predictors of cancer occurrence and
cancer-related mortality [23,25,26]. This highlights the link between the
metabolic syndrome and cancer on the one hand and cancer and lifestyle
factors like nutrition on the other. As indicated in Figure 2, restriction of
dietary CHOs would counteract this signalling cascade by normalizing
glucose and insulin levels in subjects with metabolic syndrome, in this
way acting similar to calorie restriction/fasting [61,62]. Indeed, it has been
shown in healthy subjects that CHO restriction induces hormonal and metabolic adaptions very similar to fasting [63-66]. Dietary restriction is able
to inhibit mTOR signalling through a second, energy-sensing pathway by
stimulating phosphorylation of AMP-activated protein kinase (AMPK)
[67]. In vitro, AMPK phosphorylation is sensitive to the ratio of AMP/
ATP within the cell; in vivo, however, concentrations of glucose and other
nutrients are kept fairly stable throughout calorie restriction, suggesting
that hormones such as insulin and glucagon might play a more dominant
role in regulating AMPK and thus mTOR activation [60]. This may open
a second route to mimic the positive effects of calorie restriction through
CHO restriction (Figure 2).

14.2.3 GLYCOLYSIS: BENEFICIAL FOR TUMOR CELLS

Besides the ability to grow in hypoxic environments, a high glycolytic rate
has several additional advantages for the malignant cell: First, it avoids

the production of ROS through OXPHOS. Second, the phosphometabo-
lites that accumulate during glycolysis can be processed in the pentose
phosphate pathway for biosynthesis of nucleic acids and lipids. Similarly,
overexpession of Akt induces an increased flow of pyruvate-derived citrate from the mitochondrion into the cytosol, where it is used for lipid
biosynthesis. Third, a tumor cell focusing on glycolysis no longer relies on
intact mitochondria and may evade apoptotic signalling which is linked to
mitochondrial function. In addition, the genes and pathways that up-regu-
late glycolysis are themselves anti-apoptotic [40]. Fourth, high glycolytic
activity produces high levels of lactate and H^+ ions which get transported
outside the cell where they directly promote tumor aggressiveness [68]
through invasion and metastasis, two other hallmarks of cancer. For this
purpose, glycolytic tumor cells often show overexpression of monocar-
boxylate transporters (MCTs) and/or Na^+/H^+ exchangers [69] that allow
them to effectively remove large amounts of H^+ ions. For MDA-MB-231
breast cancer cells it has been shown that lactate drives migration by acting as a chemo-attractant and enhances the number of lung metastasis in
athymic nude mice [70]. Lactate can also be taken up and used as a fuel
by some malignant cells, and oxidative tumor cells have been shown to
co-exist with glycolytic ones (both stromal and malignant) in a symbiotic
fashion [71]. In glioma cells, lactate upregulates and activates the matrix metalloproteinase (MMP)-2 which degrades the extra-cellular matrix
and basement membrane [72]. Activation of MMPs may also occur in the
microenvironment through low pH values in a similar way as discussed
for carious decay of the dentin organic matrix through lactate released
by cariogenic bacteria [73]. Acidification of the microenvironment further
induces apoptosis in normal parenchymal and stromal cells [74,75] and
therefore provides a strong selective growth advantage for tumor cells that
are resistant to low pH-induced apoptosis [76,77].

14.3 GLUCOSE AVAILABILITY AS A PROMOTER OF CANCER GROWTH

Taken together, increased glucose flux and metabolism promotes several hallmarks of cancer such as excessive proliferation, anti-apoptotic signalling, cell

cycle progression and angiogenesis. It does so, however, at the expense of substrate inflexibility compared to normal cells. It is clear that the high proliferative phenotype can only be sustained as long as a steady supply of substrates for ATP production is available. Thus, with progressive tumorigenesis, cancer cells become more and more 'addicted' to aerobic glycolysis [53] and vulnerable to glucose deprivation. Indeed, several studies have shown that malignant cells in vitro quickly lose ATP and commit apoptosis when starved of glucose [78-80]. Masur et al. showed that diabetogenic glucose concentrations (11 mM) compared to physiological ones (5.5 mM) lead to altered expression of genes that promote cell proliferation, migration and adhesion in tumor cell lines from several organs including breast, colon, prostate and bladder [81]. Adding insulin to the high-glucose medium further enhanced proliferation rates by 20-40% and promoted activation of the PI3K pathway. The question is whether altered blood glucose levels have similar effects on tumor growth in vivo. Theoretically, low blood glucose might cut some of the most hypoxic tumor cells from their diffusion-limited fuel supply. Gatenby and Gillies originally proposed this mechanism as an explanation for necrotic areas often found within tumor tissue [82], but they later revised this hypothesis based on a mathematical model that predicted only a modest decline of glucose concentrations with distance from the closest blood vessel [69]. There are, however, several lines of evidence pointing towards a strong correlation between blood glucose levels and tumor growth in vivo that might indicate other important effects mediated by glucose. For example, the reduction of plasma glucose levels in tumor-bearing animals induced through calorie restriction may be responsible, directly or indirectly, for the significantly prolonged survival compared to normal-fed controls [83,84]. In 1962, Koroljow reported the successful treatment of two patients with metastatic tumors by an insulin-induced hypoglycemic coma [85]. Hyperglycemia, on the other hand, is a predictor of poor survival in patients with various cancers [22,26,86-88] and has been positively correlated to an increased risk for developing cancer at several sites including the pancreas, esophagus, liver, colon, rectum, stomach and prostate in large cohort studies [25,89,90].

14.3.1 INDIRECT EFFECTS OF GLUCOSE AVAILABILITY

Besides delivering more glucose to the tumor tissue, hyperglycemia has two other important negative effects for the host: First, as pointed out by Ely and Krone, even modest blood glucose elevations as they typically occur after a Western diet meal competitively impair the transport of ascorbic acid into immune cells [88,91]. Ascorbic acid is needed for effective phagocytosis and mitosis, so that the immune response to malignant cells is diminished. Second, it has been shown in vitro and in vivo that hyperglycemia activates monocytes and macrophages to produce inflammatory cytokines that play an important role also for the progression of cancer [92-94] (see below). Third, high plasma glucose concentrations elevate the levels of circulating insulin and free IGF1, two potent anti-apoptotic and growth factors for most cancer cells [60]. Free IGF1 is elevated due to a decreased transcription of IGF binding protein (IGFBP)-1 in the liver mediated by insulin [95]. Due to expression of GLUT2, the β-cells of the pancreas are very sensitive to blood glucose concentration and steeply increase their insulin secretion when the latter exceeds the normal level of ~5 mM. In the typical Western diet consisting of three meals a day (plus the occasional CHO-rich snacks and drinks), this implies that insulin levels are elevated above the fasting baseline over most of the day. Both insulin and IGF1 activate the PI3K/Akt/mTOR/HIF-1α pathway by binding to the IGF1 receptor (IGF1R) and insulin receptor (IR), respectively (Figure 2). In addition, insulin stimulates the release of the pro-inflammatory cytokine interleukin (IL)-6 from human adipocytes [96]. Thus, it could be hypothesized that a diet which repeatedly elevates blood glucose levels due to a high GL provides additional growth stimuli for neoplastic cells. In this respect, Venkateswaran et al. have shown in a xenograft model of human prostate cancer that a diet high in CHO stimulated the expression of IRs and phosphorylation of Akt in tumor tissue compared to a low CHO diet [97]. In colorectal [27], prostate [24] and early stage breast cancer patients [23,98] high insulin and low IGFBP-1 levels have been associated with poor prognosis. These findings again underline the importance of controlling blood sugar and hence insulin levels in cancer patients. Dietary restriction and/or a reduced CHO intake are straightforward strategies to achieve this goal.

14.4 ALTERED NUTRITIONAL NEEDS OF CANCER PATIENTS

Cancer patients and those with metabolic syndrome share common patho-logical abnormalities. Since 1885, when Ernst Freund described signs of hyperglycemia in 70 out of 70 cancer patients [99], it has been repeatedly reported that glucose tolerance and insulin sensitivity are diminished in cancer patients even before signs of cachexia (weight loss) become evi-dent [100-102]. Both diabetes and cancer are characterized by a common pathophysiological state of chronic inflammatory signalling and associat-ed insulin resistance. In cancer patients, insulin resistance is thought to be mediated by an acute phase response that is triggered by pro-inflammatory cytokines such as tumor necrosis factor (TNF)-α [101] and IL-6 [103]. In animal and human studies, removal of the tumor resulted in improved glucose clearance, suggesting that these cytokines are secreted, at least in part, from the tumor tissue itself [104,105]. The impact on the metabo-lism of the host is illustrated in Figure 3. In the liver, the inflammatory process leads to increased gluconeogenesis that is fuelled by lactate se-creted from the tumor as well as glycerol from fatty acid breakdown and the amino acid alanine [106] from muscle proteolysis. Gluconeogenesis is an energy-consuming process and might contribute to cancer cachexia by increasing total energy expenditure. Despite increased lipolysis, hepatic production of ketone bodies is usually not enhanced in cancer patients [107,108]. This is in contrast to starvation, where the ketone bodies aceto-acetate and β-hydroxybutyrate counteract proteolysis by providing energy for the brain and muscles [109]. In muscle, glucose uptake and glycogen synthesis are inhibited already at early stages of tumor progression, while fatty acid oxidation remains at normal levels or is increased [110,111]. In the latter case, more fat has to be provided from lipolysis in the adipose tis-sue. In addition, muscles progressively lose protein to provide amino acids for hepatic synthesis of acute-phase proteins and as precursors for glu-coneogenesis. Thus, insulin resistance contributes to fat loss and muscle wasting, the two hallmarks of cancer cachexia. At the same time, it makes more glucose in the blood available for tumor cells.

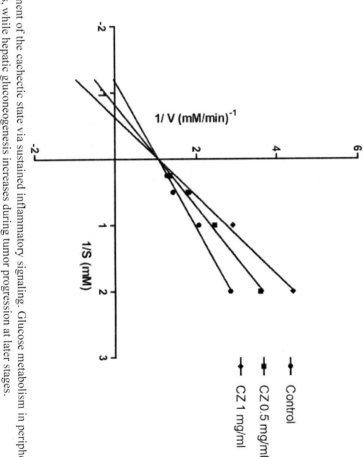

FIGURE 3: Development of the cachectic state via sustained inflammatory signaling. Glucose metabolism in peripheral tissues is impaired already at early stages, while hepatic gluconeogenesis increases during tumor progression at later stages.

14.4.1 FAT AND KETONE BODIES: ANTI-CACHECTIC EFFECTS

It therefore seems reasonable to assume that dietary carbohydrates mainly fuel malignant cells which express the insulin-independent glucose transporters GLUT1 and GLUT3, while muscle cells are more likely to benefit from an increased fat and protein intake. This was summarized as early as in 1977 by C. Young, who stated that lipid sources predominate the fuel utilization of peripheral tissue of patients with neoplastic disease compared to healthy subjects [112]. In addition, most malignant cells lack key mitochondrial enzymes necessary for conversion of ketone bodies and fatty acids to ATP [40,113,114], while myocytes retain this ability even in the cachectic state [107]. This led some authors to propose a high-fat, ketogenic diet (KD) as a strategy to selectively improve body composition of the host at the expense of the tumor [113,115,116]. The traditional KDs, which recommended protein and CHO to account, in combination, for roughly 20 E% (in the incorrect assumption that they were equivalent due to gluconeogenesis) and fat for the remaining 80 E%, have been widely used to treat childhood epilepsia since the 1920s [117]. KDs are also used to treat adiposity [118] and currently adult epilepsy [119]. In the 1980s, Tisdale and colleagues investigated the effects of a ketogenic diet consisting mainly of medium chain triglycerides (MCTs) on two aggressive animal tumor models that were known to lack the ability to utilize ketone bodies. While the diet had no effect on rats bearing the Walker 256 sarcoma [120], it decreased the cachectic weight loss in proportion to its fat content in mice bearing the mouse-specific colon carcinoma MAC16 [121]. For the latter, they further proved an anti-cachectic effect of a ketogenic diet in which the MCTs were replaced with long chain triglycerides (LCTs), although to a somewhat lesser extent [122]. Contrary to LCTs, MCTs do not require transport in chylomicrones, but readily reach the liver where they are metabolized to yield high amounts of ketone bodies. Interestingly, administration of insulin was able to reduce the weight loss similar to the ketogenic MCT diet, but at the expense of a 50% increase in tumor size, which could be counteracted by addition of β-hydroxybutyrate in the drinking water [123]. The supporting effect of insulin on tumor growth has been known since 1924, when Händel and Tadenuma described the nourishing effect of insulin on tumor tissue in an animal model [124], showing evidence that reducing insulin might reduce tumor growth.

14.4.2 CLINICAL STUDIES ON FAT AND CACHEXIA

Clinical studies investigating the anti-cachectic effects of high-fat diets are, however, rare. Fearon et al. administered a 70% MCT diet supplemented with β-hydroxybutyrate parenterally to five late-stage cachectic patients. After seven days on the diet, mean body weight had increased by 2 kg and their physical performance status had improved [125]. Nebeling et al. investigated the effects of a MCT-based ketogenic diet taken ad libitum (60% MCT oil, 20% protein, 10% CHO, 10% other fats) on body weight and glucose metabolism in two pediatric patients with advanced-stage astrocytoma. Within 7 days on the diet, blood glucose levels had decreased to normal, while glucose uptake by the tumor estimated from FDG-PET scans had decreased by an average value of 21.8%. Notably, body weight remained stable throughout the study period of 8 weeks. In a randomized controlled study, Breitkreuz et al. showed that by supplementing the normal diet of 11 under-nourished, non-diabetic patients suffering from metastatic gastro-intestinal cancers with a fat-enriched liquid supplementation for 8 weeks, it was possible to reverse the loss of body weight and lean tissue mass and to improve several quality-of-life parameters in the treatment group, while the control group continued to lose body and lean tissue weight [126]. The supplement contained 66% energy from fat, of which 45% were monounsaturated, 27% saturated (both LCT and MCT) and 28% polyunsaturated; mean energy intake ranged between 1000 and 2000 kcal/day and tended to be higher in patients receiving the additional fat drink.

14.5 THE BENEFITS OF MILD KETOSIS

The study of Breitkreuz et al. shows that ketosis might not be necessary to improve the cachectic state of cancer patients. In recent years, however, more evidence has emerged from both animal and laboratory studies indicating that cancer patients could benefit further from a very low CHO KD. In their mouse models, Tisdale et al. already noted that the KD not only attenuated the cachectic effects of the tumor, but also that the tumors grew more slowly (although they did not attribute this to a direct anti-tumor effect of β-hydroxybutyrate). Tumor growth inhibition through a KD has now been established in many animal models, is supported by a few clinical case reports, and laboratory studies have begun to reveal the underlying molecular mechanisms.

14.5.1 IN VITRO STUDIES

More than 30 years ago, Magee et al. were the first to show that treating transformed cells with various, albeit supra-physiological, concentrations of β-hydroxybutyrate causes a dose-dependent and reversible inhibition of cell proliferation [116]. Their interpretation of the results that "...ketone bodies interfere with either glucose entry or glucose metabolism..." has been confirmed and further specified by Fine et al., who connected the inhibition of glycolysis in the presence of abundant ketone bodies to the overexpression of uncoupling protein-2 (UCP-2), a mitochondrial defect occurring in many tumor cells [127]. In normal cells, abundant acetyl-CoA and citrate from the breakdown of fatty acids and ketone bodies would inhibit key enzymes of glycolysis to ensure stable ATP levels; in tumor cells, however, the same phenomenon would imply a decrease in ATP production if the compensatory ATP production in the mitochondria was impaired. For several colon and breast cancer cell lines, Fine et al. showed that the amount of ATP loss under treatment with acetoacetate was related to the level of UCP-2 expression.

Very recently, Maurer et al. demonstrated that glioma cells - although not negatively influenced by β-hydroxybutyrate - are not able to use this ketone body as a substitute for glucose when starved of the latter, contrary to benign neuronal cells [128]. This supports the hypothesis that under low glucose concentrations, ketone bodies could serve benign cells as a substitute for metabolic demands while offering no such benefit to malign cells.

14.5.2 ANIMAL STUDIES

To our knowledge, the first and—with a total of 303 rats and nine experiments - most extensive study of a KD in animals was conducted by van Ness van Alstyne and Beebe in 1913 [129]. Experiments were divided into two classes: in the first class, rats in the treatment arm were fed a CHO-free diet consisting of casein and lard for several weeks before plantation of a Buffalo sarcoma, while the control arm received either bread only or casein, lard and lactose. Rats on the CHO-free diet not only gained more weight than the controls, but also exhibited much less tumor growth and mortality rates, the differences being "... so striking as to leave no room for doubt that the diet was an important factor in enabling the rats to resist the tumor after growth had started." In a second class of experiments using either the slow-growing Jensen sarcoma or the aggressive Buffalo sarcoma, the rats were put on the CHO-free diet on the same day that the tumor was planted. This time, differences between the treatment and control groups were "... so slight that ... one is left in no doubt of the ineffectiveness of non-carbohydrate feeding begun at the time of tumor implantation." Interestingly, this parallels the observation of Fearon et al. that rats who started to receive a KD at the same day as tumor transplantation did not differ from controls in either body or tumor weight after 14 d [120]. In these rats, it was noted that despite persistent ketosis, blood glucose levels were not significantly lower than in controls which were also fed ad libitum. This stability of blood glucose, independent of ketosis, was subsequently confirmed in studies in which mice were fed ad libitum on a KD [84,114,121-123,130] although two studies reported a drop in blood glucose concentrations compared with the control group [116,131]. In the study of Magee et al., however, diet was presented as a liquid vegetable oil and energy intake was not monitored, allowing for the possibility that the animals underate voluntarily, in this way consuming a "caloric restricted KD" used in several experimental settings from the Seyfried lab [84,114,132], which was shown therein to be superior to the unrestricted KD in tumor growth control. That "caloric restriction" per se can hamper tumor growth has been impressively demonstrated already in 1942 by A. Tannenbaum in a series of comprehensive mouse models with different mouse strains and tumor induction types [133]. Throughout all experimental series, a strict restriction of food intake (impeding weight gain) several weeks before inducing tumorigenesis by application of 3,4 benzpyrene decreased the appearance rate and appearance time of tumors in the diet mice compared to the ad libitum controls. Notably, the calorie-restricted diet was composed of 53% CHOs compared to 69% in the control group. Despite a lack of data on blood glucose and ketone body levels, it could be speculated that the strict restriction of food per se (to 50-60% of the control group) induced a ketotic state and thus the ketones were - at least to some extend - responsible for the effects observed.

In Table 1, we summarize the main results of various mouse studies that determined the effects of KDs on tumor growth and host survival. The results seem to indicate an anti-tumor effect of ketosis. Freedland et al. indeed reported that the mice with the highest levels of ketone bodies had the longest survival times in a human prostate cancer xenograft model [134]. But other studies suggest that there are further possible factors to consider. Seyfried et al. used linear regression to show that plasma glucose and IGF1 levels are a better predictor of tumor growth than ketone bodies in a murine astrocytoma model [84]. Tumor growth in this as well as in a follow-up [114] study was only retarded when the KD had been restricted to induce body weight loss, again underlining the effect of caloric restriction per se. This contrasts with other studies showing growth-inhibitory effects of unrestricted or higher-caloric KDs despite neither decreases in blood glucose concentration nor body weight loss compared with a control group [130,134,135]. According to Otto et al., whose diet had been enriched in MCT and omega-3 fatty acids, fat quality might play a role in explaining these results [130]. The situation in humans might be different as well, as for example Fine et al. found no correlation between calorie intake or weight loss and disease progression in ten patients on an unrestricted KD [136] (see also below).

Concerning fat quality, Freedland et al. observed that a diet rich in corn oil might stimulate prostate cancer growth to a greater extent than one rich in saturated fat [134]. A recent study suggests, however, that tumor growth inhibition neither depends on fat quality nor ketone body levels [131]. In this case, mice injected with either murine squamous cell carcinoma or human colorectal carcinoma cells received a low CHO, high-protein diet in which ~ 60 E% was derived from protein, 10-15 E% from CHO and ~ 25 E% from fat. No systemic ketosis was measured, yet tumors grew significantly less compared with a standard diet containing 55 E% from CHO and 22 E% from the same fat source. IGF1 levels and body weight remained stable, so these findings could not be attributed to one of these factors. There was, however, a significant drop in blood glucose, insulin and lactate levels, and a positive correlation between blood lactate as well as insulin levels and tumor growth was found. The study of Venkateskwaran et al. indicates that in prostate cancer insulin and/or IGF1 play major roles in driving tumor cell proliferation [97].

The diversity of these findings should not be surprising, given the variety of mice strains, tumor cell lines, diet composition and time of diet initiation relative to tumor planting. Instead, it seems remarkable that the same basic treatment, namely drastic restriction of CHOs, apparently induces anti-tumoral effects via different pathways. Thus, it may depend on the circumstances which variables—including blood glucose, insulin, lactate, IGF1, fat quality and ketone bodies—are the best predictors of and responsible for the anti-tumor effects of very low CHO diets.

14.5.3 HUMAN STUDIES

Until now, no randomized controlled trials have been conducted to evaluate the effects of a KD on tumor growth and patient survival. It has to be noted in general, however, that any dietary intervention requiring a dramatic change of life style makes randomized studies nearly impossible —however, even prospective cohort studies are missing. There is only anecdotal evidence that such a diet might be effective as a supportive treatment. One study investigated whether a high-fat diet (80% non-nitrogenous calories from fat) would inhibit tumor cell replication compared to a high-dextrose diet (100% non-nitrogenous calories from dextrose) in 27 patients with gastro-intestinal cancers [137]. Diets were administered parenterally and cell proliferation assessed using thymidine labeling index on tumor samples. After 14 days, the authors found a non-significant trend for impaired proliferation in the high-fat group. Whether ketosis was achieved with this regime was not evaluated, but blood glucose levels were comparable in both trial groups. A very recent pilot trial demonstrated the feasibility of a low CHO up to a ketogenic regimen implemented for 12 weeks in very advanced outpatient cancer patients. Notably, severe side effects were not observed, nearly all standard blood parameters improved and some measures of quality of life changed for the better [138]. The first attempt to treat cancer patients with a long-term controlled KD was reported by L. Nebeling in 1995 for two pediatric patients with astrocytoma [139]. The results of those two cases were very encouraging and the diet was described in detail in another publication [140]. Implementing a KD with additional calorie restriction in a female patient with glioblastoma multiforme clearly demonstrated that this intervention was able to stop tumor growth [132]. This was achieved, however, on the expense of a dramatic weigh loss of 20% over the intervention period, which is no option for the majority of metastatic cancer patients being in a catabolic state. A first clinical study applying a non-restricted KD for patients with glioblastoma (ERGO-study, NHI registration number NCT00575146), which was presented at the 2010 ASCO meeting [141], showed good feasibility and suggested some anti-tumor activity. The protocol of another clinical interventional trial (RECHARGE trial, NCT00444054) treating patients with metastatic cancer by a very low CHO diet was published in 2008 [142], and preliminary data from this study presented at the 2011 ASCO-meeting showed a clear correlation between disease stability or partial remission and high ketosis, independent of weight loss and unconscious caloric restriction of the patients [136]. While a randomized study for the treatment of prostate cancer patents applying the Atkins diet (NCT00932672) is currently recruiting patients at the Duke University, another trial posted at the clinical trials database (ClinicalTrials.gov) is not yet open for recruitment (NCT01092247). Very recently, two Phase I studies applying a ketogenic diet based on KetoCal® 4:1 started recruitment at the University of Iowa, intended to treat prostate cancer patients (KETOPAN, NCT01419483) and non-small cell lung cancer (KETOLUNG, NCT01419587). Thus, in the future, several data should be available to judge whether this kind of nutrition is useful as either a supportive or even therapeutic treatment option for cancer patients.

TABLE 1: Animal studies that have investigated the effects of a KD on tumor progression and host survival

animals	n	tumor	feeding	C/P/F (E%)	major fat source	diet initiation (d)	diet duration (d)	BW vs. controls	BG vs. controls	other effects vs. controls	Ref.
C57BL/6 mice	18	B16 melanoma	ad libitum	0/0/1001	PUFA vegetable oil	0	14	-	↓ b	lower number of lung metastases b	[116]
BALB/c mice	20	Medina-Oborn-Danielson mammary tumor	restricted to 60 E% of control	30/60/5	hydrogenated vegetable oil	~14	70	↓	↓ c	mortality rate ↓ c	[83]
NMRI mice	> 15	MAC16 colon carcinoma	ad libitum	.../.../802	MCT emulsion	8	20	→	-	50% less weight loss b; left35% less tumor weight	[121]
NMRI mice	...	MAC16 colon carcinoma	ad libitum	.../.../80		14 - 21	9	→	-	36% less weight loss a 32% less tumor weight c less nitrogen output a	[123]
C57BL/6 mice	6	CT-2A mouse astrocytoma	restricted to 60 E% of control	0/8/92	lard	1	13	↓3	↓3	80% less tumor weightb; plasma IGF1 levels ↓ b,3	[84]

TABLE 1: *Cont.*

animals	n	tumor	feeding	C/P/F	major fat source	diet initiation	diet duration	BW vs. controls	BG vs. controls	other effects vs. controls	Ref.
C57BL/6 mice +	11	CT-2A mouse astrocytoma +	ad libitum	3/17/80	soy oil (Keto-Cal©)	3	> 8	-	-	no significant differences in either tumor weight, survival or vascularity	[114]
BALB/cJ SCID mice	14	U87 glioblastoma	restricted to 65-70 E% of control	3/17/80	soy oil (Keto-Cal©)	3	>8	↓ b	↓ b	65% (CT-2A)band 35% (U87)cless tumor wet weight; longer survivalb; lower number of blood vessels (both tumors)	
nu/nu mice	20	LNCaP human prostate cancer	ad libitum	10/45/45	...	14	63	↓ a	...	plasma insulin levels ↓ c; plasma IGF1 levels ↓ c; 45% less tumor volumea; 43% less tumor dry weightc; decreased levels of phosphorylated Akt (below detected limits) and insulin receptor in tumor tissue	[97]

TABLE 1: *Cont.*

animals	n	tumor	feeding	C/P/F	major fat source	diet initiation	diet duration	BW vs. controls	BG vs. controls	other effects vs. controls	Ref.
SCID mice	25	LAPC-4 human prostate cancer	9% more energy than control	0/16/84	milk fat + lard	-24	>40	-	↑ c	longer survivalb	[134];
NMRI mice	12	23132/87 human gastric adenoma	ad libitum	0/14/86	cheese + MCT + omega-3 oil	0	>16	-	-	longer survivala; tumor growth rate ↓ c; larger necrotic area in tumorsb	[130]
C3H/HeN mice 4	5	squamous cell carcinoma VII	ad libitum	16/58/26	…	-7	16	→	↓	41% less tumor volumed	[131]
Foxn1nu mice	12	LNT-229 glioma cells	ad libitum	0/13/36	flaxseed and hemp-seed oil	1	>63	-	-	no significant differences in survival, tumor growth and plasma IGF1 levels	[128]

In all but one cases, control diets contained a minimum of 40% CHO. Diet initiation refers to the time of tumor cell plantation.
SCID = Severe Combined Immunodeficiency; C/P/F = ratio of CHO:protein:fat; E% = percent of energy; BW = body weight; BG = blood glucose
1 plus not further specified pellets on days 5, 8 and 11/2 plus 3 mg/ml beta-hydroxybutyrate in drinking water/3 controls were fed a KD ad libitum, not high-CHO/4 similar results for Rag2M mice bearing human colorectal HCT-116 tumors/a $p < 0.005$; b $p < 0.01$; c $p < 0.05$; d $p < 0.1$

14.6 IS THERE A ROLE FOR CARBOHYDRATE RESTRICTION IN THE PREVENTION OF CANCER?

"Prevention of cancer" can refer to either the inhibition of carcinogenesis per se or—once that cells made the transition to malignancy—the sufficient delay of tumor growth, so that it remains undetected and asymptomatic during a subject's lifespan. There is evidence that even modest CHO restriction may influence both of these mechanisms positively through various pathways. The IGF1R-IR pathway has already been discussed: once a potentially carcinogenic somatic mutation has occurred, the probability for carcinogenesis of a cell that is borderline between apoptosis and malignancy might be raised by high levels of insulin and IGF1 in the micro-environment. Once a cell became malignant, high insulin and IGF1 levels might accelerate proliferation and progression towards a more aggressive, glycolytic phenotype. In rats treated with the carcinogen N-methyl-N-nitrosourea, it has been shown that lowering the CHO content of the diet from 60 E% to 40 E% with a simultaneous increase in protein was sufficient to lower postprandial insulin levels as well as decrease the appearance rate of tumors from (18.2 ± 1.3)%/wk to (12.9 ± 1.4)%/wk ($p < 0.05$), however with no statistically significant effect on tumor latency and weight measured after 10 wk [143]. Similarly, a recent study reported that NOP mice, which normally have a 70 - 80% chance of developing breast cancer over their lifetime due to genetic mutations, stayed tumor-free at 1 year of age when their calories from CHO were limited to 15%, while almost half of those on a 55% CHO diet developed tumors [131]. Notably, only 3 out of 11 mice in the 15% CHO group died with having a tumor compared to 7 out of 10 in the 55% CHO group; at death, significantly lower plasma insulin levels had been measured for the low CHO group. These results support the epidemiological [25,29,31,32] and in vitro [81,144] findings that high CHO diets, in particular those including high GI foods, promote mammary tumorigenesis via the sustained action of insulin.

Lower insulin levels may further increase the chance of intermittent ketosis, in particular if CHO restriction is combined with exercise, calorie restriction or intermittent fasting. Seyfried and Shelton [40] pointed out the possibility of ketone bodies to help in cancer prevention through their ability to protect the mitochondria from inflammation and ROS. Being more satiating than low-fat diets [145,146], a low CHO diet would make it easier to avoid caloric overconsumption or to implement intermittent fasting as an additional lifestyle change [147].

14.6.1 AVOIDANCE OF CHRONIC INFLAMMATION

Another potential benefit of low CHO diets might lie in their influence upon inflammatory processes that take place within various tissues. Inflammation is a well-established driver of early tumorigenesis and accompanies most, if not all cancers [148]. Chronic, 'smouldering' inflammation can both cause and develop along with neoplasia. There is evidence that chronic intake of easily digestible CHOs is able to promote such an inflammatory state in leukocytes and endothelial cells [94]. In obese individuals [149] and healthy subjects who underwent eccentric exercise training [150], the inflammatory state was further augmented postprandially through a high CHO intake, but not through high-fat, low CHO meals in the latter study. Maybe more importantly, even moderate CHO restriction has been shown to effectively target several important markers of atherosclerosis and type II diabetes, both of which are associated with chronic inflammation [151-157]. Forsythe et al. showed that in overweight individuals with dyslipidemia a very low CHO diet had a more favorable effect than a low fat diet in reducing several markers of inflammation [158]. Given these findings, it can be hypothesized that a diet with a low GL positively affects cancer risk through reducing postprandial hyperglycemia and the associated inflammatory response.

In this context, it is important to note that a low CHO diet offers further possibilities to target inflammation through omission or inclusion of certain foods. Usually, CHO restriction is not only limited to avoiding sugar and other high-GI foods, but also to a reduced intake of grains. Grains can induce inflammation in susceptible individuals due to their content of omega-6 fatty acids, lectins and gluten [159,160]. In particular gluten might play a key role in the pathogenesis of auto-immune and inflammatory disorders and some malignant diseases. In the small intestine, gluten triggers the release of zonulin, a protein that regulates the tight junctions between epithelial cells and therefore intestinal, but also blood-brain barrier function. Recent evidence suggests that overstimulation of zonulin in susceptible individuals could dysregulate intercellular communication promoting tumorigenesis at specific organ sites [161].

Paleolithic-type diets, that by definition exclude grain products, have been shown to improve glycemic control and cardiovascular risk factors more effectively than typically recommended low-fat diets rich in whole grains [162]. These diets are not necessarily very low CHO diets, but focus on replacing high-GI modern foods with fruits and vegetables, in this way reducing the total GL. This brings us back to our initial perception of cancer as a disease of civilization that has been rare among hunter-gatherer societies until they adopted the Western lifestyle. Although there are certainly many factors contributing to this phenomenon, the evidence presented in this review suggests that reduction of the high CHO intake that accounts for typically > 50 E% in the Western diet may play its own important role in cancer prevention and outcome.

14.7 CONCLUSIONS

We summarize our main findings from the literature regarding the role of dietary CHO restriction in cancer development and outcome.

1. Most, if not all, tumor cells have a high demand on glucose compared to benign cells of the same tissue and conduct glycolysis even in the presence of oxygen (the Warburg effect). In addition, many cancer cells express insulin receptors (IRs) and show hyperactivation of the IGF1R-IR pathway. Evidence exists that chronically elevated blood glucose, insulin and IGF1 levels facilitate tumorigenesis and worsen the outcome in cancer patients.

2. The involvement of the glucose-insulin axis may also explain the association of the metabolic syndrome with an increased risk for several cancers. CHO restriction has already been shown to exert favorable effects in patients with the metabolic syndrome. Epidemiological

and anthropological studies indicate that restricting dietary CHOs could be beneficial in decreasing cancer risk.

3. Many cancer patients, in particular those with advanced stages of the disease, exhibit altered whole-body metabolism marked by increased plasma levels of inflammatory molecules, impaired glycogen synthesis, increased proteolysis and increased fat utilization in muscle tissue, increased lipolysis in adipose tissue and increased gluconeogenesis by the liver. High fat, low CHO diets aim at accounting for these metabolic alterations. Studies conducted so far have shown that such diets are safe and likely beneficial, in particular for advanced stage cancer patients.

4. CHO restriction mimics the metabolic state of calorie restriction or—in the case of KDs—fasting. The beneficial effects of calorie restriction and fasting on cancer risk and progression are well established. CHO restriction thus opens the possibility to target the same underlying mechanisms without the side-effects of hunger and weight loss.

5. Some laboratory studies indicate a direct anti-tumor potential of ketone bodies. During the past years, a multitude of mouse studies indeed proved anti-tumor effects of KDs for various tumor types, and a few case reports and pre-clinical studies obtained promising results in cancer patients as well. Several registered clinical trials are going to investigate the case for a KD as a supportive therapeutic option in oncology.

REFERENCES

1. Levine I: Cancer among the American Indians and its bearing upon the ethnological distribution of the disease. J Cancer Res Clin Oncol 1910, 9:422-435.
2. Orenstein AJ: Freedom Of Negro Races From Cancer. Br Med J 1923, 2:342.
3. Prentice G: Cancer Among Negroes. Br Med J 1923, 2:1181.
4. Brown GM, Cronk LB, Boag TJ: The occurrence of cancer in an Eskimo. Cancer 1952, 5:142-143.
5. Eaton SB, Konner M, Shostak M: Stone agers in the fast lane: chronic degenerative diseases in evolutionary perspective. Am J Med 1988, 84:739-749.

6. Carrera-Bastos P, Fontes-Villalba M, O'Keefe JH, Lindeberg S, Cordain L: The western diet and lifestyle and diseases of civilization. Research Reports in Clinical Cardiology 2011, 2:15-35.

7. Cordain L, Miller JB, Eaton SB, Mann N: Macronutrient estimations in hunter-gatherer diets. Am J Clin Nutr 2000, 72:1589-1592.

8. Hu Y, Shang H, Tong H, Nehlich O, Liu W, Zhao C, Yu J, Wang C, Trinkaus E, Richards MP: Stable isotope dietary analysis of the Tianyuan 1 early modern human. Proc Natl Acad Sci USA 2009, 106:10971-10974.

9. Richards MP: A brief review of the archaeological evidence for Palaeolithic and Neolithic subsistence. Eur J Clin Nutr 2002, 56:16.

10. Ströhle A, Hahn A: Diets of modern hunter-gatherers vary substantially in their carbohydrate content depending on ecoenvironments: results from an ethnographic analysis. Nutrition Research 2011, 31:429-435.

11. Weinberg SL: The diet-heart hypothesis: a critique. J Am Coll Cardiol 2004, 43:731-733.

12. Henderson ST: High carbohydrate diets and Alzheimer's disease. Med Hypotheses 2004, 62:689-700.

13. Seneff S, Wainwright G, Mascitelli L: Nutrition and Alzheimer's disease: the detrimental role of a high carbohydrate diet. Eur J Intern Med 2011, 22:134-140.

14. Chiu CJ, Milton RC, Gensler G, Taylor A: Dietary carbohydrate intake and glycemic index in relation to cortical and nuclear lens opacities in the Age-Related Eye Disease Study. Am J Clin Nutr 2006, 83:1177-1184.

15. Chiu CJ, Hubbard LD, Armstrong J, Rogers G, Jacques PF, Chylack LT Jr, Hankinson SE, Willett WC, Taylor A: Dietary glycemic index and carbohydrate in relation to early age-related macular degeneration. Am J Clin Nutr 2006, 83:880-886.

16. Kaushik S, Wang JJ, Flood V, Tan JS, Barclay AW, Wong TY, Brand-Miller J, Mitchell P: Dietary glycemic index and the risk of age-related macular degeneration. Am J Clin Nutr 2008, 88:1104-1110.

17. Dessein PH, Shipton EA, Stanwix AE, Joffe BI, Ramokgadi J: Beneficial effects of weight loss associated with moderate calorie/carbohydrate restriction, and increased proportional intake of protein and unsaturated fat on serum urate and lipoprotein levels in gout: a pilot study. Ann Rheum Dis 2000, 59:539-543.

18. Roe CM, Fitzpatrick AL, Xiong C, Sieh W, Kuller L, Miller JP, Williams MM, Kopan R, Behrens MI, Morris JC: Cancer linked to Alzheimer disease but not vascular dementia. Neurology 2010, 74:106-112.

19. Boffetta P, Nordenvall C, Nyren O, Ye W: A prospective study of gout and cancer. Eur J Cancer Prev 2009, 18:127-132.

20. Braun S, Bitton-Worms K, Leroith D: The Link between the Metabolic Syndrome and Cancer. Int J Biol Sci 2011, 7:1003-1015.

21. Cheung N, Shankar A, Klein R, Folsom AR, Couper DJ, Wong TY: Age-related macular degeneration and cancer mortality in the atherosclerosis risk in communities study. Arch Ophthalmol 2007, 125:1241-1247.

22. Derr RL, Ye X, Islas MU, Desideri S, Saudek CD, Grossman SA: Association between hyperglycemia and survival in patients with newly diagnosed glioblastoma. J Clin Oncol 2009, 27:1082-1086.

23. Goodwin PJ, Ennis M, Pritchard KI, Trudeau ME, Koo J, Madarnas Y, Hartwick W, Hoffman B, Hood N: Fasting insulin and outcome in early-stage breast cancer: results of a prospective cohort study. J Clin Oncol 2002, 20:42-51.

24. Ma J, Li H, Giovannucci E, Mucci L, Qiu W, Nguyen PL, Gaziano JM, Pollak M, Stampfer MJ: Prediagnostic body-mass index, plasma C-peptide concentration, and prostate cancer-specific mortality in men with prostate cancer: a long-term survival analysis. Lancet Oncol 2008, 9:1039-1047.

25. Stattin P, Bjor O, Ferrari P, Lukanova A, Lenner P, Lindahl B, Hallmans G, Kaaks R: Prospective study of hyperglycemia and cancer risk. Diabetes Care 2007, 30:561-567.

26. Weiser MA, Cabanillas ME, Konopleva M, Thomas DA, Pierce SA, Escalante CP, Kantarjian HM, O'Brien SM: Relation between the duration of remission and hyperglycemia during induction chemotherapy for acute lymphocytic leukemia with a hyperfractionated cyclophosphamide, vincristine, doxorubicin, and dexamethasone/methotrexate-cytarabine regimen. Cancer 2004, 100:1179-1185.

27. Wolpin BM, Meyerhardt JA, Chan AT, Ng K, Chan JA, Wu K, Pollak MN, Giovannucci EL, Fuchs CS: Insulin, the insulin-like growth factor axis, and mortality in patients with nonmetastatic colorectal cancer. J Clin Oncol 2009, 27:176-185.

28. Yuhara H, Steinmaus C, Cohen SE, Corley DA, Tei Y, Buffler PA: Is Diabetes Mellitus an Independent Risk Factor for Colon Cancer and Rectal Cancer? Am J Gastroenterol 2011.

29. Augustin LS, Dal Maso L, La Vecchia C, Parpinel M, Negri E, Vaccarella S, Kendall CW, Jenkins DJ, Francesch S: Dietary glycemic index and glycemic load, and breast cancer risk: a case-control study. Ann Oncol 2001, 12:1533-1538.

30. Melnik BC, John SM, Schmitz G: Over-stimulation of insulin/IGF1 signaling by Western diet may promote diseases of civilization: lessons learnt from Laron syndrome. Nutr Metab (Lond) 2011, 8:41.

31. Sieri S, Pala V, Brighenti F, Pellegrini N, Muti P, Micheli A, Evangelista A, Grioni S, Contiero P, Berrino F, Krogh V: Dietary glycemic index, glycemic load, and the risk of breast cancer in an Italian prospective cohort study. Am J Clin Nutr 2007, 86:1160-1166.

32. Wen W, Shu XO, Li H, Yang G, Ji BT, Cai H, Gao YT, Zheng W: Dietary carbohydrates, fiber, and breast cancer risk in Chinese women. Am J Clin Nutr 2009, 89:283-289.

33. Braunstein A: Wratschebnaje obosrnije. 1921, 7:291.

34. Bierich R: Über die Beteiligung des Bindegewebes an der experimentellen Krebsbildung. Virchows Archiv f Pathol Anatom und Physiol 1922, 23:1-19.

35. Bierich R: Über die Vorgänge Beim Einwuchern der Krebszellen. Wien Klin Wochenschr 1927, 6:1599-1603.

36. Warburg O: Über den Stoffwechsel der Carzinomzelle. Klinische Wochenschrift 1925, :534-536.

37. Warburg O, Posener K, Negelein E: Über den Stoffwechsel der Carcinomzelle. Biochem Zeitschr 1924, :309-344.

38. Warburg O, Wind F, Negelein E: Über den Stoffwechsel der Tumoren im Körper. Klinische Wochenschrift 1926, :828-832.

39. Hanahan D, Weinberg RA: Hallmarks of cancer: the next generation. Cell 2011, 144:646-674.
40. Seyfried TN, Shelton LM: Cancer as a metabolic disease. Nutr Metab (Lond) 2010, 7:7.
41. Warburg O: On respiratory impairment in cancer cells. Science 1956, 124:269-270.
42. Pelicano H, Xu RH, Du M, Feng L, Sasaki R, Carew JS, Hu Y, Ramdas L, Hu L, Keating MJ, et al.: Mitochondrial respiration defects in cancer cells cause activation of Akt survival pathway through a redox-mediated mechanism. J Cell Biol 2006, 175:913-923.
43. Robey RB, Hay N: Mitochondrial hexokinases, novel mediators of the antiapoptotic effects of growth factors and Akt. Oncogene 2006, 25:4683-4696.
44. Robey RB, Hay N: Is Akt the "Warburg kinase"?-Akt-energy metabolism interactions and oncogenesis. Semin Cancer Biol 2009, 19:25-31.
45. Young CD, Anderson SM: Sugar and fat - that's where it's at: metabolic changes in tumors. Breast Cancer Res 2008, 10:202.
46. Deberardinis RJ, Lum JJ, Thompson CB: Phosphatidylinositol 3-kinase-dependent modulation of carnitine palmitoyltransferase 1A expression regulates lipid metabolism during hematopoietic cell growth. J Biol Chem 2006, 281:37372-37380.
47. Berwick DC, Hers I, Heesom KJ, Moule SK, Tavare JM: The identification of ATP-citrate lyase as a protein kinase B (Akt) substrate in primary adipocytes. J Biol Chem 2002, 277:33895-33900.
48. Schwertfeger KL, McManaman JL, Palmer CA, Neville MC, Anderson SM: Expression of constitutively activated Akt in the mammary gland leads to excess lipid synthesis during pregnancy and lactation. J Lipid Res 2003, 44:1100-1112.
49. Laplante M, Sabatini DM: mTOR signaling at a glance. J Cell Sci 2009, 122:3589-3594.
50. Mamane Y, Petroulakis E, LeBacquer O, Sonenberg N: mTOR, translation initiation and cancer. Oncogene 2006, 25:6416-6422.
51. Sun Q, Chen X, Ma J, Peng H, Wang F, Zha X, Wang Y, Jing Y, Yang H, Chen R, et al.: Mammalian target of rapamycin up-regulation of pyruvate kinase isoenzyme type M2 is critical for aerobic glycolysis and tumor growth. Proc Natl Acad Sci USA 2011, 108:4129-4134.
52. Zha X, Sun Q, Zhang H: mTOR upregulation of glycolytic enzymes promotes tumor development. Cell Cycle 2011, 10:1015-1016.
53. Koppenol WH, Bounds PL, Dang CV: Otto Warburg's contributions to current concepts of cancer metabolism. Nat Rev Cancer 2011, 11:325-337.
54. Cully M, You H, Levine AJ, Mak TW: Beyond PTEN mutations: the PI3K pathway as an integrator of multiple inputs during tumorigenesis. Nat Rev Cancer 2006, 6:184-192.
55. Choi NC, Fischman AJ, Niemierko A, Ryu JS, Lynch T, Wain J, Wright C, Fidias P, Mathisen D: Dose-response relationship between probability of pathologic tumor control and glucose metabolic rate measured with FDG PET after preoperative chemoradiotherapy in locally advanced non-small-cell lung cancer. Int J Radiat Oncol Biol Phys 2002, 54:1024-1035.
56. Kunkel M, Reichert TE, Benz P, Lehr HA, Jeong JH, Wieand S, Bartenstein P, Wagner W, Whiteside TL: Overexpression of Glut-1 and increased glucose metabolism

in tumors are associated with a poor prognosis in patients with oral squamous cell carcinoma. Cancer 2003, 97:1015-1024.

57. Bentzen SM, Gregoire V: Molecular imaging-based dose painting: a novel paradigm for radiation therapy prescription. Semin Radiat Oncol 2011, 21:101-110.

58. LeRoith D: Can endogenous hyperinsulinaemia explain the increased risk of cancer development and mortality in type 2 diabetes: evidence from mouse models. Diabetes Metab Res Rev 2010, 26:599-601.

59. Huang XF, Chen JZ: Obesity, the PI3K/Akt signal pathway and colon cancer. Obes Rev 2009, 10:610-616.

60. Pollak M: Insulin and insulin-like growth factor signalling in neoplasia. Nat Rev Cancer 2008, 8:915-928.

61. Fontana L, Partridge L, Longo VD: Extending healthy life span--from yeast to humans. Science 2010, 328:321-326.

62. Lee C, Longo VD: Fasting vs dietary restriction in cellular protection and cancer treatment: from model organisms to patients. Oncogene 2011, 30:3305-3316.

63. Bloom WL, Azar GJ: Similarities Of Carbohydrate Deficiency And Fasting. I. Weight Loss, Electrolyte Excretion, And Fatigue. Arch Intern Med 1963, 112:333-337.

64. Fery F, Bourdoux P, Christophe J, Balasse EO: Hormonal and metabolic changes induced by an isocaloric isoproteinic ketogenic diet in healthy subjects. Diabete Metab 1982, 8:299-305.

65. Klein S, Wolfe RR: Carbohydrate restriction regulates the adaptive response to fasting. Am J Physiol 1992, 262:E631-636.

66. Azar GJ, Bloom WL: Similarities Of Carbohydrate Deficiency And Fasting. Ii. Ketones, Nonesterified Fatty Acids And Nitrogen Excretion. Arch Intern Med 1963, 112:338-343.

67. Jiang W, Zhu Z, Thompson HJ: Dietary energy restriction modulates the activity of AMP-activated protein kinase, Akt, and mammalian target of rapamycin in mammary carcinomas, mammary gland, and liver. Cancer Res 2008, 68:5492-5499.

68. Walenta S, Wetterling M, Lehrke M, Schwickert G, Sundfor K, Rofstad EK, Mueller-Klieser W: High lactate levels predict likelihood of metastases, tumor recurrence, and restricted patient survival in human cervical cancers. Cancer Res 2000, 60:916-921.

69. Gatenby RA, Smallbone K, Maini PK, Rose F, Averill J, Nagle RB, Worrall L, Gillies RJ: Cellular adaptations to hypoxia and acidosis during somatic evolution of breast cancer. Br J Cancer 2007, 97:646-653.

70. Bonuccelli G, Tsirigos A, Whitaker-Menezes D, Pavlides S, Pestell RG, Chiavarina B, Frank PG, Flomenberg N, Howell A, Martinez-Outschoorn UE, et al.: Ketones and lactate "fuel" tumor growth and metastasis: Evidence that epithelial cancer cells use oxidative mitochondrial metabolism. Cell Cycle 2010, 9:3506-3514.

71. Semenza GL: Tumor metabolism: cancer cells give and take lactate. J Clin Invest 2008, 118:3835-3837.

72. Baumann F, Leukel P, Doerfelt A, Beier CP, Dettmer K, Oefner PJ, Kastenberger M, Kreutz M, Nickl-Jockschat T, Bogdahn U, et al.: Lactate promotes glioma migration by TGF-beta2-dependent regulation of matrix metalloproteinase-2. Neuro Oncol 2009, 11:368-380.

73. Chaussain-Miller C, Fioretti F, Goldberg M, Menashi S: The role of matrix metalloproteinases (MMPs) in human caries. J Dent Res 2006, 85:22-32.

74. Williams AC, Collard TJ, Paraskeva C: An acidic environment leads to p53 dependent induction of apoptosis in human adenoma and carcinoma cell lines: implications for clonal selection during colorectal carcinogenesis. Oncogene 1999, 18:3199-3204.

75. Park HJ, Lyons JC, Ohtsubo T, Song CW: Acidic environment causes apoptosis by increasing caspase activity. Br J Cancer 1999, 80:1892-1897.

76. Gatenby RA, Gawlinski ET, Gmitro AF, Kaylor B, Gillies RJ: Acid-mediated tumor invasion: a multidisciplinary study. Cancer Res 2006, 66:5216-5223.

77. Fang JS, Gillies RD, Gatenby RA: Adaptation to hypoxia and acidosis in carcinogenesis and tumor progression. Semin Cancer Biol 2008, 18:330-337.

78. Demetrakopoulos GE, Linn B, Amos H: Rapid loss of ATP by tumor cells deprived of glucose: contrast to normal cells. Biochem Biophys Res Commun 1978, 82:787-794.

79. Priebe A, Tan L, Wahl H, Kueck A, He G, Kwok R, Opipari A, Liu JR: Glucose deprivation activates AMPK and induces cell death through modulation of Akt in ovarian cancer cells. Gynecol Oncol 2011, 122:389-95.

80. Shim H, Chun YS, Lewis BC, Dang CV: A unique glucose-dependent apoptotic pathway induced by c-Myc. Proc Natl Acad Sci USA 1998, 95:1511-1516.

81. Masur K, Vetter C, Hinz A, Tomas N, Henrich H, Niggemann B, Zanker KS: Diabetogenic glucose and insulin concentrations modulate transcriptome and protein levels involved in tumour cell migration, adhesion and proliferation. Br J Cancer 2011, 104:345-352.

82. Gatenby RA, Gillies RJ: Why do cancers have high aerobic glycolysis? Nat Rev Cancer 2004, 4:891-899.

83. Santisteban GA, Ely JT, Hamel EE, Read DH, Kozawa SM: Glycemic modulation of tumor tolerance in a mouse model of breast cancer. Biochem Biophys Res Commun 1985, 132:1174-1179.

84. Seyfried TN, Sanderson TM, El-Abbadi MM, McGowan R, Mukherjee P: Role of glucose and ketone bodies in the metabolic control of experimental brain cancer. Br J Cancer 2003, 89:1375-1382.

85. Koroljow S: Two cases of malignant tumors with metastases apparently treated successfully with hypoglycemic coma. Psychiatr Q 1962, 36:261-270.

86. McGirt MJ, Chaichana KL, Gathinji M, Attenello F, Than K, Ruiz AJ, Olivi A, Quinones-Hinojosa A: Persistent outpatient hyperglycemia is independently associated with decreased survival after primary resection of malignant brain astrocytomas. Neurosurgery 2008, 63:286-291.

87. Maestu I, Pastor M, Gomez-Codina J, Aparicio J, Oltra A, Herranz C, Montalar J, Munarriz B, Reynes G: Pretreatment prognostic factors for survival in small-cell lung cancer: a new prognostic index and validation of three known prognostic indices on 341 patients. Ann Oncol 1997, 8:547-553.

88. Krone CA, Ely JT: Controlling hyperglycemia as an adjunct to cancer therapy. Integr Cancer Ther 2005, 4:25-31.

89. Jee SH, Ohrr H, Sull JW, Yun JE, Ji M, Samet JM: Fasting serum glucose level and cancer risk in Korean men and women. Jama 2005, 293:194-202.

90. Ikeda F, Doi Y, Yonemoto K, Ninomiya T, Kubo M, Shikata K, Hata J, Tanizaki Y, Matsumoto T, Iida M, Kiyohara Y: Hyperglycemia increases risk of gastric cancer posed by Helicobacter pylori infection: a population-based cohort study. Gastroenterology 2009, 136:1234-1241.

91. Ely JT, Krone CA: Glucose and cancer. N Z Med J 2002, 115:U123.

92. Shanmugam N, Reddy MA, Guha M, Natarajan R: High glucose-induced expression of proinflammatory cytokine and chemokine genes in monocytic cells. Diabetes 2003, 52:1256-1264.

93. Wen Y, Gu J, Li SL, Reddy MA, Natarajan R, Nadler JL: Elevated glucose and diabetes promote interleukin-12 cytokine gene expression in mouse macrophages. Endocrinology 2006, 147:2518-2525.

94. Dandona P, Chaudhuri A, Ghanim H, Mohanty P: Proinflammatory effects of glucose and anti-inflammatory effect of insulin: relevance to cardiovascular disease. Am J Cardiol 2007, 99:15B-26B.

95. Rajaram S, Baylink DJ, Mohan S: Insulin-like growth factor-binding proteins in serum and other biological fluids: regulation and functions. Endocr Rev 1997, 18:801-831.

96. LaPensee CR, Hugo ER, Ben-Jonathan N: Insulin stimulates interleukin-6 expression and release in LS14 human adipocytes through multiple signaling pathways. Endocrinology 2008, 149:5415-5422.

97. Venkateswaran V, Haddad AQ, Fleshner NE, Fan R, Sugar LM, Nam R, Klotz LH, Pollak M: Association of diet-induced hyperinsulinemia with accelerated growth of prostate cancer (LNCaP) xenografts. J Natl Cancer Inst 2007, 99:1793-1800.

98. Goodwin PJ, Ennis M, Pritchard KI, Trudeau ME, Koo J, Hartwick W, Hoffma B, Hood N: Insulin-like growth factor binding proteins 1 and 3 and breast cancer outcomes. Breast Cancer Res Treat 2002, 74:65-76.

99. Freund E: Zur Diagnose des Carcinoms. Wien med Bl 1885, 1:268-269.

100. Lundholm K, Holm G, Schersten T: Insulin resistance in patients with cancer. Cancer Res 1978, 38:4665-4670.

101. McCall JL, Tuckey JA, Parry BR: Serum tumour necrosis factor alpha and insulin resistance in gastrointestinal cancer. Br J Surg 1992, 79:1361-1363.

102. Marat D, Noguchi Y, Yoshikawa T, Tsuburaya A, Ito T, Kondo J: Insulin resistance and tissue glycogen content in the tumor-bearing state. Hepatogastroenterology 1999, 46:3159-3165.

103. Makino T, Noguchi Y, Yoshikawa T, Doi C, Nomura K: Circulating interleukin 6 concentrations and insulin resistance in patients with cancer. Br J Surg 1998, 85:1658-1662.

104. Yoshikawa T, Noguchi Y, Matsumoto A: Effects of tumor removal and body weight loss on insulin resistance in patients with cancer. Surgery 1994, 116:62-66.

105. Permert J, Ihse I, Jorfeldt L, von Schenck H, Arnquist HJ, Larsson J: Improved glucose metabolism after subtotal pancreatectomy for pancreatic cancer. Br J Surg 1993, 80:1047-1050.

106. Waterhouse C, Jeanpretre N, Keilson J: Gluconeogenesis from alanine in patients with progressive malignant disease. Cancer Res 1979, 39:1968-1972.

107. Rich AJ, Wright PD: Ketosis and nitrogen excretion in undernourished surgical patients. JPEN J Parenter Enteral Nutr 1979, 3:350-354.

108. Conyers RA, Need AG, Rofe AM, Potezny N, Kimber RJ: Nutrition and cancer. Br Med J 1979, 1:1146.

109. Owen OE, Morgan AP, Kemp HG, Sullivan JM, Herrera MG, Cahill GF Jr: Brain metabolism during fasting. J Clin Invest 1967, 46:1589-1595.

110. Gambardella A, Paolisso G, D'Amore A, Granato M, Verza M, Varricchio M: Different contribution of substrates oxidation to insulin resistance in malnourished elderly patients with cancer. Cancer 1993, 72:3106-3113.

111. Korber J, Pricelius S, Heidrich M, Muller MJ: Increased lipid utilization in weight losing and weight stable cancer patients with normal body weight. Eur J Clin Nutr 1999, 53:740-745.

112. Young VR: Energy metabolism and requirements in the cancer patient. Cancer Res 1977, 37:2336-2347.

113. Tisdale MJ, Brennan RA: Loss of acetoacetate coenzyme A transferase activity in tumours of peripheral tissues. Br J Cancer 1983, 47:293-297.

114. Zhou W, Mukherjee P, Kiebish MA, Markis WT, Mantis JG, Seyfried TN: The calorically restricted ketogenic diet, an effective alternative therapy for malignant brain cancer. Nutr Metab (Lond) 2007, 4:5.

115. Conyers RA, Need AG, Durbridge T, Harvey ND, Potezny N, Rofe AM: Cancer, ketosis and parenteral nutrition. Med J Aust 1979, 1:398-399.

116. Magee BA, Potezny N, Rofe AM, Conyers RA: The inhibition of malignant cell growth by ketone bodies. Aust J Exp Biol Med Sci 1979, 57:529-539.

117. Freeman JM, Kossoff EH: Ketosis and the ketogenic diet, 2010: advances in treating epilepsy and other disorders. Adv Pediatr 2010, 57:315-329.

118. Westman EC, Feinman RD, Mavropoulos JC, Vernon MC, Volek JS, Wortman JA, Yancy WS, Phinney SD: Low-carbohydrate nutrition and metabolism. Am J Clin Nutr 2007, 86:276-284.

119. Kossoff EH, Dorward JL: The modified Atkins diet. Epilepsia 2008, 49(Suppl 8):37-41.

120. Fearon KC, Tisdale MJ, Preston T, Plumb JA, Calman KC: Failure of systemic ketosis to control cachexia and the growth rate of the Walker 256 carcinosarcoma in rats. Br J Cancer 1985, 52:87-92.

121. Tisdale MJ, Brennan RA, Fearon KC: Reduction of weight loss and tumour size in a cachexia model by a high fat diet. Br J Cancer 1987, 56:39-43.

122. Tisdale MJ, Brennan RA: A comparison of long-chain triglycerides and medium-chain triglycerides on weight loss and tumour size in a cachexia model. Br J Cancer 1988, 58:580-583.

123. Beck SA, Tisdale MJ: Effect of insulin on weight loss and tumour growth in a cachexia model. Br J Cancer 1989, 59:677-681.

124. Händel M, Tadeuma K: Über die Beziehung des Geschwulstwachstums zur Ernährung und zum Stoffwechsel. II. Mitteilung. Versuche zur Frage der Bedeutung der Kohlenhydrate für das Wachstum des Rattencarcinoms. Klin Wochenschr 1924,: 288-293.

125. Fearon KC, Borland W, Preston T, Tisdale MJ, Shenkin A, Calman KC: Cancer cachexia: influence of systemic ketosis on substrate levels and nitrogen metabolism. Am J Clin Nutr 1988, 47:42-48.

126. Breitkreutz R, Tesdal K, Jentschura D, Haas O, Leweling H, Holm E: Effects of a high-fat diet on body composition in cancer patients receiving chemotherapy: a randomized controlled study. Wien Klin Wochenschr 2005, 117:685-692.
127. Fine EJ MA, Quadros EV, Sequeira JM, Feinman RD: Acetoacetate reduces growth and ATP concentration in cancer cell lines which over-express uncoupling protein 2. Cancer Cell international 2009, 9:14:11.
128. Maurer GD, Brucker DP, Baehr O, Harter PN, Hattingen E, Walenta S, Mueller-Klieser W, Steinbach JP, Rieger J: Differential utilization of ketone bodies by neurons and glioma cell lines: a rationale for ketogenic diet as experimental glioma therapy. BMC Cancer 2011, 11:315.
129. van Ness van Alstyne E, Beebe SP: Diet studies in transplantable tumors. I. The effect of non-carbohydrate diet upon the growth of transplantable sarcoma in rats. J Med Res 1913, :217-232.
130. Otto C, Kaemmerer U, Illert B, Muehling B, Pfetzer N, Wittig R, Voelker HU, Thiede A, Coy JF: Growth of human gastric cancer cells in nude mice is delayed by a ketogenic diet supplemented with omega-3 fatty acids and medium-chain triglycerides. BMC Cancer 2008, 8:122.
131. Ho VW, Leung K, Hsu A, Luk B, Lai J, Shen SY, Minchinton AI, Waterhouse D, Bally MB, Lin W, et al.: A Low Carbohydrate, High Protein Diet Slows Tumor Growth and Prevents Cancer Initiation. Cancer Res 2011.
132. Zuccoli G, Marcello N, Pisanello A, Servadei F, Vaccaro S, Mukherjee P, Seyfried TN: Metabolic management of glioblastoma multiforme using standard therapy together with a restricted ketogenic diet: Case Report. Nutr Metab (Lond) 2010, 7:33.
133. Tannenbaum A: The Genesis and Growth of Tumors. II. Effects of Caloric Restriction per se. Cancer Res 1942, 2:460-467.
134. Freedland SJ, Mavropoulos J, Wang A, Darshan M, Demark-Wahnefried W, Aronson WJ, Cohen P, Hwang D, Peterson B, Fields T, et al.: Carbohydrate restriction, prostate cancer growth, and the insulin-like growth factor axis. Prostate 2008, 68:11-19.
135. Masko EM, Thomas JA, Antonelli JA, Lloyd JC, Phillips TE, Poulton SH, Dewhirst MW, Pizzo SV, Freedland SJ: Low-carbohydrate diets and prostate cancer: how low is "low enough"? Cancer Prev Res (Phila) 2010, 3:1124-1131.
136. Fine EJ, Segal-Isaacson CJ, Feinman RD, Herszkopf S, Romano M, Tomuta N, Bontempo A, Sparano JA: A pilot safety and feasibility trial of a reduced carbohydrate diet in patients with advanced cancer. J Clin Oncol 2011., 29(suppl; abstr e13573)
137. Rossi-Fanelli F, Franchi F, Mulieri M, Cangiano C, Cascino A, Ceci F, Muscaritoli M, Seminara P, Bonomo L: Effect of energy substrate manipulation on tumour cell proliferation in parenterally fed cancer patients. Clin Nutr 1991, 10:228-232.
138. Schmidt M, Pfetzer N, Schwab M, Strauss I, Kammerer U: Effects of a ketogenic diet on the quality of life in 16 patients with advanced cancer: A pilot trial. Nutr Metab (Lond) 2011, 8:54.
139. Nebeling LC, Miraldi F, Shurin SB, Lerner E: Effects of a ketogenic diet on tumor metabolism and nutritional status in pediatric oncology patients: two case reports. J Am Coll Nutr 1995, 14:202-208.
140. Nebeling LC, Lerner E: Implementing a ketogenic diet based on medium-chain triglyceride oil in pediatric patients with cancer. J Am Diet Assoc 1995, 95:693-697.

141. Rieger J, Baehr O, Hattingen E, Maurer G, Coy J, Weller M, Steinbach J: The ERGO trial: A pilot study of a ketogenic diet in patients with recurrent glioblastoma. J Clin Oncol (Meeting Abstracts) 2010, 28:e12532.
142. Fine EJ, Segal-Isaacson CJ, Feinman R, Sparano J: Carbohydrate restriction in patients with advanced cancer: a protocol to assess safety and feasibility with an accompanying hypothesis. Commun Oncol 2008, 5:22-26.
143. Moulton CJ, Valentine RJ, Layman DK, Devkota S, Singletary KW, Wallig MA, Donovan SM: A high protein moderate carbohydrate diet fed at discrete meals reduces early progression of N-methyl-N-nitrosourea-induced breast tumorigenesis in rats. Nutr Metab (Lond) 2010, 7:1.
144. Osborne CK, Bolan G, Monaco ME, Lippman ME: Hormone responsive human breast cancer in long-term tissue culture: effect of insulin. Proc Natl Acad Sci USA 1976, 73:4536-4540.
145. Jonsson T, Granfeldt Y, Erlanson-Albertsson C, Ahren B, Lindeberg S: A paleolithic diet is more satiating per calorie than a mediterranean-like diet in individuals with ischemic heart disease. Nutr Metab (Lond) 2010, 7:85.
146. Nickols-Richardson SM, Coleman MD, Volpe JJ, Hosig KW: Perceived hunger is lower and weight loss is greater in overweight premenopausal women consuming a low-carbohydrate/high-protein vs high-carbohydrate/low-fat diet. J Am Diet Assoc 2005, 105:1433-1437.
147. Mavropoulos JC, Isaacs WB, Pizzo SV, Freedland SJ: Is there a role for a low-carbohydrate ketogenic diet in the management of prostate cancer? Urology 2006, 68:15-18.
148. Mantovani A, Allavena P, Sica A, Balkwill F: Cancer-related inflammation. Nature 2008, 454:436-444.
149. Gonzalez F, Minium J, Rote NS, Kirwan JP: Altered tumor necrosis factor alpha release from mononuclear cells of obese reproductive-age women during hyperglycemia. Metabolism 2006, 55:271-276.
150. Depner CM, Kirwan RD, Frederickson SJ, Miles MP: Enhanced inflammation with high carbohydrate intake during recovery from eccentric exercise. Eur J Appl Physiol 2010, 109:1067-1076.
151. Rudnick PA, Taylor KW: Effect Of Prolonged Carbohydrate Restriction On Serum-Insulin Levels In Mild Diabetes. Br Med J 1965, 1:1225-1228.
152. Garg A, Bantle JP, Henry RR, Coulston AM, Griver KA, Raatz SK, Brinkley L, Chen YD, Grundy SM, Huet BA, et al.: Effects of varying carbohydrate content of diet in patients with non-insulin-dependent diabetes mellitus. Jama 1994, 271:1421-1428.
153. Accurso A, Bernstein RK, Dahlqvist A, Draznin B, Feinman RD, Fine EJ, Gleed A, Jacobs DB, Larson G, Lustig RH, et al.: Dietary carbohydrate restriction in type 2 diabetes mellitus and metabolic syndrome: time for a critical appraisal. Nutr Metab (Lond) 2008, 5:9.
154. Perez-Guisado J, Munoz-Serrano A, Alonso-Moraga A: Spanish Ketogenic Mediterranean Diet: a healthy cardiovascular diet for weight loss. Nutr J 2008, 7:30.
155. Volek JS, Phinney SD, Forsythe CE, Quann EE, Wood RJ, Puglisi MJ, Kraemer WJ, Bibus DM, Fernandez ML, Feinman RD: Carbohydrate restriction has a more favorable impact on the metabolic syndrome than a low fat diet. Lipids 2009, 44:297-309.

156. Jonsson T, Granfeldt Y, Ahren B, Branell UC, Palsson G, Hansson A, Soderstrom M, Lindeberg S: Beneficial effects of a Paleolithic diet on cardiovascular risk factors in type 2 diabetes: a randomized cross-over pilot study. Cardiovasc Diabetol 2009, 8:35.
157. Elhayany A, Lustman A, Abel R, Attal-Singer J, Vinker S: A low carbohydrate Mediterranean diet improves cardiovascular risk factors and diabetes control among overweight patients with type 2 diabetes mellitus: a 1-year prospective randomized intervention study. Diabetes Obes Metab 2010, 12:204-209.
158. Forsythe CE, Phinney SD, Fernandez ML, Quann EE, Wood RJ, Bibus DM, Kraemer WJ, Feinman RD, Volek JS: Comparison of low fat and low carbohydrate diets on circulating fatty acid composition and markers of inflammation. Lipids 2008, 43:65-77.
159. Cordain L: Cereal grains: humanity's double-edged sword. World Rev Nutr Diet 1999, 84:19-73.
160. Cordain L, Toohey L, Smith MJ, Hickey MS: Modulation of immune function by dietary lectins in rheumatoid arthritis. Br J Nutr 2000, 83:207-217.
161. Fasano A: Zonulin and its regulation of intestinal barrier function: the biological door to inflammation, autoimmunity, and cancer. Physiol Rev 2011, 91:151-175.
162. Klonoff DC: The beneficial effects of a Paleolithic diet on type 2 diabetes and other risk factors for cardiovascular disease. J Diabetes Sci Technol 2009, 3:1229-1232.

This chapter was originally published under the Creative Commons Attribution License. Klement, R. J., and Kämmerer, U. Is There a Role for Carbohydrate Restriction in the Treatment and Prevention of Cancer? Nutrition & Metabolism 2011: 8(75), doi:10.1186/1743-7075-8-75.

PART IV

RECENT DEVELOPMENTS AND FUTURE TRENDS IN CLINICAL NUTRITION

CHAPTER 15

PARENTERAL NUTRITION ADDITIVE SHORTAGES: THE SHORT-TERM, LONG-TERM AND POTENTIAL EPIGENETIC IMPLICATIONS IN PREMATURE AND HOSPITALIZED INFANTS

CORRINE HANSON, MELISSA THOENE, JULIE WAGNER,
DEAN COLLIER, KASSANDRA LECCI,
and ANN ANDERSON-BERRY

15.1 INTRODUCTION

Product shortages in the healthcare system can have a significant impact on the care provided to patients. In the case of premature or ill infants, high nutrient needs and a lack of nutrient stores make the appropriate administration of nutrition essential. At birth, the clamping of the umbilical cord immediately disrupts the delivery of nutrients from the placenta, which places these infants into a situation that makes adequate provision of nutrients extremely important and challenging. Though the preferred method of feeding, enteral feedings are often delayed in the premature infant due to the fragility and medical complications associated with prematurity. Management of co-morbid conditions, such as patent ductus arteriosis, chronic lung disease and feeding intolerance frequently involve restriction of fluids and delays in enteral feeding advancement. As a result, these cases usually remain dependent on parenteral nutrition (PN) for the first few weeks of life; however, those with complications, such as necrotizing enterocolitis, may require sole PN for much longer time periods. In the infant with congenital anomalies, such as gastroschisis, trachea-esophageal fistula or bowel disease, feedings may not be feasible for weeks or even months. There is growing evidence that inadequate nutrition in the first few weeks of life results in growth failure and poor long-term neurodevelopmental outcomes [1,2]. Due to concern for current shortages of parenteral nutrition (PN) micronutrient additives, the purpose of this paper is to review the potential effect of these shortages on premature and newborn infants and to present a case study of nutrient deficiency resulting from this shortage.

15.2 CURRENT SHORTAGES AND TPN MANAGEMENT STRATEGIES

According the American Society for Enteral and Parenteral nutrition (ASPEN), all PN products, aside from dextrose and water, have been in short supply at some point since the spring of 2010 (see Table 1) [3]. At the time of this writing, a number of PN products continue to be unavailable or in short supply. The current status of these and other drug products can be accessed at the Food and Drug Administration web site [4].

TABLE 1: Parenteral Shortages 2010–2012.

Amino Acids	Ascorbic Acid	Calcium Chloride
Calcium Gluconate	Chromium	Copper
Cyanocobalamin	Fat Emulsions	L-cysteine
Magnesium Sulfate	Multivitamins (MVI)	Phytonadione (vitamin K)
Potassium Acetate	Potassium Phosphate	Selenium
Sodium Acetate	Sodium phosphate	Trace Elements
Vitamin A	Zinc	

ASPEN has provided timely and comprehensive advice to clinicians for dealing with PN product shortages. Recommendations for conserving products during shortages of electrolytes, vitamins and minerals are included in Table 2.

TABLE 2: ASPEN Recommendations for Conservation of PN Products.

1. Consider oral or enteral administration

2. Prioritize patients, saving supplies for those most vulnerable patients

3. Eliminate adding injectable electrolytes/minerals to enteral nutrition products

4. Minimize the use of additives to daily maintenance IV fluids

5. Reevaluate replacement algorithms or treatment protocols

6. Carefully evaluate alternative supplies of individual and multiple electrolyte products that are available, including standardized, commercially available PN products

In a recent survey conducted by ASPEN, 25% of respondents stated their hospitals are in short supply of pediatric multi-dose products, and 28% indicated they are in short supply of single-dose products, such as selenium. When asked what actions were being employed in response to these shortages, 70% reported giving multivitamins (MVI) only three times per week, 28% were giving half the recommended dose daily, 27% were giving no MVI and 9% were giving adult MVI to pediatric patients [3].

Product shortages are not new and have historically been documented to cause morbidity and mortality. The omission of vitamins from PN has been associated with death as far back as 1989, when three people at a large university medical center died from refractory lactic acidosis caused by receiving thiamine-deficient PN [5]. In 1997, three additional patients receiving thiamine-free TPN due to a national shortage developed lactic acidosis, and later, in 1998, a case report of Wernicke encephalopathy and beriberi due to a multivitamin shortage was published [6]. Due to the historical documentation of such adverse outcomes in adults, we sought documentation of the potentially adverse effects in high-risk, premature infants.

15.3 NUTRITIONAL NEEDS OF PRETERM INFANTS AND POTENTIAL EFFECT OF SHORTAGES OF PN COMPONENTS

15.3.1 PROTEINS AND AMINO ACIDS

Per kilogram, premature infants have among the highest protein needs of any population during the lifecycle. Adequate protein provision of up to 4–4.5 g/kg/day is required for very low birthweight infants to match intra-uterine accretion rates and to promote appropriate growth [7,8]. Adequate growth during Neonatal Intensive Care Unit (NICU) hospitalization is essential to reduce the risk for negative outcomes associated with growth restriction, including chronic lung disease, cerebral palsy, neurological impairment and rehospitalization after discharge [3,9]. The early administration of parenteral protein helps to offset the nutritional deficits that begin with preterm birth and continue throughout the infant's hospitalization [10]. Early administration of PN that meets protein goals has been associated with improvements in both short-term [11] and long-term growth [1]. In contrast, infants not receiving early administration of amino acids have been found to have suboptimal head growth at 18 months of age [1]. Restrictions in head circumference growth are especially concerning, given the association between poor head growth and decreased neurode-velopmental outcomes [12]. Likewise, goal provisions of both protein and energy during the first week of life may positively influence 18-month developmental outcomes [13]. Furthermore, shortages of individual amino acids can have a profound effect on premature infant outcomes. For example, supplementation of neonatal PN with cysteine has been associated with improved nitrogen balance, which may support appropriate growth for both weight and head circumference [14,15]. The addition of cysteine may also help to lower the pH of the PN mixture. This allows increased amounts of calcium and phosphorus to be provided with a decreased risk for mineral precipitation, further promoting adequate bone mineralization and growth [16]. Consequently, shortages of amino acid formulations impacting early and adequate provision of protein in this population can have significant long-term ramifications.

15.3.2 LIPIDS

Fat provision is essential for life, but most specifically for premature infants to promote normal growth and development. Fat is the most calorically-dense nutrient and aids in the development of cells, the eye and the brain. Without lipid provision to PN-dependent infants, essential fatty acid deficiency (EFAD) develops quickly as there are reports as early as the second day of life [17]. EFAD may result in failure to thrive, dermatitis, thrombocytopenia, susceptibility to infection and poor would healing [17]. Fat-free PN as the primary source of nutrition may further result in suboptimal calorie provision and associated growth restriction. Increased total caloric intake in the first week of life has been associated with improved Bailey MDI scores in a preterm infant population [13].

15.3.3 MINERALS

In addition to macronutrient shortages, micronutrient shortages have the potential to significantly impact the health of infants. One PN additive that is commonly used among the premature infant population is calcium gluconate. Although higher in aluminum content than other available PN calcium salts, calcium gluconate is often the additive of choice due to its favorable solubility curves, allowing for higher calcium and phosphorus administration. Like protein, calcium and phosphorus needs in premature infants remain high. Approximately 80% of total body calcium, phosphorus and magnesium at birth are accrued within the last trimester of pregnancy. Consequently, infants born prematurely have inadequately mineralized bones and require higher weight-based provisions of calcium and phosphorus compared to infants born at term [8]. Adequate magnesium provision is also necessary to promote bone growth, as hypomagnesaemia may hinder calcium absorption. In addition, many common medications used for NICU infants can decrease calcium and magnesium absorption, including diuretics, steroids and anti-convulsants [8,18]. It has been well-documented that premature infants receiving inadequate amounts of calcium and phosphorus from PN have higher incidences of osteopenia and elevated levels of serum alkaline phosphatase, which may indicate poor bone mineralization and rapid bone turnover [19]. Clinical manifestations of poorly mineralized bone will vary depending on the degree of bone mineralization. Bone fractures may develop in these infants as a result and may negatively affect the stability of the chest wall, which can lead to atelectasis or an increased risk of chronic lung disease [14].

15.3.4 TRACE ELEMENTS

Only two trace elements are recommended on the initial day of PN; zinc and selenium. Other trace elements are not thought to be needed until after two weeks of age [14]. Zinc is a cofactor in more than 300 metabolic processes and supports protein and nucleic acid synthesis, immune function, gene expression and growth. Two-thirds of the total body zinc is transferred from mother to fetus during the last trimester of pregnancy and serum levels of zinc decline progressively in infants on zinc-free PN [20]. As a result, ill neonates are at a high risk of developing zinc deficiency if adequate supplementation cannot be provided. Additionally, most commercially-available trace element formulations contain insufficient zinc to meet the needs of the preterm infant. Therefore, supplemental zinc must be added to PN, creating an additional mechanism for shortages.

Selenium is a component of glutathione peroxidase, a compound which protects against free radical injury. Premature infants are often exposed to high levels of oxygen and resulting oxidative stress. It has been speculated, though not proven, that selenium could be an important contributing factor in the pathogenesis of disorders, such as bronchopulmonary dysplasia [21]. Most of the placental transfer of selenium occurs after the 36th week of gestation [20]; hence, most premature infants will be born selenium-depleted. Serum selenium concentrations have been shown to decrease quickly in infants treated for respiratory distress syndrome who receive selenium-free or selenium-deficient PN [22]. A 2009 Cochrane review of selenium supplementation suggested that the currently recommended dose of selenium (2 µg/kg/day) for preterm infants receiving parenteral nutrition is inadequate to maintain selenium concentrations, so a dose of 3 µg/kg/day may be more appropriate to achieve concentrations found in healthy breast-fed infants [23].

As current shortages make it difficult to provide even the previously recommended amounts, implementing new evidence-based recommendations for increased nutrient dosing becomes nearly impossible.

Inadequate provision of many other trace elements also poses nutritional risks for premature infants. For example, both rapid growth and limited stores make premature infants at risk for copper deficiency, which can result in osteoporosis, neutropenia or hypochromatic anemia [17]. Like zinc and selenium, accretion of these nutrients occurs primarily during the last trimester of pregnancy, so adequate provision is essential.

15.3.5 VITAMINS

Premature infants require higher amounts of most vitamins when compared to term infants, due to increased nutrient losses or increased requirements for growth. Recent studies have documented nutrient deficiencies, specifically vitamin D deficiency, are highly prevalent in preterm births [24–27]. Vitamin D supplementation during infancy is associated with increased bone mass in childhood [28]. Consequently, deficiency and inadequate supplementation may result in rickets or craniotabes [29]. Recent research has also expanded our understanding of vitamin D status during infancy to include health benefits beyond bone status. Poor vitamin D status during early infancy is now thought to be associated with other negative health outcomes, such as type 1 diabetes [30,31], and pulmonary problems, such as respiratory tract infections or wheezing later in childhood [32–34]. The current recommendation for parenteral vitamin D intake is 400 IU/day [8] which is the amount included in 5 mL in most pediatric PN MVI formulations. Concerning, however, is that PN pediatric MVI dosing is weight-based according to the manufacturer instructions; so many low birth weight infants receive less than 5 mL (400 IU Vitamin D) daily. These dosing practices, combined with product shortages, may make adequate administration of vitamin D challenging in infants dependent on PN. Monitoring the vitamin D status of newborns is additionally challenging, as 25(OH)D levels are not an accurate marker of vitamin D status in the newborn population. In 2006, Singh et al. showed that a biologically inactive

C-3 epimer of vitamin D is present in high levels in the bloodstream of infants up to one year of age and may lead to an overestimation of vitamin D status in infants and concerns regarding vitamin D overdosing in others [35].

Administration of vitamin E is recommended immediately after birth in premature infants, as some older studies suggest a reduction in incidence and severity of intraventricular hemorrhage. A plasma target of >1 mg/dL by 24 h of life, and 2 mg/dL by three days of life has been recommended to reduce IVH [14,36,37]. These levels should be attainable with the administration of current PN MVI formulations, which would provide 2.8 mg/kg/day of vitamin E if given daily. However, limiting the amount of MVI provided to premature infants, as many institutions are now being forced to do, could negatively impact serum levels.

Vitamin A is necessary in premature infants for normal lung growth and for maintaining the integrity of the respiratory epithelial track. Preterm infants are born with essentially no hepatic reserves of Vitamin A, so levels of vitamin A at birth are reflectively low [38]. Therefore, Vitamin A needs to be provided consistently from PN to promote adequate intake. However, a 2011 study demonstrated that despite a policy to introduce intravenous-lipid supplemented PN by day of life two, only 11% of infants consistently met the recommended daily intake of vitamin A during the first two weeks of life [39]. Considering inadequate provision despite the best efforts, it remains concerning that many PN-dependent infants are receiving reduced MVI dosing due to current shortages. The role of vitamin A in preventing neonatal chronic lung disease has consistently been documented, including evidence that intramuscular supplementation of vitamin A in extremely low birthweight infants improves respiratory outcomes [38,40]. A meta-analysis of low birthweight infants demonstrated that either enteral or parenteral supplementation with vitamin A reduced the risk of both death and oxygen requirement at one month of age, and the risk of oxygen requirement at 36 weeks corrected gestational age [38]. This practice may be limited, since intramuscular injections are considered painful; however, current product shortages of the vitamin injections would inhibit this practice from being initiated in NICUs targeting bronchopulmonary dysplasia (BPD). In addition to its role in lung integrity, vitamin A appears critical in the development of ocular photoreceptors.

During the third trimester of pregnancy, the ocular content of rhodopsin (of which vitamin A is an essential component) increases 10-fold [39]. For the NICU hospitalized infant, an adequate substrate in the form of vitamin A needs to be available to support this process in the extrauterine environment. Recommended PN administration of vitamins and minerals discussed above are given in Table 3. Vitamin levels provided by current MVI dosing guidelines are provided in Table 4.

TABLE 3: Recommended PN Administration of Select Nutrients *.

	Birth weight <1.5 kg	Term Infants
Calcium	3 mEq/kg/day	2 mEq/kg/day
Zinc	1000–3000 µg/kg/day	250 µg/day <3 months
		100 µg/day >3 months
Selenium	1.3–4.5 µg/kg/day	2.0 µg/day
Vitamin A	700–1500 IU/day	2300 IU
Vitamin D	400 IU/day	400 IU/day
Vitamin E	6–12 IU/kg/day	7 IU/day

* Adapted from [16].

TABLE 4: Vitamin Levels Provided by Current Dosing of Pediatric MVI.

	Per 1.5 mL MVI (<1000 g)	Per 3.25 mL MVI (1001–2500 g)	Per 5 mL MVI (>2500 g)
Vitamin C (mg)	24	5.2	80
Vitamin A (IU)	690	1495	2300
Vitamin D (IU)	120	260	400
Thiamine (B1) (mg)	0.36	0.78	1.2
Riboflavin (B2) (mg)	0.42	0.91	1.4
Pyridoxine (B6) (mg)	0.3	0.65	1
Niacin (mg)	5.1	11.1	17
Dexpanthenol (mg)	1.5	3.3	5
VitaminE (IU)	2.1	4.6	7
Vitamin K (mg)	0.06	0.13	0.2
Folic Acid (µg)	42	91	140
Biotin (µg)	6	13	20
B12 (µg)	0.3	0.65	1

15.3.6 EPIGENETIC RAMIFICATIONS OF EARLY NEONATAL NUTRITION

In addition to the acute problems from inadequate nutrient provision during the NICU stay, accumulating evidence implies that the early prenatal period is critical for influencing disease risk for a range of disorders that may develop later in life. There is considerable evidence suggesting that the risk of developing non-communicable diseases can be altered by modifying influences of early-life environment, which includes nutritional factors. This programming appears to be largely independent of genomic sequences and is likely to be mediated by epigenetic mechanisms. Epigenetic programming during development is widely believed to have a long-lasting effect on the health of a newborn [41]. Epigenetic changes are modification to the DNA, which can be caused by various factors, including the environment, which do not change the underlying sequence.

Studies have demonstrated that infants born prematurely have decreased insulin sensitivity when compared with those born at term [42,43]. In one study of preterm vs. term infants and insulin sensitivity, all of the infants born prematurely had inadequate protein intake in the first month of life, which was proposed as a trigger to an epigenetic modification of genes involved in glucose regulation [42]. Supplementation with vitamin D during infancy has been reported to confer protection against beta-cell regulated autoimmune disorders [44,45]. A potentially very important activity of vitamin D receptor agonists is their capacity to induce in vitro and in vivo tolerogenic dendrite cells, which are able to enhance suppressor T-cells that, in turn, inhibit T-cell responses. Failure of tolerance mechanisms may lead to auto-reactive T-cell activation and to induction of autoimmune diseases [46]. In a birth-cohort study published in 2001, Hypponen et al. found that vitamin D supplementation during the first year of life is associated with a lower risk of type-1 diabetes [47]. This prospective study followed 12,055 infants born in Finland and collected data in the first year of life regarding vitamin D supplementation practices; later in life, data was collected on the diagnosis of type I diabetes. At this time in Finland, the recommended level of Vitamin D supplementation for infants was 2000 IU daily, and infants in the study were classified as follows:

receiving daily supplementation of less than 2000 IU, within 2000 IU or over 2000 IU. Higher vitamin D supplementation in infancy was associated with a decreased frequency of Type 1 diabetes later in life when adjusted for neonatal, anthropometric and social characteristics. Infants who regularly took the recommended dose of 2000 IU vitamin D per day had a relative risk (RR) of 0.22 (95% CI: 0.05–0.89) compared to those who regularly received less than the recommended amount. Children suspected of having rickets during the first year of life had a RR of 3.0 (95% CI: 1.0–9.0) compared with those without such a suspicion [31]. These results are consistent with the findings of the EURODIAB study in 1999, which was a large multicenter and population-based case-control study on early risk factors of childhood onset Type I diabetes. Vitamin D supplementation in early infancy to prevent rickets in seven different European regions was also associated with a decreased risk for childhood-onset, insulin-dependent diabetes. The favorable association with vitamin D supplementation persisted after adjustment for birth weight, duration of breast feeding, maternal age and study center [30]. Additionally, vitamin D supplementation in infancy has also been associated with a decreased risk of pre-eclampsia later in life [47]. Consideration of the potential for early nutrition interventions to have long-term health outcome implications is crucial when designing nutrition support regimens for the premature infant population.

15.3.7 POTENTIAL COST OF SHORTAGES

Poor outcomes attributable to PN shortages can quickly become costly to both an infant's health and associated healthcare costs. In 2007, the Journal of Pediatrics compiled data regarding health care costs associated with initial hospitalization for premature infants. The data clearly showed a monetary cost increase for all premature births compared to term births, but this cost was four-to-seven-times higher for low birthweight infants with complications like chronic lung disease or intraventricular hemorrhage. Additionally, 15% of all premature or low birthweight infants were given a diagnosis of slow growth, malnutrition or small for gestational age. The cost for these categorized infants was nearly $450 million [48]. Despite high health care costs, complications associated with inadequate nutrition from PN shortages can have a much more devastating toll on infant health. Complications, such as intraventricular hemorrhages or developmental delay, may impact life-long ability and care requirements. Similarly, chronic diseases pose increased risks for infections and infant mortality. Adequate provision of nutrients from PN is essential to help preserve the health integrity of these infants, but unfortunately, PN shortages have the potential to do the opposite.

15.3.8 CASE STUDY

At our care facility, one infant on prolonged PN-developed selenium deficiency with associated skin symptoms. This infant was born at an estimated gestational age of approximately 26 weeks with a birth weight of 790 g. The infant developed a bowel perforation within the first few weeks of life and required surgery, with a resulting jejunostomy placement. The infant required both sole and partial PN for most of his extensive hospital stay, and was approximately four months of age when able to take full enteral feedings. Due to current shortages, no selenium was available to add to the PN formulation. The infant developed dry, scaly skin and a selenium level was checked around three months of life secondary to skin symptoms and recent PN additive shortages. The selenium level was reported from the laboratory as 11 µg/L, which is well below the normal range for serum selenium of 23–190 µg/L. Conditions, such as macrocytosis and fatal cardiomyopathy, have been reported when selenium levels fall below 16 µg/L [23]. Once enteral feedings were established, 25 µg of oral selenium was supplemented every other day, because no parenteral selenium was available. By discharge around five months of life, the infant was on calorically-dense full enteral feedings and his skin symptoms had resolved, so at this point selenium supplementation was discontinued.

15.3.9 POTENTIAL SOLUTIONS:

As is evident from Table 2, whenever possible during a shortage of PN products, prioritization of resources is crucial in ensuring that the most vulnerable populations receive critical products. Additional strategies to potentially maximize the nutrition status of premature infants during PN product shortages should be explored. For instance, our care facility was forced to reduce pediatric PN MVI to tri-weekly provision to conserve supplies. With the concern for inadequate nutrient provision to our extremely and very low birthweight infants, we increased the weight-based MVI dosing. For example, infants receiving 1.5 mL of PN MVI would receive 3.25 mL tri-weekly. Though this is not a documented strategy, it does allow for a higher administration of nutrients while conserving available local resources.

15.4 CONCLUSION

This review demonstrates the potential short-term and long term epigenetic impacts that current PN shortages can have on premature and ill infants. Clinicians must, therefore, make decisions using current evidence and clinical judgment to ensure avoidance of poor outcomes in situations where adequate administration of all essential nutrients is not possible.

REFERENCES

1. Poindexter, B.B.; Langer, J.C.; Dusick, A.M.; Ehrenkranz, R.A. National Institute of Child Health and Human Development Neonatal Research Network. Early provision of parenteral amino acids in extremely low birth weight infants: Relation to growth and neurodevelopmental outcome. J. Pediatr. 2006, 148, 300–305.
2. Ehrenkranz, R.A.; Dusick, A.M.; Vohr, B.R.; Wright, L.L.; Wrage, L.A.; Poole, W.K. Growth in the neonatal intensive care unit influences neurodevelopmental and growth outcomes of extremely low birth weight infants. Pediatrics 2006, 117, 1253–1261.
3. Mirtallo, J.M.; Holcombe, B.; Kochevar, M.; Guenter, P. Parenteral nutrition product shortages: The A.S.P.E.N. strategy. Nutr. Clin. Pract. 2012, 27, 385–391.
4. FDA. U.S. Food and Drug Administration. Available online: http://www.fda.gov/Drugs/ DrugSafety/DrugShortages/default.htm (accessed on 5 December 2012).
5. Centers for Disease Control (CDC). Deaths associated with thiamine-deficient total parenteral nutrition. MMWR Morb. Mortal. Wkly. Rep. 1989, 38, 43–46.

6. Hahn, J.S.; Berquist, W.; Alcorn, D.M.; Chamberlain, L.; Bass, D. Wernicke encephalopathy and beriberi during total parenteral nutrition attributable to multivitamin infusion shortage. Pediatrics 1998, 101, E10.

7. Kleinman, R. Pediatric Nutrition Handbook, 6th ed.; American Academy of Pediatrics: Elk Grove, IL, USA, 2009.

8. Nutrition of the Premature Infant: Scenitific Basis and Practical Guidelines; Tsang, R.C., Uauy, R., Koletzki, B., Zlotkin, S.H., Eds.; Digital Education Publishing Inc.: Cincinnati, OH, USA, 2005.

9. Dusick, A.M.; Poindexter, B.B.; Ehrenkranz, R.A.; Lemons, J.A. Growth failure in the preterm infant: Can we catch up? Semin. Perinatol. 2003, 27, 302–310.

10. Pieltain, C.; Habibi, F.; Rigo, J. Early nutrition, postnatal growth retardation and outcome of VLBW infants. Arch. Pediatr. 2007, 14, S11–S15.

11. Berry, M.A.; Abrahamowicz, M.; Usher, R.H. Factors associated with growth of extremely premature infants during initial hospitalization. Pediatrics 1997, 100, 640–646.

12. Hack, M.; Breslau, N.; Weissman, B.; Aram, D.; Klein, N.; Borawski, E. Effect of very low birth weight and subnormal head size on cognitive abilities at school age. N. Engl. J. Med. 1991, 325, 231–237.

13. Stephens, B.E.; Walden, R.V.; Gargus, R.A.; Tucker, R.; Mckinley, L.; Mance, M.; Nye, J.; Vohr, B.R. First-week protein and energy intakes are associated with 18-month developmental outcomes in extremely low birth weight infants. Pediatrics 2009, 123, 1337–1343.

14. Schanler, R. UpToDate. Available online: http//www.uptodate.com (accessed on 1 October 2012).

15. Soghier, L.M.; Brion, L.P. Cysteine, cystine or N-acetylcysteine supplementation in parenterally fed neonates. Cochrane Database Syst. Rev. 2006, CD004869; doi:10.1002/14651858. CD004869.pub2.

16. Greene, H.L.; Hambidge, K.M.; Schanler, R.; Tsang, R.C. Guidelines for the use of vitamins, trace elements, calcium, magnesium, and phosphorus in infants and children receiving total parenteral nutrition: Report of the subcommittee on pediatric parenteral nutrient requirements from the committee on clinical practice issues of the american society for clinical nutrition. Am. J. Clin. Nutr. 1988, 48, 1324–1342.

17. Groh-Wargo, S.; Thompson, M.; Hovasi Cox, J. Nutrition Care for High Risk Newborns, 3rd ed.; Precept Press, Inc.: Chicago, IL, USA, 2000.

18. Koo, W.W. Parenteral nutrition-related bone disease. J. Parenter. Enteral. Nutr. 1992, 16, 386–394.

19. Prestridge, L.L.; Schanler, R.J.; Shulman, R.J.; Burns, P.A.; Laine, L.L. Effect of parenteral calcium and phosphorus therapy on mineral retention and bone mineral content in very low birth weight infants. J. Pediatr. 1993, 122, 761–768.

20. Burjonrappa, S.C.; Miller, M. Role of trace elements in parenteral nutrition support of the surgical neonate. J. Pediatr. Surg. 2012, 47, 760–771.

21. Falciglia, H.S.; Johnson, J.R.; Sullivan, J.; Hall, C.F.; Miller, J.D.; Riechmann, G.C.; Galciglia, G.A. Role of antioxidant nutrients and lipid peroxidation in premature

infants with respiratory distress syndrome and bronchopulmonary dysplasia. Am. J. Perinatol. 2003, 20, 97–107.

22. Daniels, L.; Gibson, R.; Simmer, K. Randomised clinical trial of parenteral selenium supplementation in preterm infants. Arch. Dis. Child. 1996, 74, F158–F164.

23. Darlow, B.A.; Austin, N.C. Selenium supplementation to prevent short-term morbidity in preterm neonates. Cochrane Database Syst. Rev. 2003, CD003312; doi:10.1002/14651858.CD003312.

24. Shah, M.D.; Shah, S.R. Nutrient deficiencies in the premature infant. Pediatr. Clin. North. Am. 2009, 56, 1069–1083.

25. Hanson, C.; Armas, L.; Lyden, E.; Anderson-Berry, A. Vitamin D status and associations in newborn formula-fed infants during initial hospitalization. J. Am. Diet. Assoc. 2011, 111, 1836–1843.

26. Merewood, A.; Mehta, S.D.; Grossman, X.; Chen, T.C.; Mathieu, J.S.; Holick, M.F.; Bauchner, H. Widespread vitamin D deficiency in urban Massachusetts newborns and their mothers. Pediatrics 2010, 125, 640–647.

27. Basile, L.A.; Taylor, S.N.; Wagner, C.L.; Quinones, L.; Hollis, B.W. Neonatal vitamin D status at birth at latitude 32 degrees 72′: Evidence of deficiency. J. Perinatol. 2007, 27, 568–571.

28. Zamora, S.A.; Rizzoli, R.; Belli, D.C.; Slosman, D.O.; Bonjour, J.P. Vitamin D supplementation during infancy is associated with higher bone mineral mass in prepubertal girls. J. Clin. Endocrinol. Metab. 1999, 84, 4541–4544.

29. Yorifuji, J.; Yorifuji, T.; Ṭachibana, K.; Nagai, S.; Kawai, M.; Momoi, T.; Nagasaka, H.; Hatayama, H.; Nakahata, T. Craniotabes in normal newborns: The earliest sign of subclinical vitamin D deficiency. J. Clin. Endocrinol. Metab. 2008, 93, 1784–1788.

30. The EURODIAB substudy 2 study group. Vitamin D supplement in early childhood and risk for type I (insulin-dependent) diabetes mellitus. Diabetologia 1999, 42, 51–54.

31. Hypponen, E.; Laara, E.; Reunanen, A.; Jarvelin, M.R.; Virtanen, S.M. Intake of vitamin D and risk of type 1 diabetes: A birth-cohort study. Lancet 2001, 358, 1500–1503.

32. Ginde, A.A.; Mansbach, J.M.; Camargo, C.A., Jr. Association between serum 25-hydroxyvitamin D level and upper respiratory tract infection in the third national health and nutrition examination survey. Arch. Intern. Med. 2009, 169, 384–390.

33. Erkkola, M.; Kaila, M.; Nwaru, B.I.; Kronberg-Kipplia, C.; Ahonen, S.; Nevalainen, J.; Veijola, R.; Pekkanen, J.; Ilonen, J.; Simell, O.; Knip, M.; Virtanen, S.M. Maternal vitamin D intake during pregnancy is inversely associated with asthma and allergic rhinitis in 5-year-old children. Clin. Exp. Allergy 2009, 39, 875–882.

34. Camargo, C.A., Jr.; Rifas-Shiman, S.L.; Litonjua, A.A.; Rich-Edwards, J.W.; Weiss, S.T.; Gold, D.R.; Kleinmann, K.; Gillman, M.W. Maternal intake of vitamin D during pregnancy and risk of recurrent wheeze in children at 3 y of age. Am. J. Clin. Nutr. 2007, 85, 788–795.

35. Singh, R.J.; Taylor, R.L.; Reddy, G.S.; Grebe, S.K. C-3 epimers can account for a significant proportion of total circulating 25-hydroxyvitamin D in infants, compli-

cating accurate measurement and interpretation of vitamin D status. J. Clin. Endocrinol. Metab. 2006, 91, 3055–3061.

36. Brion, L.P.; Bell, E.F.; Raghuveer, T.S. Vitamin E supplementation for prevention of morbidity and mortality in preterm infants. Cochrane Database Syst. Rev. 2003, CD003665; doi:10.1002/ 14651858.CD003665.

37. Brion, L.P.; Bell, E.F.; Raghuveer, T.S.; Soghier, L. What is the appropriate intravenous dose of vitamin E for very-low-birth-weight infants? J. Perinatol. 2004, 24, 205–207.

38. Darlow, B.A.; Graham, P.J. Vitamin A supplementation to prevent mortality and short- and long-term morbidity in very low birthweight infants. Cochrane Database Syst. Rev. 2007, CD000501; doi:10.1002/14651858.CD000501.pub2.

39. Mactier, H.; Mokaya, M.M.; Farrell, L.; Edwards, C.A. Vitamin A provision for preterm infants: Are we meeting current guidelines? Arch. Dis. Child. 2011, 96, F286–F289.

40. Tyson, J.E.; Wright, L.L.; Oh, W.; Kennedy, K.A.; Mele, L.; Ehenkranz, R.A.; Stoll, B.J.; Lemons, J.A.; Stevenson, D.K.; Bauer, C.R.; Korones, S.B.; Fanaroff, A.A. Vitamin A supplementation for extremely-low-birth-weight infants. National Institute of Child Health and Human Development Neonatal Research Network. N. Engl. J. Med. 1999, 340, 1962–1968.

41. Bocheva, G.; Boyadjieva, N. Epigenetic regulation of fetal bone development and placental transfer of nutrients: Progress for osteoporosis. Interdiscip. Toxicol. 2011, 4, 167–172.

42. Regan, F.M.; Cutfield, W.S.; Jefferies, C.; Robinson, E.; Hofman, P.L. The impact of early nutrition in premature infants on later childhood insulin sensitivity and growth. Pediatrics 2006, 118, 1943–1949.

43. Mathai, S.; Cutfield, W.S.; Derraik, J.G.; Dalziel, S.R.; Harding, J.E.; Robinson, E.; Biggs, J.; Jefferies, C.; Hofman, P.L. Insulin sensitivity and beta-cell function in adults born preterm and their children. Diabetes 2012, 61, 2479–2483.

44. Stene, L.C.; Ulriksen, J.; Magnus, P.; Joner, G. Use of cod liver oil during pregnancy associated with lower risk of type I diabetes in the offspring. Diabetologia 2000, 43, 1093–1098.

45. Staples, J.A.; Ponsonby, A.L.; Lim, L.L.; McMichael, A.J. Ecologic analysis of some immune-related disorders, including type 1 diabetes, in australia: Latitude, regional ultraviolet radiation, and disease prevalence. Environ. Health Perspect. 2003, 111, 518–523.

46. Adorini, L. Intervention in autoimmunity: The potential of vitamin D receptor agonists. Cell. Immunol. 2005, 233, 115–124.

47. Hypponen, E.; Hartikainen, A.L.; Sovio, U.; Jarvelin, M.R.; Pouta, A. Does vitamin D supplementation in infancy reduce the risk of pre-eclampsia? Eur. J. Clin. Nutr. 2007, 61, 1136–1139; doi:10.1038/sj.ejcn.1602625.

48. Russell, R.B.; Green, N.S.; Steiner, C.A.; Meikle, S.; Howse, J.L.; Pochman, K.; Dias, T.; Potetz, L.; Davidoff, M.J.; Damus, K.; Petrini, J.R. Cost of hospitalization for preterm and low birth weight infants in the united states. Pediatrics 2007, 120, e1–e9.

This chapter was originally published under the Creative Commons Attribution License. Hanson, C., Thoene, M., Wagner, J., Collier, D., Lecci, K., and Anderson-Berry, A. Parenteral Nutrition Additive Shortages: The Short-Term, Long-Term and Potential Epigenetic Implications in Premature and Hospitalized Infants. Nutrients 2012: 4(12); 1977-1988. doi:10.3390/nu4121977.

CHAPTER 16

AN OBSERVATIONAL STUDY REVEALS THAT NEONATAL VITAMIN D IS PRIMARILY DETERMINED BY MATERNAL CONTRIBUTIONS: IMPLICATIONS OF A NEW ASSAY ON THE ROLES OF VITAMIN D FORMS

SPYRIDON N. KARRAS, ILTAF SHAH,
ANDREA PETROCZI, DIMITRIOS G. GOULIS, HELEN BILI,
FOTINI PAPADOPOULOU, VIKENTIA HARIZOPOULOU,
BASIL C. TARLATZIS, and DECLAN P. NAUGHTON

16.1 INTRODUCTION

Vitamin D insufficiency and deficiency has been associated with a wide spectrum of diseases, ranging from neurological disorders to chronic inflammatory conditions [1]. The resurgence of rickets in some Western countries highlights the potential risks of not gaining sufficient vitamin D through diet, supplementation or exposure to sunlight [2,3]. Vitamin D deficiency is frequently defined as serum concentrations less than 20 ng/mL with concentrations between 21–29 ng/mL treated as insufficiency and greater than 30 ng/mL as sufficient [4-7]. Recent studies attest to widespread insufficiency of vitamin D in many Western nations, namely the UK, USA and other European countries, including Greece [5,6,8]. Vitamin D deficiency during pregnancy has been associated with maternal morbidity, including gestational diabetes [9] and an increased rate of caesarean section [10]. Likewise, for the neonate, there is a putative association with being small-for-gestational age (SGA) [11]. Finally, as far as children are concerned, impaired neurocognitive development [12] and skeletal problems, such as reduced bone mineral content [13] have been reported.

A recent report details the importance of maternal circulating vitamin D concentrations in determining neonatal circulating vitamin D [14]. The authors compared the contributions of genetic factors to maternal vitamin D levels and found that 19% of neonatal circulating vitamin D levels are predicted by the latter with genetics having little influence. The recent report of a lack of significant relationship between circulating 25(OH)D and the highly active $1\alpha,25\text{-}(OH)_2D$ concentrations in a meta-analysis of mother-neonate studies suggest that measurement of vitamin D concentrations should go beyond the routinely measured 25(OH)D forms [15]. Many studies have relied on questionable assays to assess concentrations of the various forms of vitamin D [16,17]. Given the complexities involved in rigorous assessment of vitamin D analogues, a novel assay was recently introduced to differentiate and quantify the circulating precursors and active forms from biologically inactive epimers [18,19]. It is envisaged that the role of vitamin D in disease prevention and treatment can be further elucidated with the accurate measurement of all forms of vitamin D, including epimers.

The primary aim of this study was to determine serum (mothers) and umbilical cord (neonates) concentrations of all vitamin D forms [single-hydroxylated [$25(OH)D_2$, $25(OH)D_3$], double-hydroxylated [$1\alpha,25(OH)_2D_2$, $1\alpha,25(OH)_2D_3$], epimers [$3\text{-epi-}25(OH)D_2$, $3\text{-epi-}25(OH)D_3$]], in a Northern Greece cohort of pregnant women at term and their neonates, by applying a novel highly specific and accurate assay. A secondary aim was to predict neonatal vitamin D concentrations by means of maternal parameters.

16.2 SUBJECTS AND METHODS

16.2.1 SUBJECTS

The study was conducted from January 2011 until December 2011. Pregnant women were recruited from the Maternity Unit of the First Department of Obstetrics and Gynaecology, Aristotle University, Thessaloniki, Greece. Inclusion criterion was full-term pregnancy (37th -42th gestational week). Maternal exclusion criteria were primary hyperparathyroidism, secondary osteoporosis, liver disease, hyperthyroidism, nephrotic syndrome, inflammatory bowel disease, rheumatoid arthritis, osteomalacia, morbid obesity, diabetes in pregnancy, age < 18 year and use of medications affecting calcium (Ca) or vitamin D status. Neonatal exclusion criteria were being small-for-gestational age (SGA) and presence of severe congenital anomaly. Informed consent was obtained from all mothers. The protocol received approval from the Bioethics Committee of Aristotle University of Thessaloniki, Greece.

16.2.2 DEMOGRAPHICS AND DIET

At enrolment, demographic and social characteristics were recorded. Ca and vitamin D dietary intake during the last month of pregnancy were assessed through a validated, semi- quantitative, food frequency questionnaire that includes 150 foods and beverages [20]. For each dietary item, participants were asked to report their frequency of consumption and portion size. From these data, calculations were made for estimations of consumed quantities (in g per day) and total energy intake (in kcal per day), on the basis of a food composition database, modified to accommodate the particularities of the Greek diet [21].

16.2.3 BIOCHEMICAL AND HORMONAL ASSAYS

Blood samples were obtained from mothers by antecubital venipuncture 30–60 minutes before delivery. Umbilical cord blood was collected immediately after clamping, from the umbilical vein. Serum and umbilical cord specimens were stored at -20°C prior to analysis for the following parameters: Ca, phosphorus (P), parathyroid hormone (PTH), vitamin D_2, vitamin D_3, 25(OH)D_2, 25(OH)D_3, 1α,25(OH)$_2D_2$, 1α,25(OH)$_2D_3$, 3-epi-25(OH)D_2 and 3-epi-25(OH)D_3. Serum Ca and P determinations were performed using the Cobas INTEGRA clinical chemistry system (D-68298; Roche Diagnostics, Mannheim, Germany). The inter- and intra-assay coefficients of variation (CVs) were 0.99% and 3.5% for Ca, and 1.3% and 2.5% for P, respectively. PTH determinations were performed using the electrochemiluminescence immunoassay ECLIA (Roche Diagnostics GmbA, Mannheim, Germany). Reference range for PTH was 15–65 pg/mL, functional sensitivity 6.0 pg/mL, within-run precision 0.6 - 2.8% and total precision 1.6 - 3.4%. Using the novel assay, a total of eight forms of vitamin D were quantified by liquid chromatography tandem mass spectrometry (LC-MS/MS) with lower limits of quantification (LLOQ) as follows: vitamin D_2 (0.5 ng/mL), vitamin D_3 (0.5 ng/mL), 25(OH)D2 (0.5 ng/mL), 25(OH)D_3 (0.5 ng/mL), 1α,25(OH)$_2D_2$ (0.015 ng/mL), 1α,25(OH)$_2D_3$ (0.015 ng/mL), 3-epi-25(OH)D_2 (0.01 ng/mL) and 3-epi-25(OH)D_3 (0.015 ng/mL). Briefly, the assay involves a chiral column in tandem with a rapid resolution microbore column along with liquid-liquid extraction. The method is fully validated using quality controls at four different concentration levels (QCL, QCM, QCH, LLOQ). Quality controls were calculated after chromatographically separating the epimers, isobars and other analogues. The same concentrations were recovered from spiked quality controls prepared in house. The accuracy of the assay was also double checked using DEQAS and Chromsystem quality controls. Full method validation parameters have been reported previously [18,19]. Maternal vitamin D deficiency was defined as serum concentrations ≤20 ng/mL, insufficiency as 21–29 ng/mL and sufficiency as ≥30 ng/mL.

16.2.4 UVB MEASUREMENTS

Ultraviolet B (UVB) radiation includes wavelengths from 280 to 320 nm. UVB data for the broad geographical region of Thessaloniki, Greece were collected from the Section of Applied and Environmental Physics, Aristotle University of Thessaloniki. Daily integral of effective UVB radiation from sunrise to sunset (from 09:00 to 16:00) was used as the most representative parameter for UVB exposure. These hours were selected as they represent the beginning and the end of the working time for the majority of the population. Individual sunlight exposure was recorded for each participant during that period. Finally, mean UVB exposure during the previous 45 days (daily integral) before blood sample collection (estimated mean half-life of vitamin D) was calculated for each participant.

16.2.5 STATISTICAL ANALYSIS

The dependent variables (DV) were the concentrations of circulating vitamin D_2 and D_3 in neonates. Adjusted body mass index (BMI) was calculated by adjusting the pre-delivery weight with the average expected weight gain based on the mother's pre-pregnancy BMI. In cases below the limit of quantification (BLQ), a conservative zero value was imputed. Owing to large within group variances, vitamin D concentrations between mothers and neonates were compared using Wilcoxon Signed Rank test. ANOVA was used to compare the circulating vitamin D concentrations in neonates of mothers with deficient, insufficient and sufficient vitamin D status. To determine the explained variances by the independent variables (IV) in predicting the DV (neonatal serum vitamin D_2 and D_3, separately), two hierarchical linear regression analyses were used. In both models, in order to control for random differences between mothers (e.g. maternal age, number of previous live birth, UVB exposure and vitamin D), these variables were entered in the first block, followed by serum concentrations of $25OHD_2$ and D_3, along with their corresponding epimers, individually.

Meeting assumptions for the regression models were defined as follows: Durbin-Watson statistics (d) between 1.5 and 2.5 for auto-correlation of residuals and Variance Inflating Factor (VIF)<5 for multi-colinearity, along with satisfactory normal P-P plot of regressions standardized residual. The level of significance was set as $p < 0.05$. All statistical analyses were conducted in SPSS v19 (SPSS Inc, Chicago, Ill).

16.3 RESULTS

The sample consisted of 60 pairs of Caucasian mothers and their neonates. Mean maternal age was 32.8 ± 5.2 years, 40% with previous live birth (31.7% primiparous and 8.3% multiparous). The mean pre-conception BMI was 22.2 ± 3.3 kg/m^2 (range 16.1 - 31.6), adjusted BMI was 22.4 ± 4.3 kg/m^2 (range 13.5 - 35.5). Thirty-six women were on Ca supplementation (range 250 – 1000 mg per day, with 32 on 500 mg per day) and none were on vitamin D supplementation. Of the 60 neonates, 67% were female. PTH, Ca, P concentrations of mothers and neonates, along with the estimated daily average intake of Ca and vitamin D, and UVB exposure are presented in Table 1.

16.3.1 MATERNAL AND NEONATAL VITAMIN 25(OH)D CONCENTRATIONS

Mothers had slightly, but not statistically significantly, higher concentrations of circulating vitamin D [25(OH)D$_2$ and 25(OH)D$_3$] compared to neonates (17.9 ± 13.2 vs. 15.9 ± 13.6 ng/mL, W=771.0, p=0.289) (Figure 1). The proportions of the mothers with sufficient, insufficient and deficient 25(OH)D concentrations are shown in Figure 2A. The frequency distribution revealed 40 women below 20 ng/mL, with a further 11 between 21–29 ng/mL, leaving a minority in the sufficient range. Notably, whilst the pattern of neonatal 25(OH)D concentration roughly followed the same of the mothers in the deficient and insufficient mother groups, it varied widely resembling uniform distribution in the group of mothers with sufficient vitamin D status. Although thresholds for neonatal serum vitamin D sufficiency are yet to be established, the frequency distribution of neonatal 25(OH)D concentrations (Figure 2B), followed the pattern of the maternal circulating levels, with the majority of the values being concentrated at the low end of the spectrum. The mean neonatal 25(OH)D concentrations in the three maternal groups were significantly different [12.5±8.7 vs. 19.2±9.1 vs. 26.6±26.3 ng/mL, F(2,59)=4.914, p =0.011] for neonates of mothers in the deficient, insufficient and sufficient group, respectively. This overall result was due to a difference between the deficient and sufficient groups (p =0.012), but not due to other comparisons (deficient vs. insufficient, p=0.279 and insufficient vs. sufficient, p=0.413).

TABLE 1: Measures of PTH, Ca, P concentrations of mothers and neonates, and daily average intake of Ca, vitamin D

	Mother		Neonates	
	Range	Mean±SD	Range	Mean±SD
Vitamin D[a] intake (µg/day)	0.35-5781.00	421.97±1206.130	-	-
Ca intake[a] (mg/day)	111.0-1935.40	786.10±360.240	-	-
UVB (wh/m²)	0.01-0.36	0.20±0.11	-	-
PTH (mg/dL)[b]	19.00-85.40	36.91±15.15	1.20-17.90	6.99±2.78
Ca (mg/dL)[c]	4.20-9.60	8.56±0.75	8.90-11.80	10.32±0.62
P (pg/mL)[c]	1.40-5.00	3.58±0.63	4.30-7.10	5.73±0.58

[a] mother n = 58.
[b] mother n = 59, neonate n = 57.
[c] mother n = 60, neonate n = 57.

16.3.2 PROPORTIONS OF VITAMIN D FORMS

Mean concentrations of vitamin D forms in mothers and neonates are illustrated in Figure 1. As far as the $1\alpha,25(OH)_2D_2$ and $1\alpha,25(OH)_2D_3$ forms are concerned, only $1\alpha,25(OH)_2D_3$ was measured in mothers, at a very low concentration (0.06±0.06 ng/mL). The $1\alpha,25(OH)_2D_2$ form was below the limit of quantitation. In line with previous reports [15], no significant relationship was observed between maternal circulating forms [$25(OH)D_3$] and the highly active $1\alpha,25(OH)_2D_3$ concentrations (r=-0.011, p=0.931).

The epimer concentrations (Figure 1) were similar in mothers and neonates (4.8 ± 7.8 vs. 4.5 ± 4.7 ng/mL, W=1015.0, p=0.462). Notably, 24.7% and 22.2% of the measured vitamin D forms were for inactive epimer forms for mothers and neonates, respectively. The 25(OH)D$_3$ concentrations were higher compared to 25(OH)D$_2$ levels ($75.6 \pm 22.2\%$ in mothers and $75.9 \pm 23.9\%$ in neonates); thus, the ratios of 25(OH)D$_3$: 25(OH)D$_2$ were 3:1, approximately, for both mother and neonates. A positive correlation (r=0.543, p<0.001) was detected between maternal and neonatal 25(OH)D concentrations, whereas inactive [3-epi-25(OH)D] concentrations showed a weaker correlation (r=0.268, p=0.038) (Figure 3). The 25(OH)D and inactive [3-epi-25(OH)D] concentrations were positively correlated in the mothers (r=0.528, p<0.001) but not in the neonates (r=0.142, p=0.414). There was no significant correlation between $1\alpha,25(OH)_2D_3$ and 3-epi-25(OH)D concentrations.

16.3.3 MATERNAL PREDICTORS OF NEONATAL VITAMIN D CONCENTRATIONS

The hierarchical linear regression models for predicting neonatal 25(OH)D concentrations are detailed in Table 2. In the majority of analyses, assumptions were met as defined. In the independent models (Table 2), the neonatal 25(OH)D$_2$ concentrations were best predicted from maternal characteristics ($R^2=0.253$), whereas 25(OH)D$_3$ was strongly linked to maternal vitamin D forms ($R^2=0.478$). Maternal serum concentrations of PTH, Ca and P together only explained a small proportion of the neonatal 25(OH)D$_2$ ($R^2=0.046$) and an even smaller part of the 25(OH)D$_3$ ($R^2=0.013$). Neonatal vitamin D concentrations were calculated as the sum of 25(OH)D$_2$ and 25(OH)D$_3$. Circulating neonatal vitamin D concentrations in newborns followed the pattern of predicting 25(OH)D$_3$, with maternal 25(OH)D$_2$ and 25(OH)D$_3$ explaining 32.1% of the neonatal vitamin D variance and epimer forms contributing an additional 11.9%. Therefore, all four maternal vitamin D forms combined [25(OH)D$_2$, 25(OH)D$_3$, 3-epi-25(OH)D$_2$, 3-epi-25(OH)D$_3$] explained 44% of the neonatal vitamin D concentrations when controlled for other maternal characteristics such as age, UVB exposure, vitamin D and Ca intake and Ca, P and PTH concentrations.

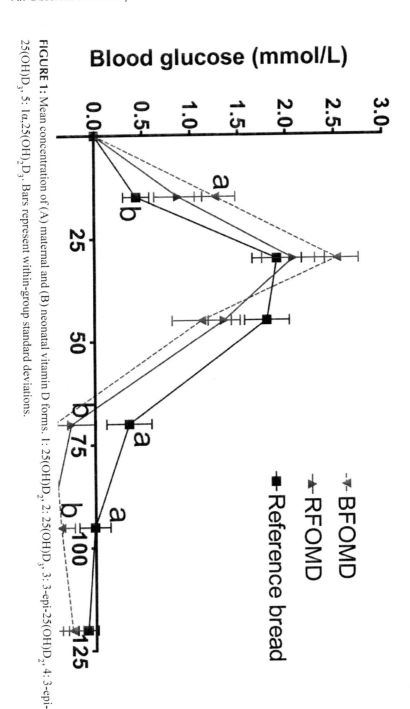

FIGURE 1: Mean concentration of (A) maternal and (B) neonatal vitamin D forms. 1: 25(OH)D$_2$, 2: 25(OH)D$_3$, 3: 3-epi-25(OH)D$_2$, 4: 3-epi-25(OH)D$_3$, 5: 1α,25(OH)$_2$D$_3$. Bars represent within-group standard deviations.

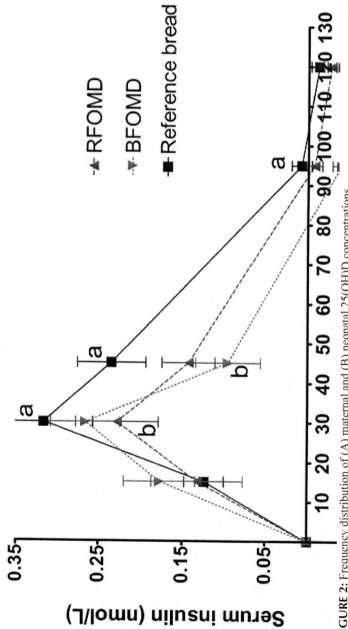

FIGURE 2: Frequency distribution of (A) maternal and (B) neonatal 25(OH)D concentrations.

On the contrary, $1\alpha,25(OH)_2D_3$ did not make a contribution to the neonatal vitamin D concentrations. Predicting 25(OH)D in neonates, mother's age showed statistical significance for the coefficients (β = -0.343). For $25(OH)D_2$, mother's $25(OH)D_2$ concentrations showed statistical significance for the coefficients (β = 0.218) and 3-epi-25(OH)D_3 (β = 0.596). These standardized β values can be used for weighting each individual's measures on the IVs to obtain individual predicted score on the DV, respectively. Mother's age was independent of vitamin D intake (r=-0.093, p=0.483), negatively correlated with UVB exposure (r=-0.304, p=0.019) and weakly negatively correlated with Ca intake (r=-0.244, p=0.062).

16.4 DISCUSSION

16.4.1 MATERNAL AND NEONATAL VITAMIN 25(OH)D CONCENTRATIONS

The potential impact of vitamin D deficiency during pregnancy on maternal and neonatal health has attracted much interest in recent years. It has been suggested that maintaining adequate maternal stores of vitamin D during pregnancy is of vital importance for both mothers and neonates to ensure skeletal and extra-skeletal health.

The results of this study come mainly from a population of pregnant women with vitamin D deficiency or insufficiency. Although the study was not designed for this purpose, a high prevalence of maternal vitamin D insufficiency and deficiency was detected, in a sunny European area, such as Northern Greece. A similar pattern of distribution between maternal and neonatal 25(OH)D concentrations was observed, with 25(OH)D_3 being the most abundant circulating vitamin D form in both mothers and neonates. These results reflect previous reports of widespread vitamin D deficiency and insufficiency in Europe and the USA. However, the known cross-reactivity of many assays with the epimer forms suggests that levels reported in previous studies are overestimations. Furthermore, the conundrum of a mismatch between levels of the usually quantified circulating

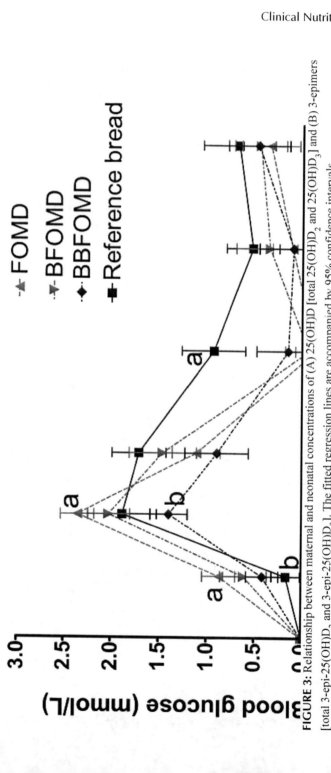

FIGURE 3: Relationship between maternal and neonatal concentrations of (A) 25(OH)D [total 25(OH)D_2 and 25(OH)D_3] and (B) 3-epimers [total 3-epi-25(OH)D_2 and 3-epi-25(OH)D_3]. The fitted regression lines are accompanied by 95% confidence intervals.

forms (25OHD) and the active form ($1\alpha,25\text{-(OH)}_2D$) [15] have been confirmed in this study, as no relationship was observed between $25(OH)D_3$ and $1\alpha,25(OH)_2D_3$ once epimers have been differentiated.

TABLE 2: Hierarchical linear regression model for predicting neonatal 25(OH)D concentrations

Step	IV (Maternal)	DV: Neonatal $25(OHD)_2$			DV: Neonatal $25(OH)D_3$		
		R^2	ΔR^2	SD β	R^2	ΔR^2	SD β
1	UVB exposure			-0.243			-0.121
	Age			-0.343*			-0.227 *
	Adjusted BMI			-0.172			0.032
	Vitamin D intake			0.082			0.143
	Ca intake	0.207	0.207 *	0.222	0.096	0.096	-0.018
2	Serum PTH			0.043			0.046
	Serum Ca			-0.267			0.169
	Serum P	0.253	0.046	-0.011	0.109	0.013	-0.161
3	$25(OH)D_2$	0.254	0.002	0.040	0.267	0.158 **	0.271*
4	$25(OH)D_3$	0.302	0.048	0.272	0.438	0.171 ***	0.218
5	Epi-$25(OH)D_2$	0.303	0.000	0.124	0.518	0.080 **	-0.091
6	Epi-$25(OH)D_3$	0.309	0.006	-0.179	0.586	0.068**	0.596 **
7	$1\alpha,25(OH)_2D_3$	0.329	0.020	-0.147	0.587	0.001	0.032

*$p<0.05$; ** $p<0.01$, *** $p<0.001$. BMI: body mass index, Ca: calcium, DV: dependent variable, IV: independent variable, P: phosphorus, PTH: parathyroid hormone, SD: standard deviation, UVB: ultraviolet B.

At this time, there is no documented benefit in measuring $25(OH)D_2$ and $25(OH)D_3$, separately; serum total 25(OH)D has been designated as the functional indicator of vitamin D status [22]. However, the ability to accurately measure serum concentrations of $25(OH)D_2$ and $25(OH)D_3$ brings new potential to both observational and intervention studies. On a physiological basis, it could be hypothesised that maternal vitamin D active forms have an impact on the newborn, which, to a great extent, depends on the mother to form its dynamic vitamin D equilibrium. Therefore, these findings confirm current concerns regarding the maintenance of adequate maternal vitamin D status during pregnancy, since the reflection of maternal concentrations of these forms explains 32.1% in neonates. It should be noted that data on $25(OH)D_2$ and $25(OH)D_3$ concentrations exclude epimer forms; thus, caution should be paid when comparing them to other studies [8].

Given that vitamin D_2 is the only high-dose preparation available in many countries, potential differences in the ability of assays to accurately detect $25(OH)D_2$ and $25(OH)D_3$ are of clinical importance, in cases where supplementation is suggested. Moreover, when $25(OH)D$ results are reported as $25(OH)D_2$ and $25(OH)D_3$, vitamin D_2 administration does reduce serum $25(OH)D_3$ concentrations [23]. Until the physiologic impact of this reduction, if any, is clarified by future studies, a low $25(OH)D_3$ value in the setting of ergocalciferol supplementation does not constitute vitamin D deficiency. LC-MS/MS and the potential of accurate measurement of both bioactive forms of vitamin D could offer a valuable tool in daily practice, in order to avoid data misinterpretation, especially in conditions like pregnancy.

16.4.2 PROPORTIONS OF VITAMIN D FORMS

The findings of this study, using a novel assay with the ability not just to exclude but also to measure vitamin D epimers demonstrated that epimers comprise approximately 25% of the measured vitamin D concentrations in both mothers and neonates, following similar patterns of distribution. The presence of both 3-epi-$25(OH)D_2$ and 3-epi-$25(OH)D_3$ forms have been previously reported in infants [24]. Our group has demonstrated the presence of 3-epi-$25(OH)D_3$ form, in a small cohort of healthy adults [18]. These results were further confirmed in a larger study, in adults [25]. The present study is the first to quantify concentrations of the 3-epi-$25(OH)D_2$ in both mothers and neonates. Large inter-individual variances in the epimer content were noted in vitamin D concentrations, ranging between 0% and 100% with 63.8% of the mothers and 67.8% of the neonates showing epimer to total circulating concentration of 25% or less. Thus, the epimer-adjusted concentration is only applicable to conclusions at the aggregated level (i.e. mothers, neonates) and should not be used for making judgments at the individual level, unless 3-epi-25(OH)D$_2$ and 3-epi-25(OH)D3 are clearly separated and excluded from the 25(OH)D measurements. On the other hand, based on present results, it becomes evident that 1α,25(OH)$_2$D$_2$ and 1α,25(OH)$_2$D$_3$ have minor contributions to the sum of vitamin D measurements in both mothers and infants.

Based on these findings, it could be hypothesized that assays that do not separate the 3-epi forms or have significant cross-reactivity with the epimer will, most likely, report erroneously high concentrations for both infants and adults, as 3-epi constitutes a substantial fraction of total 25(OH)D. This assay limitation should be considered by clinicians measuring vitamin D status in infants and mothers. LC-MS/MS, by measuring vitamin D isoforms separately, provides a 'clear-cut' view of vitamin D status. By excluding epimer concentrations, it appears that the mean vitamin D concentration in term pregnancies is considerably below the sufficiency threshold. Although the sample size of the present study was small for drawing conclusions, the accurate measurement of active vitamin D metabolites could offer a valuable tool in the establishment of a novel, realistic view of vitamin D status during pregnancy.

16.4.3 MATERNAL PREDICTORS OF NEONATAL VITAMIN D CONCENTRATIONS

Based on our primary results, regarding the accurate proportions of vitamin D metabolites in maternal circulation, we further investigated if there is an ability to predict neonatal 25(OH)D concentrations from maternal parameters. Our analysis showed that, apart from being a reliable marker of vitamin D maternal status, 25(OH)D comprises a significant parameter in predicting neonatal 25(OH)D$_3$ concentrations, which constitutes the major neonatal vitamin D form. The addition of certain maternal parameters could offer additional prognostic value in this process, specifically in neonatal 25(OH)D$_2$ concentrations. The additional analytical capacity enhances the predictive power with the epimers contributing 11.9% to an overall 44% explained variances in active vitamin D concentrations in neonates. This result significantly exceeded previous reports of 19% in a twin study, which investigated genetic versus maternal vitamin D concentrations in determining offspring vitamin D concentrations [14]. Overall, the above findings regarding maternal vitamin D concentrations and other parameters could be useful in daily clinical practice, as a part of a predictive model for neonatal vitamin D concentrations, based on maternal parameters, which could contribute to the appropriate management of the major health issue of maternal vitamin deficiency during pregnancy.

16.4.4 ADVANTAGES AND DISADVANTAGES

The present study has three major advantages. First, the data incorporate specific and accurate measurement of seven out of eight forms of vitamin D, including vitamin D_2 and D_3, hydroxylated derivatives and epimer forms. To the best of our knowledge, these data are unique to the literature on pregnancy. Second, as routine assays do not allow differentiation among the full range of different vitamin D forms, this novel assay allowed for a very detailed approach to the complex vitamin D metabolism in the mother - newborn bipole. Third, the study allowed the control for maternal characteristics such as age, UVB exposure, dietary intake and PTH, Ca and P concentrations, which afforded separating the explained variances for the active vitamin D concentrations over and above the shared variances by maternal characteristics. In combination, we were able to explain 56.1% in the variances in neonatal 25(OH)D concentrations. Limitations of the study were its rather small sample size and its cross-sectional design, which prevented prospective data to be collected throughout pregnancy. Moreover, measurement of vitamin D-binding protein (VDBP), a significant parameter of vitamin D dynamics in pregnancy, was not feasible.

16.5 CONCLUSIONS

This study provided evidence for i) maternal and neonatal vitamin 25(OH)D concentrations in a sunny European area, which proved to be sub-optimal, ii) 3-epi-25(OH)D_3 and 3-epi-25(OH)D_2 forms in both mothers and neonates, which contribute approximately 25% to the total vitamin D concentrations and iii) a relationship between maternal and neonatal concentrations leading to a prediction model. The accurate assay highlights a considerable proportion of vitamin D exists as epimers and there is a lack of correlation between the circulating and active forms. These results underscore the need for accurate measurements to appraise vitamin D status. The results, based on specific and accurate measurement, revealed that maternal characteristics and active forms of vitamin D, along with their epimers explain 56% of neonatal vitamin D concentrations. Further investigation, based on accurate measurements of vitamin D metabolites, is warranted to establish optimal concentrations during pregnancy, in an attempt to prevent maternal morbidity and developmental deficiencies.

REFERENCES

1. Zhang R, Naughton DP: Vitamin D in health and disease: Current perspectives.

2. Nutr J 2010, 9:65.

3. Haris N, Wall AP, Sangster M, Paton RW: The presentation of rickets to orthopaedic clinics: return of the English disease. Acta Orthop Belg 2011, 77:239-245.

4. Munns CF, Simm PJ, Rodda CR, Garnett SP, Zacharin MR, Ward LM, Geddes J, Cherian S, Zurynski Y, Cowell CTY, APSU Vitamin D Study Group: Incidence of vitamin D deficiency rickets among Australian children: an Australian Paediatric Surveillance Unit study. Med J Australia 2012, 196:466-468.

5. Holick MF: Vitamin D deficiency. N Engl J Med 2007, 357:266-281.

6. Holick MF, Siris ES, Binkley N, Beard MK, Khan A, Katzer JT, Petruschke RA, Chen E, de Papp AE: Prevalence of vitamin D inadequacy among postmenopausal North American women receiving osteoporosis therapy. J Clin Endocrinol Metab 2005, 90:3215-3224.

7. Lips P, Hosking D, Lippuner K, Norquist JM, Wehren L, Maalouf G, Ragi-Eis S, Chandler J: The prevalence of vitamin D inadequacy amongst women with osteoporosis: an international epidemiological investigation. J Intern Med 2006, 260:245-254.

8. Thomas KK, Lloyd-Jones DM, Thadhani RI, Shaw AC, Deraska DJ, Kitch BT, Vamvakas EC, Dick IM, Prince RL, Finkelstein JS: Hypovitaminosis D in medical in patients. N Engl J Med 1998, 338:777-783.

9. Nicolaidou P, Hatzistamatiou Z, Papadopoulou A, Kaleyias J, Floropoulou E, Lagona E, Tsagris V, Costalos C, Antsaklis A: Low vitamin D status in mother-newborn pairs in Greece. Calcif Tissue Int 2006, 78:337-342.

10. Poel YHM, Hummel P, Lips P, Stam F, Van Der Ploeg T, Simsek S: Vitamin D and gestational diabetes: A systematic review and meta-analysis. E J Int Med 2012, 23:465-469.

11. Scholl TO, Chen X, Stein P: Maternal vitamin D status and delivery by caesarean. Nutrients 2012, 4:319-330.

12. Burris HH, Rifas-Shiman SL, Camargo CA, Litonjua AA, Huh SY, Rich-Edwards JW, Gillman MW: Plasma 25-hydroxyvitamin D during pregnancy and small-for-gestational age in black and white infants. Ann Epidem 2012, 22:581-586.

13. Whitehouse AJO, Holt BJ, Serralha M, Holt PG, Kusel MMH, Hart PH: Maternal serum vitamin D levels during pregnancy and offspring neurocognitive development. Pediatrics 2012, 129:485-493.

14. Javaid MK, Crozier SR, Harvey NC, Gale CR, Dennison EM, Boucher BJ, Arden NK, Godfrey KM, Cooper C, Princess Anne Hospital Study Group: Maternal vitamin D status during pregnancy and childhood bone mass at age 9 years: a longitudinal study. Lancet 2006, 367:36-43.

15. Novakovic B, Galati JC, Chen A, Morley R, Craig JM, Saffery R: Maternal vitamin D predominates over genetic factors in determining neonatal circulating vitamin D concentrations. Am J Clin Nutr 2012, 96:188-195.

16. Papapetrou PD: The interrelationship of serum 1,25-dihydroxyvitamin D, 25- dihydroxyvitamin D and 24,25-dihydroxyvitamin D in pregnancy at term: a meta- analysis. Hormones 2010, 9:136-144.

17. Farrell CJL, Martin S, McWhinney B, Straub I, Williams P, Herrman M: State-of-the-art vitamin D assays: a comparison of automated immunoassays with liquid chromatography–tandem mass spectrometry methods. Clin Chem 2012, 58:531-542.

18. Carter GD: 25-Hydroxyvitamin D: a difficult analyte. Clin Chem 2012, 58:486-488.

19. Shah I, James R, Barker J, Petroczi A, Naughton DP: Misleading measures in Vitamin D analysis: a novel LC-MS/MS assay to account for epimers and isobars. Nutr J 2011, 10:46.

20. Shah I, Petroczi A, Naughton DP: Method for simultaneous analysis of eight analogues of vitamin D using liquid chromatography tandem mass spectrometry. Chem Central J 2012, 6:112.

21. Gnardellis C, Trichopoulou A, Katsouyanni K, Polychronopoulos E, Rimm EB, Trichopoulos D: Reproducibility and validity of an extensive semi-quantitative food frequency questionnaire among Greek school teachers. Epidemiology 1995, 6:74-77.

22. Trichopoulou A, Georga K: Composition tables of foods and Greek dishes. Athens, Greece: Parisianos; 2004.

23. Standing Committee on the Scientific Evaluation of Dietary Reference Intakes Food and Nutrition Board, Institute of Medicine: DRI Dietary Reference Intakes for calcium phosphorus, magnesium, vitamin D and fluoride. Washington, DC: National Academy Press; 1997. OpenURL

24. Binkley N, Gemar D, Ramamurthy R: Daily versus monthly oral vitamin D2 and D3: Effect on serum 25(OH)D concentration. J Bone Miner Res 2007, 22(1):S215.

25. Singh RJ, Taylor RL, Reddy GS, Grebe SK: C-3 epimers can account for a significant proportion of total circulating 25-hydroxyvitamin D in infants, complicating accurate measurement and interpretation of vitamin D status. J Clin Endocrinol Metab 2006, 91:3055-3061.
26. Lensmeyer G, Poquette M, Wiebe D, Binkley N: The C-3 epimer of 25-hydroxyvitamin D(3) is present in adult serum. J Clin Endocrinol Metab 2012, 97:163-168.

This chapter was originally published under the Creative Commons Attribution License. Karras, S. N., Shah, I., Petroczi, A., Goulis, D. G., Bill, H., Papadopoulou, F., Harizopoulou, V., Tarlatzis, B. C., and Naughton, D. P. An Observational Study Reveals that Neonatal Vitamin D Is Primarily Determined by Maternal Contributions: Implications of a New Assay on the Roles of Vitamin D Forms. Nutrition Journal 2013: 12(77). doi:10.1186/1475-2891-12.77.

WEIGHT SCIENCE: EVALUATING THE EVIDENCE FOR A PARADIGM SHIFT

LINDA BACON and LUCY APHRAMOR

17.1 INTRODUCTION

Concern regarding "overweight" and "obesity" is reflected in a diverse range of policy measures aimed at helping individuals reduce their body mass index (BMI) [1]. Despite attention from the public health establishment, a private weight loss industry estimated at $58.6 billion annually in the United States [1], unprecedented levels of body dissatisfaction [2] and repeated attempts to lose weight [3,4], the majority of individuals are unable to maintain weight loss over the long term and do not achieve the putative benefits of improved morbidity and mortality [5]. Concern has arisen that this weight focused paradigm is not only ineffective at producing thinner, healthier bodies, but also damaging, contributing to food and body preoccupation, repeated cycles of weight loss and regain, distraction from other personal health goals and wider health determinants, reduced self-esteem, eating disorders, other health decrement, and weight stigmatization and discrimination [6-8]. As evidence-based competencies are more firmly embedded in health practitioner standards, attention has been given to the ethical implications of recommending treatment that may be ineffective or damaging [5,9].

A growing trans-disciplinary movement called Health at Every Size[SM] (HAES)[2] shifts the focus from weight management to health promotion. The primary intent of HAES is to support improved health behaviors for people of all sizes without using weight as a mediator; weight loss may or may not be a side effect.

HAES is emerging as standard practice in the eating disorders field: The Academy for Eating Disorders, Binge Eating Disorder Association, Eating Disorder Coalition, International Association for Eating Disorder Professionals, and National Eating Disorder Association explicitly support this approach [10]. Civil rights groups including the National Association to Advance Fat Acceptance and the Council on Size and Weight Discrimination also encourage HAES. An international professional organization, the Association for Size Diversity and Health, has developed, composed of individual members across a wide span of professions who are committed to HAES principles.

17.1.2 HEALTH AT EVERY SIZE: A REVIEW OF RANDOMIZED CONTROLLED TRIALS

Several clinical trials comparing HAES to conventional obesity treatment have been conducted. Some investigations were conducted before the name "Health at Every Size" came into common usage; these earlier studies typically used the terms "non-diet" or "intuitive eating" and included an explicit focus on size acceptance (as opposed to weight loss or weight maintenance). A Pub Med search for "Health at Every Size" or "intuitive eating" or "non-diet" or "nondiet" revealed 57 publications. Randomized controlled trials (RCTs) were vetted from these publications, and additional RCTs were vetted from their references. Only studies with an explicit focus on size acceptance were included.

Evidence from these six RCTs indicates that a HAES approach is associated with statistically and clinically relevant improvements in physiological measures (e.g. blood pressure, blood lipids), health behaviors (e.g. physical activity, eating disorder pathology) and psychosocial outcomes (e.g, mood, self-esteem, body image) [11-20]. (See Table 1.) All studies indicate significant improvements in psychological and behavioral outcomes;

TABLE 1: Randomized controlled HAES studies reported in peer-reviewed journals

Investigation	Group type[a] (n)	Population	Number of treatment sessions	Follow-up (number of weeks post treatment)	Attrition	Improvements			Decrements
						Physio-logic	Health behaviors	Psycho-social	
Provencher, et al., 2009[17] and 2007[20]	HAES (n = 48); social support (n = 48); control (n = 48)	Over-weight and obese women	15	26	8%; 19%; 21%	Not evaluated	Eating behaviors	Not evaluated	None
Bacon et al., 2005 [11] and 2002[19]	HAES (n = 39); diet (n = 39)	Obese women, chronic dieters	30	52	8%; 42%	LDL, systolic blood pressure	Activity, binge eating	Self esteem, depression, body dissatisfaction, body image, interoceptive awareness	None
Rapaport et al., 2000[16]	Modified cogni-tive-behavioral treatment (n=37); cogni-tive behavioral treatment (n= 38)	Over-weight and obese women	10	52	16%; 16%	Total choles-terol[b], LDL cholesterol[b], systolic blood pressure[b], diastolic blood pressure	Activity[b], di-etary quality[b]	Emotional well-being[b], distress[b]	None

TABLE 1: *Cont.*

Investigation	Group type[a] (n)	Population	Number of treatment sessions	Follow-up (number of weeks post-treatment)	Attrition	Improvements			Decrements
						Physio-logic	Health behaviors	Psycho-social	
Ciliska, 1998[12]	Psycho-educational (n = 29); education only (n = 26), waitlist control (n = 23)	Obese women	12	52	14%; 23%; 41%	Diastolic blood pressure	Binge eating	Self-esteem, body dissat-isfact-ion, depression	None
Goodrick et al., 1998[13]	Nondiet (n = 62); diet (n = 65); wait-list control (n = 58)	Over-weight and obese women, binge-eaters	50	78	Not reported	Not evaluated	Binge eating, exercise[b]	Not evaluated	None
Tanco, et al., 1998[14]	Cognitive group treatment (n = 20); weight loss (n = 21); waitlist control (n = 19)	Obese women	8	26	10%; 10%; 32%	Not evaluate	Not evaluated	Depression, anxiety, eating-related psycho-pathology, perception of self-control	None

[a] HAES group listed first and in bold. (The names reflect those used in the publication.)
[b] Improvement in HAES group, but not statistically different from the control.

improvements in self-esteem and eating behaviors were particularly note-worthy [11-14,16,17,19,20]. Four studies additionally measured metabol-ic risk factors and three of these studies indicated significant improvement in at least some of these parameters, including blood pressure and blood lipids [11,12,16,17,19,20]. No studies found adverse changes in any vari-ables.

A seventh RCT reported at a conference also found significantly posi-tive results [18], as did a non-randomized controlled study [21] and five studies conducted without a control [22-26].

All of the controlled studies showed retention rates substantially higher than, or, in one instance, as high, as the control group, and all of the uncontrolled studies also showed high retention rates. Given the well-documented recidivism typical of weight loss programs [5,27,28] and the potential harm that may arise[29,30], this aspect is particularly noteworthy.

17.2 ASSUMPTIONS UNDERLYING THE CONVENTIONAL (WEIGHT-FOCUSED) PARADIGM

Dieting and other weight loss behaviors are popular in the general popu-lation and widely encouraged in public health policy and health care practice as a solution for the "problem" of obesity. There is increas-ing concern about the endemic misrepresentation of evidence in these weight management policies [5,8]. Researchers have demonstrated ways in which bias and convention interfere with robust scientific reasoning such that obesity research seems to "enjoy special immunity from ac-cepted standards in clinical practice and publishing ethics" [5,8,31]. This section discusses the assumptions that underlie the current weight-fo-cused paradigm, presenting evidence that contests their scientific merit and challenges the value of promoting weight management as a public health measure.

17.2.1 ASSUMPTION: ADIPOSITY POSES SIGNIFICANT MORTALITY RISK

Evidence: Except at statistical extremes, body mass index (BMI)—or amount of body fat—only weakly predicts longevity [32]. Most epidemiological studies find that people who are overweight or moderately obese live at least as long as normal weight people, and often longer [32-35]. Analysis of the National Health and Nutrition Examination Surveys I, II, and III, which followed the largest nationally representative cohort of United States adults, determined that greatest longevity was in the overweight category [32]. As per the report, published in the Journal of the American Medical Association and reviewed and approved by the Centers for Disease Control and Prevention and the National Cancer Institute, "[this] finding is consistent with other results reported in the literature." Indeed, the most comprehensive review of the research pooled data for over 350,000 subjects from 26 studies and found overweight to be associated with greater longevity than normal weight [36]. More recently, Janssen analyzed data in the elderly (among whom more than 70 percent of all deaths occur)—also from 26 published studies—and similarly found no evidence of excess mortality associated with overweight [37]. The Americans' Changing Lives study came to a similar conclusion, indicating that "when socioeconomic and other risk factors are controlled for, obesity is not a significant risk factor for mortality; and... for those 55 or older, both overweight and obesity confer a significant decreased risk of mortality." [38] The most recent analysis, published in the New England Journal of Medicine, concluded that overweight was associated with increased risk, but only arrived at this conclusion after restricting the analysis by excluding 78 percent of the deaths [39]. They also used a reference category much narrower than the entire "normal weight" category used by most other studies, which also contributed to making the relative risk for overweight higher.

There is a robust pattern in the epidemiological literature that has been named the "obesity paradox" [40,41]: obesity is associated with longer survival in many diseases. For example, obese persons with type 2 diabetes [42], hypertension [43,44], cardiovascular disease[41,45], and chronic kidney disease [46] all have greater longevity than thinner people with these conditions [47-49]. Also, obese people who have had heart attacks, coronary bypass[50], angioplasty[51] or hemodialysis [52] live longer than thinner people with these histories [49]. In addition, obese senior citizens live longer than thinner senior citizens [53].

The idea that "this is the first generation of children that may have a shorter life expectancy than their parents" is commonly expressed in scientific journals [54] and popular press articles [55], even appearing in Congressional testimony by former Surgeon General Richard Carmona [56] and a 2010 report from the White House Task Force on Childhood Obesity[57]. When citation is provided, it refers to an opinion paper published in the New England Journal of Medicine [54], which offered no statistical evidence to support the claim. Life expectancy increased dramatically during the same time period in which weight rose (from 70.8 years in 1970 to 77.8 years in 2005) [58]. Both the World Health Organization and the Social Security Administration project life expectancy will continue to rise in coming decades [59,60].

17.2.2 ASSUMPTION: ADIPOSITY POSES SIGNIFICANT MORBIDITY RISK

Evidence: While it is well established that obesity is associated with increased risk for many diseases, causation is less well-established. Epidemiological studies rarely acknowledge factors like fitness, activity, nutrient intake, weight cycling or socioeconomic status when considering connections between weight and disease. Yet all play a role in determining health risk. When studies do control for these factors, increased risk of disease disappears or is significantly reduced [61]. (This is less true at statistical extremes.) It is likely that these other factors increase disease risk at the same time they increase the risk of weight gain.

Consider weight cycling as an example. Attempts to lose weight typically result in weight cycling, and such attempts are more common among obese individuals [62]. Weight cycling results in increased inflammation, which in turn is known to increase risk for many obesity-associated diseases [63]. Other potential mechanisms by which weight cycling contributes to morbidity include hypertension, insulin resistance and dyslipidemia [64]. Research also indicates that weight fluctuation is associated with poorer cardiovascular outcomes and increased mortality risk [64-68]. Weight cycling can account for all of the excess mortality associated with obesity in both the Framingham Heart Study [69] and the National Health and Nutrition Examination Survey (NHANES) [70]. It may be, therefore, that the association between weight and health risk can be better attributed to weight cycling than adiposity itself [63].

As another example, consider type 2 diabetes, the disease most highly associated with weight and fat distribution. There is increasing evidence that poverty and marginalization are more strongly associated with type 2 diabetes than conventionally-accepted risk factors such as weight, diet or activity habits [30,71-73]. A large Canadian report produced in 2010, for example, found that low income was strongly associated with diabetes even when BMI (and physical activity) was accounted for [73]. Also, much evidence suggests that insulin resistance is a product of an underlying metabolic disturbance that predisposes the individual to increased fat storage due to compensatory insulin secretion [61,74-78]. In other words, obesity may be an early symptom of diabetes as opposed to its primary underlying cause.

Hypertension provides another example of a condition highly associated with weight; research suggests that it is two to three times more common among obese people than lean people [79]. To what extent hypertension is caused by adiposity, however, is unclear. That BMI correlates more strongly with blood pressure than percent body fat [80] indicates that the association between BMI and blood pressure results from higher lean mass as opposed to fat mass. Also, the association may have more to do with the weight cycling that results from trying to control weight than the actual weight itself [48,81,82]. One study conducted with obese individuals determined that weight cycling was strongly positively associated with incident hypertension [82]. Another study showed that obese women who had dieted had high blood pressure, while those who had never been on a diet had normal blood pressure [67]. Rat studies also show that obese rats that have weight cycled have very high blood pressures compared to obese rats that have not weight cycled [83,84]. This finding could also explain the weak association between obesity and hypertension in cultures where dieting is uncommon[48,85]. Additionally, it is well documented that obese people with hypertension live significantly longer than thinner people with hypertension [43,86-88] and have a lower risk of heart attack, stroke, or early death [45]. Rather than identifying health risk, as it does in thinner people, hypertension in heavier people may simply be a requirement for pumping blood through their larger bodies [89].

It is also notable that the prevalence of hypertension dropped by half between 1960 and 2000, a time when average weight sharply increased, declining much more steeply among those deemed overweight and obese than among thinner individuals [90]. Incidence of cardiovascular disease also plummeted during this time period and many common diseases now emerge at older ages and are less severe [90]. (The notable exception is diabetes, which showed a small, non-significant increase during this time period [90].) While the decreased morbidity can at least in part be attributed to improvements in medical care, the point remains that we are simply not seeing the catastrophic disease consequences predicted to result from the "obesity epidemic."

17.2.3 ASSUMPTION: WEIGHT LOSS WILL PROLONG LIFE

Evidence: Most prospective observational studies suggest that weight loss increases the risk of premature death among obese individuals, even when the weight loss is intentional and the studies are well controlled with regard to known confounding factors, including hazardous behavior and underlying diseases [91-96]. Recent review of NHANES, for example, a nationally representative sample of ethnically diverse people over the age of fifty, shows that mortality increased among those who lost weight [97].

While many short-term weight loss intervention studies do indicate improvements in health measures, because the weight loss is always accompanied by a change in behavior, it is not known whether or to what extent the improvements can be attributed to the weight loss itself. Liposuction studies that control for behavior change provide additional information about the effects of weight (fat) loss itself. One study which explicitly monitored that there were no changes in diet and activity for 10-12 weeks post abdominal liposuction is a case in point. Participants lost an average of 10.5 kgs but saw no improvements in obesity-associated metabolic abnormalities, including blood pressure, triglycerides, cholesterol, or insulin sensitivity [98]. (Note that liposuction removes subcutaneous fat, not the visceral fat that is more highly associated with disease, and these results should be interpreted carefully.)

In most studies on type 2 diabetes, the improvement in glycemic control is seen within days, before significant weight or fat is lost. Evidence also challenges the assumption that weight loss is associated with improvement in long-term glycemic control, as reflected in HbA1c values [99,100]. One review of controlled weight-loss studies for people with type 2 diabetes showed that initial improvements were followed by a deterioration back to starting values six to eighteen months after treatment, even when the weight loss was maintained [101].

Furthermore, health benefits associated with weight loss rarely show a dose response (in other words, people who lose small amounts of weight generally get as much health benefit from the intervention as those who lose larger amounts).

These data suggest that the behavior change as opposed to the weight loss itself may play a greater role in health improvement.

17.2.4 ASSUMPTION: ANYONE WHO IS DETERMINED CAN LOSE WEIGHT AND KEEP IT OFF THROUGH APPROPRIATE DIET AND EXERCISE

Evidence: Long-term follow-up studies document that the majority of individuals regain virtually all of the weight that was lost during treatment, regardless of whether they maintain their diet or exercise program [5,27]. Consider the Women's Health Initiative, the largest and longest randomized, controlled dietary intervention clinical trial, designed to test the current recommendations. More than 20,000 women maintained a low-fat diet, reportedly reducing their calorie intake by an average of 360 calories per day [102] and significantly increasing their activity [103]. After almost eight years on this diet, there was almost no change in weight from starting point (a loss of 0.1 kg), and average waist circumference, which is a measure of abdominal fat, had increased (0.3 cm) [102].

A panel of experts convened by the National Institutes of Health determined that "one third to two thirds of the weight is regained within one year [after weight loss], and almost all is regained within five years." [28] More recent review finds one-third to two-thirds of dieters regain more weight than was lost on their diets; "In sum," the authors report, "there is little support for the notion that diets lead to lasting weight loss or health benefits [5]." Other reviews demonstrate the unreliability of conventional claims of sustained weight loss [104,105]. There is a paucity of long term data regarding surgical studies, but emerging data indicates gradual post-surgery weight regain as well [106,107]. Weight loss peaks about one year postoperative, after which gradual weight regain is the norm.

17.2.5 ASSUMPTION: THE PURSUIT OF WEIGHT LOSS IS A PRACTICAL AND POSITIVE GOAL

Evidence: As discussed earlier, weight cycling is the most common result of engaging in conventional dieting practices and is known to increase morbidity and mortality risk. Research identifies many other contraindications to the pursuit of weight loss. For example, dieting is known to reduce bone mass, increasing risk for osteoporosis [108-111]; this is true even in an obese population, though obesity is typically associated with reduced risk for osteoporosis[108]. Research also suggests that dieting is associated with increased chronic psychological stress and cortisol production, two factors known to increase disease risk [112]. Also, there is emerging evidence that persistent organic pollutants (POPs), which bioaccumulate in adipose tissue and are released during its breakdown, can increase risk of various chronic diseases including type 2 diabetes [113,114], cardiovascular disease [115] and rheumatoid arthritis [116]; two studies document that people who have lost weight have higher concentration of POPs in their blood [117,118]. One review of the diabetes literature indicates "that obese persons that (sic) do not have elevated POPs are not at elevated risk of diabetes, suggesting that the POPs rather than the obesity per se is responsible for the association" [114].

Positing the value of weight loss also supports widespread anxiety about weight [119,120]. Evidence from the eating disorder literature indicates an emphasis on weight control can promote eating disordered behaviors [7]. Prospective studies show that body dissatisfaction is associated with binge eating and other eating disordered behaviors, lower levels of physical activity and increased weight gain over time [121,122]. Many studies also show that dieting is a strong predictor of future weight gain [66,123-128].

Another unintended consequence of the weight loss imperative is an increase in stigmatization and discrimination against fat individuals. Discrimination based on weight now equals or exceeds that based on race or gender [129]. Extensive research indicates that stigmatizing fat demotivates, rather than encourages, health behavior change [130]. Adults who face weight stigmatization and discrimination report consuming increased quantities of food [131-134], avoiding exercise [133,135-137], and postponing or avoiding medical care (for fear of experiencing stigmatization) [138]. Stigmatization and bias on the part of health care practitioners is well-documented, resulting in lower quality care [139,140].

17.2.6 ASSUMPTION: THE ONLY WAY FOR OVERWEIGHT AND OBESE PEOPLE TO IMPROVE HEALTH IS TO LOSE WEIGHT

Evidence: That weight loss will improve health over the long-term for obese people is, in fact, an untested hypothesis. One reason the hypothesis is untested is because no methods have proven to reduce weight long-term for a significant number of people. Also, while normal weight people have lower disease incidence than obese individuals, it is unknown if weight loss in individuals already obese reduces disease risk to the same level as that observed in those who were never obese [91,93].

As indicated by research conducted by one of the authors and many other investigators, most health indicators can be improved through changing health behaviors, regardless of whether weight is lost [11]. For example, lifestyle changes can reduce blood pressure, largely or completely independent of changes in body weight [11,141-143]. The same can be said for blood lipids [11,143-145]. Improvements in insulin sensitivity and blood lipids as a result of aerobic exercise training have been documented even in individuals who gained body fat during the intervention [145,146].

17.2.7 ASSUMPTION: OBESITY-RELATED COSTS PLACE A LARGE BURDEN ON THE ECONOMY, AND THIS CAN BE CORRECTED BY FOCUSED ATTENTION TO OBESITY TREATMENT AND PREVENTION

Evidence: The health cost attributed to obesity in the United States is currently estimated to be $147 billion annually [147] and this cost estimate has been used to justify efforts at obesity treatment and prevention. Although this estimate has been granted credence by health experts, the word "estimate" is important to note: as the authors state, most of the cost changes are not "statistically different from zero." Also, the estimate fails to account for many potentially confounding variables, among them physical activity, nutrient intake, history of weight cycling, degree of discrimination, access to (quality) medical care, etc. All are independently correlated with both weight and health and could play a role in explaining the costs associated with having a BMI over 30. Nor does it account for costs associated with unintended consequences of positing the value of a weight focus, which may include eating disorders, diet attempts, weight cycling, reduced self-esteem, depression, and discrimination.

Because BMI is considered a risk factor for many diseases, obese persons are automatically relegated to greater testing and treatment, which means that positing BMI as a risk factor results in increased costs, regardless of whether BMI itself is problematic. Yet using BMI as a proxy for health may be more costly than addressing health directly. Consider, for example, the findings of a study which examined the "healthy obese" and the "unhealthy normal weight" populations [148]. The study identified six different risk factors for cardiometabolic health and included subjects in the "unhealthy" group if they had two or more risk factors, making it a more stringent threshold of health than that used in categorizing metabolic syndrome or diabetes. The study found a substantial proportion of the overweight and obese population, at every age, who were healthy and a substantial proportion of the "normal weight" group who were unhealthy. Psychologist Deb Burgard examined the costs of overlooking the normal weight people who need treatment and over-treating the obese people who do not (personal communication, March 2010). She found that BMI profiling overlooks 16.3 million "normal weight" individuals who are not healthy and identifies 55.4 million overweight and obese people who are not ill as being in need of treatment (see Table 2). When the total population is considered, this means that 31 percent of the population is misidentified when BMI is used as a proxy for health.

TABLE 2: Cost of Using BMI as a Proxy for Health[a]

		Abnormal cardiometabolic profile	Normal cardiometabolic profile	TOTAL
Untreated	"Normal" weight (BMI = 18.5 - 24.9)	23.5% (16.3 million people)[b]	76.5% (53.0 million people)	100% (69.3 million people)
Treated	"Overweight" (BMI = 25.0 - 29.9)	48.7% (34.1 million people)	51.3% (35.9 million people)[c]	100% (70.0 million people)
	"Obese" (BMI ≥ 30.0)	68.3% (42.0 million people)	31.7% (19.5 million people)[c]	100% (61.5 million people)
TOTAL		46% 92.4 million people	54% 108.4 million people	100% 200.8 million people

[a]Based on study by Wildman et al. [148].
[b]False negative: 16.3 million of 92.4 million (17.6%) who have abnormal cardiometabolic profile are overlooked
[c]False positive: 55.4 million of 131.5 million (42%) are identified as ill who are not

The weight bias inherent in BMI profiling may actually result in higher costs and sicker people. As an example, consider a 2009 study published in the American Journal of Public Health (96). The authors compared people of similar age, gender, education level, and rates of diabetes and hypertension, and examined how often they reported feeling sick over a 30-day period. Results indicated that body image had a much bigger impact on health than body size. In other words, two equally fat women would have very different health outcomes, depending on how they felt about their bodies. Likewise, two women with similar body insecurities would have similar health outcomes, even if one were fat and the other thin. These results suggest that the stigma associated with being fat is a major contributor to obesity-associated disease. BMI and health are only weakly related in cultures where obesity is not stigmatized, such as in the South Pacific [48,149].

17.3 HEALTH AT EVERY SIZE: SHIFTING THE PARADIGM FROM WEIGHT TO HEALTH

This section explains the rationale supporting some of the significant ways in which the HAES paradigm differs from the conventional weight-focused paradigm. The following topics are addressed:

1. HAES encourages body acceptance as opposed to weight loss or weight maintenance;
2. HAES supports reliance on internal regulatory processes, such as hunger and satiety, as opposed to encouraging cognitively-imposed dietary restriction; and
3. HAES supports active embodiment as opposed to encouraging structured exercise.

17.3.1 ENCOURAGING BODY ACCEPTANCE

Conventional thought suggests that body discontent helps motivate beneficial lifestyle change [150,151]. However, as discussed previously in the section on the pursuit of weight loss, evidence suggests the opposite: promoting body discontent instead induces harm [122,133,134,152], resulting in less favorable lifestyle choices. A common aphorism expressed in the HAES community is that "if shame were effective motivation, there wouldn't be many fat people." Mounting evidence suggests this belief is unfounded and detrimental[8,152]. Promoting one body size as more favorable than another also has ethical consequences [120], contributing to shaming and discrimination.

Compassion-focused behavior change theory emerging from the eating disorders field suggests that self-acceptance is a cornerstone of self-care, meaning that people with strong self-esteem are more likely to adopt positive health behaviors [153,154]. The theory is borne out in practice: HAES research shows that by learning to value their bodies as they are right now, even when this differs from a desired weight or shape or generates ambivalent feelings, people strengthen their ability to take care of themselves and sustain improvements in health behaviors [8,11].

Critics of HAES express concern that encouraging body acceptance will lead individuals to eat with abandon and disregard dietary considerations, resulting in weight gain. This has been disproven by the evidence; no randomized controlled HAES study has resulted in weight gain, and all studies that report on dietary quality or eating behavior indicate improvement or at least maintenance [11,14-23]. This is in direct contrast to dieting behavior, which is associated with weight gain over time [66,123-128].

17.3.2 SUPPORTING INTUITIVE EATING

Conventional recommendations view conscious efforts to monitor and restrict food choices as a necessary aspect of eating for health or weight control [155]. The underlying belief is that cognitive monitoring is essential for keeping appetite under control and that without these injunctions people would make nutritionally inadvisable choices, including eating to excess. The evidence, however, disputes the value of encouraging external regulation and restraint as a means for weight control: several large scale studies demonstrate that eating restraint is actually associated with weight gain over time [66,123-126].

In contrast, HAES teaches people to rely on internal regulation, a process dubbed intuitive eating [156], which encourages them to increase awareness of their body's response to food and learn how to make food choices that reflect this "body knowledge." Food is valued for nutritional, psychological, sensual, cultural and other reasons. HAES teaches people to make connections between what they eat and how they feel in the short- and medium-term, paying attention to food and mood, concentration, energy levels, fullness, ease of bowel movements, comfort eating, appetite, satiety, hunger and pleasure as guiding principles.

The journey towards adopting intuitive eating is typically a process one engages in over time. Particularly for people with a long history of dieting, other self-imposed dietary restriction, or body image concerns, it can feel very precarious to let go of old habits and attitudes and risk trying new ways of relating to food and self. Coming to eat intuitively happens gradually as old beliefs about food, nutrition and eating are challenged, unlearned and replaced with new ones.

A large popular literature has accumulated that supports individuals in developing intuitive eating skills [8,156-160]. (Intuitive eating is also known in the literature as "attuned eating" or "mindful eating." Note that intuitive eating is sometimes promoted as a means to weight loss and in that context is inconsistent with a HAES approach.)

There is considerable evidence that intuitive eating skills can be learned [11,18,161], and that intuitive eating is associated with improved nutrient intake [162], reduced eating disorder symptomatology [17,18,163-165] - and not with weight gain [11,13,16-18]. Several studies have found intuitive eating to be associated with lower body mass [162,163,166,167].

17.3.3 SUPPORTING ACTIVE EMBODIMENT

HAES encourages people to build activity into their day-to-day routines and focuses on helping people find enjoyable ways of being active. The goal is to promote well-being and self-care rather than advising individuals to meet set guidelines for frequency and intensity of exercise. Active living is promoted for a range of physical, psychological and other synergistic benefits which are independent of weight loss. Myths around weight control and exercise are explicitly challenged. Physical activity is also used in HAES as a way of healing a sense of body distrust and alienation from physicality that may be experienced when people are taught to over-ride embodied internal signals in pursuit of externally derived goals, such as commonly occurs in dieting. In addition, some HAES programs have used physical activity sessions, along with other activities such as art and relaxation, to further a community development agenda, creating volunteer, training and employment opportunities and addressing issues of isolation, poor self-esteem and depression among course participants.

17.4 CLINICAL ETHICS

There are serious ethical concerns regarding the continued use of a weight-centered paradigm in current practice in relation to beneficence and non-maleficence. Beneficence concerns the requirement to effect treatment benefit. There is a paucity of literature to substantiate that the pursuit of weight control is beneficial, and a similar lack of evidence to support that weight loss is maintained over the long term or that programs aimed at prevention of weight gain are successful. Nonmaleficence refers to the requirement to do no harm. Much research suggests damage results from a weight-centered focus, such as weight cycling and stigmatization. Consideration of several dimensions of ethical practice—veracity, fidelity, justice and a compassionate response—suggests that the HAES paradigm shift may be required for professional ethical accountability [168].

17.5 PUBLIC HEALTH ETHICS

The new public health ethics advocates scrutiny of the values and structure of medical care, recognizing that the remedy to poor health and health inequalities does not lie solely in individual choices.

This ethicality has been adopted by HAES in several ways. HAES academics have highlighted the inherent limitations of an individualistic approach to conceptualizing health. Individual self-care is taken as a starting point for HAES programs, but, unlike more conventional interventions, the HAES ethos recognizes the structural basis of health inequities and understands empowerment as a process that effects collective change in advancing social justice [169]. HAES advocates have also stressed the need for action to challenge the thinness privilege and to better enable fat people's voices to be heard in and beyond health care [8,170].

The hallmark theme of the new public health agenda is that it emphasizes the complexity of health determinants and the need to address systemic health inequities in order to improve population-wide health outcomes and reduce health disparities, making use of the evidence on the strong relationship between a person's social positioning and their health. For example, research since the 1950s has documented huge differences in cardiac health between and across socioeconomic gradients which has come to be recognized as arising from disparities in social standing and is articulated as the status syndrome [171]. Since weight tracks closely with socioeconomic class, obesity is a particularly potent marker of social disparity [172].

There is extensive research documenting the role of chronic stress in conditions conventionally described as obesity-associated, such as hypertension, diabetes and coronary heart disease [173]. These conditions are mediated through increased metabolic risk seen as raised cholesterol, raised blood pressure, raised triglycerides and insulin resistance. The increase in metabolic risk can in part be explained by a change in eating, exercise and drinking patterns attendant on coping with stress. However, changes in health behaviors do not fully account for the metabolic disturbances. Instead, stress itself alters metabolism independent of a person's lifestyle habits [174]. Thus, it has been suggested that psychological distress is the antecedent of high metabolic risk [175], which indicates the need to ensure health promotion policies utilize strategies known to reduce, rather than increase, psychological stress. In addition to the impact of chronic stress on health, an increasing body of international research, discussed earlier, recognizes particular pathways through which weight stigmatization and discrimination impact on health, health-seeking behaviors, and quality of health care [125-133].

Policies which promote weight loss as feasible and beneficial not only perpetuate misinformation and damaging stereotypes [176], but also contribute to a healthist, moralizing discourse which mitigates against socially-integrated approaches to health [155,168,177,178]. While access to size acceptance practitioners can ameliorate the harmful effects of discrimination in health care for individuals, systemic change is required to address the iatrogenic consequences of institutional size discrimination in and beyond health care, discrimination that impacts on people's opportunities and health.

Quite aside from the ethical arguments underscoring inclusive, non-discriminatory health care and civil rights, there are plausible metabolic pathways through which reducing weight stigma, by reducing inequitable social processes, can help alleviate the burden of poor health.

17.6 CONCLUSION

From the perspective of efficacy as well as ethics, body weight is a poor target for public health intervention. There is sufficient evidence to recommend a paradigm shift from conventional weight management to Health at Every Size. More research that considers the unintended consequences of a weight focus can help to clarify the associated costs and will better allow practitioners to challenge the current paradigm. Continued research that includes larger sample sizes and more diverse populations and examines how best to deliver a Health at Every Size intervention, customized to specific populations, is called for.

We propose the following guidelines, which are supported by the Association for Size Diversity and Health (ASDAH), to assist professionals in implementing HAES. Our proposed guidelines are modified, with permission, from guidelines developed by the Academy for Eating Disorders for working with children [7].

- Interventions should meet ethical standards. They should focus on health, not weight, and should be referred to as "health promotion" and not marketed as "obesity prevention." Interventions should be careful to avoid weight-biased stigma, such as using language like "overweight" and "obesity."
- Interventions should seek to change major determinants of health that reside in inequitable social, economic and environmental factors, including all forms of stigma and oppression.
- Interventions should be constructed from a holistic perspective, where consideration is given to physical, emotional, social, occupational, intellectual, spiritual, and ecological aspects of health.
- Interventions should promote self-esteem, body satisfaction, and respect for body size diversity.
- Interventions should accurately convey the limited impact that lifestyle behaviors have on overall health outcomes.

- Lifestyle-oriented elements of interventions that focus on physical activity and eating should be delivered from a compassion-centered approach that encourages self-care rather than as prescriptive injunctions to meet expert guidelines.
- Interventions should focus only on modifiable behaviors where there is evidence that such modification will improve health. Weight is not a behavior and therefore not an appropriate target for behavior modification.
- Lay experience should inform practice, and the political dimensions of health research and policy should be articulated.

These guidelines outline ways in which health practitioners can shift their practice towards a HAES approach and, in so doing, uphold the tenets of their profession in providing inclusive, effective, and ethical care consistent with the evidence base.

REFERENCES

1. Marketdata Enterprises: The U.S. Weight Loss & Diet Control Market (10th Edition). Lynbrook 2009.
2. Monteath SA, McCabe MP: The influence of societal factors on female body image. J Soc Psychol 1997, 137:708-727.
3. Neumark-Sztainer D, Rock CL, Thornquist MD, Cheskin LJ, Neuhouser ML, Barnett MJ: Weight-control behaviors among adults and adolescents: Associations with dietary intake. Prev Med 2000, 30:381-391.
4. Jeffery RW, Adlis SA, Forster JL: Prevalence of dieting among working men and women: The Healthy Worker Project. Health Psychol 1991, 10:274-281.
5. Mann T, Tomiyama AJ, Westling E, Lew AM, Samuels B, Chatman J: Medicare's Search for Effective Obesity Treatments: Diets Are Not the Answer. Am Psychol 2007, 62:220-233.
6. Neumark-Sztainer D: Preventing obesity and eating disorders in adolescents: what can health care providers do? J Adolesc Health 2009, 44:206-213.
7. Daníelsdóttir S, Burgard D, Oliver-Pyatt W: AED Guidelines for Childhood Obesity Prevention Programs. Academy of Eating Disorders; 2009.
8. Bacon L: Health at Every Size: The Surprising Truth About Your Weight. Second edition. Dallas: BenBella Books; 2010.
9. Schmidt H, Voigt K, Wikler D: Carrots, Sticks, and Health Care Reform -- Problems with Wellness Incentives. N Engl J Med 2009, 362:e3.
10. Medical News Today: Eating Disorder Organizations Join Forces To Urge Focus On Health And Lifestyle Rather Than Weight. 2009.
11. Bacon L, Stern J, Van Loan M, Keim N: Size acceptance and intuitive eating improve health for obese, female chronic dieters. J Am Diet Assoc 2005, 105:929-936.

12. Ciliska D: Evaluation of two nondieting interventions for obese women. West J Nurs Res 1998, 20:119-135.

13. Goodrick GK, Poston WSC II, Kimball KT, Reeves RS, Foreyt JP: Nondieting versus dieting treatment for overweight binge-eating women. J Consult Clin Psychol 1998, 66:363-368.

14. Tanco S, Linden W, Earle T: Well-being and morbid obesity in women: A controlled therapy evaluation. Int J Eat Disord 1998, 23:325-339.

15. Miller WC, Wallace JP, Eggert KE, Lindeman AK: Cardiovascular risk reduction in a self-taught, self-administered weight loss program called the nondiet diet. Med Exerc Nutr Health 1993, 2:218-223.

16. Rapoport L, Clark M, Wardle J: Evaluation of a modified cognitive-behavioural programme for weight management. Int J Obes 2000, 24:1726-1737.

17. Provencher V, Begin C, Tremblay A, Mongeau L, Corneau L, Dodin S, Boivin S, Lemieux S: Health-at-every-size and eating behaviors: 1-year follow-up results of a size acceptance intervention. J Am Diet Assoc 2009, 109:1854-1861.

18. Mensinger J, Close H, Ku J: Intuitive eating: A novel health promotion strategy for obese women. Paper presented at American Public Health Association. Philadelphia, PA 2009.

19. Bacon L, Keim N, Van Loan M, Derricote M, Gale B, Kazaks A, Stern J: Evaluating a "Non-diet" Wellness Intervention for Improvement of Metabolic Fitness, Psychological Well-Being and Eating and Activity Behaviors. Int J Obes 2002, 26:854-865.

20. Provencher V, Bégin C, Tremblay A, Mongeau L, Boivin S, Lemieux S: Short-term effects of a "health-at-every-size" approach on eating behaviors and appetite ratings. Obesity (Silver Spring) 2007, 15:957-966.

21. Steinhardt M, Bezner J, Adams T: Outcomes of a traditional weight control program and a nondiet alternative: a one-year comparison. J Psychol 1999, 133:495-513.

22. Carrier KM, Steinhardt MA, Bowman S: Rethinking traditional weight management programs: A 3-year follow-up evaluation of a new approach. J Psychol 1993, 128:517-535.

23. Omichinski L, Harrison KR: Reduction of dieting attitudes and practices after participation in a non-diet lifestyle program. J Can Diet Assoc 1995, 56:81-85.

24. Polivy J, Herman CP: Undieting: A program to help people stop dieting. Int J Eat Disord 1992, 11:261-268.

25. Roughan P, Seddon E, Vernon-Roberts J: Long-term effects of a psychologically based group programme for women preoccupied with body weight and eating behaviour. Int J Obes 1990, 14:135-147.

26. Higgins L, Gray W: Changing the body image concern and eating behaviour of chronic dieters: the effects of a psychoeducational intervention. Psychol and Health 1998, 13:1045-1060.

27. Miller WC: How effective are traditional dietary and exercise interventions for weight loss? Med Sci Sports Exerc 1999, 31:1129-1134.

28. National Institutes of Health (NIH): Methods for voluntary weight loss and control (Technology Assessment Conference Panel). Ann Intern Med 1992, 116:942-949.

29. Gregg EW, Gerzoff RB, Thompson TJ, Williamson DF: Intentional weight loss and death in overweight and obese U.S. adults 35 years of age and older. Ann Intern Med 2003, 138:383-389.

30. Wamala S, Lynch J, Horsten M: Education and the Metabolic Syndrome in Women. Diabetes Care 1999, 22:1999-2003.
31. Aphramor L: Validity of claims made in weight management research: a narrative review of dietetic articles. Nutr J 2010, 9:30.
32. Flegal KM, Graubard BI, Williamson DF, Gail MH: Excess deaths associated with underweight, overweight, and obesity. JAMA 2005, 293:1861-1867.
33. Durazo-Arvizu R, McGee D, Cooper R, Liao Y, Luke A: Mortality and optimal body mass index in a sample of the US population. Am J Epidemiol 1998, 147:739-749.
34. Troiano R, Frongillo E Jr, Sobal J, Levitsky D: The relationship between body weight and mortality: A quantitative analysis of combined information from existing studies. Int J Obes Relat Metab Disord 1996, 20:63-75.
35. Flegal K, Graubard B, Williamson D, Gail M: Supplement: Response to "Can Fat Be Fit". Sci Am 2008, 297:5-6.
36. McGee DL: Body mass index and mortality: a meta-analysis based on person-level data from twenty-six observational studies. Ann Epidemiol 2005, 15:87-97.
37. Janssen I, Mark AE: Elevated body mass index and mortality risk in the elderly. Obes Rev 2007, 8:41-59.
38. Lantz PM, Golberstein E, House JS, Morenoff J: Socioeconomic and behavioral risk factors for mortality in a national 19-year prospective study of U.S. adults. Soc Sci Med 2010, 70:1558-1566.
39. Berrington de Gonzalez A, Hartge P, Cerhan JR, Flint AJ, Hannan L, MacInnis RJ, Moore SC, Tobias GS, Anton-Culver H, Freeman LB, et al.: Body-mass index and mortality among 1.46 million white adults. N Engl J Med 2010, 363:2211-2219.
40. Childers D, Allison D: The 'obesity paradox': a parsimonious explanation for relations among obesity, mortality rate and aging? Int J Obes (Lond) 2010, 34:1231-1238.
41. Morse S, Gulati R, Reisin E: The obesity paradox and cardiovascular disease. Curr Hypertens Rep 2010, 12:120-126.
42. Ross C, Langer RD, Barrett-Connor E: Given diabetes, is fat better than thin? Diabetes Care 1997, 20:650-652.
43. Barrett-Connor E, Khaw K: Is hypertension more benign when associated with obesity? Circulation 1985, 72:53-60.
44. Barrett-Connor EL: Obesity, atherosclerosis and coronary artery disease. Ann Intern Med 1985, 103:1010-1019.
45. Kang X, Shaw LJ, Hayes SW, Hachamovitch R, Abidov A, Cohen I, Friedman JD, Thomson LE, Polk D, Germano G, Berman DS: Impact of body mass index on cardiac mortality in patients with known or suspected coronary artery disease undergoing myocardial perfusion single-photon emission computed tomography. J Am Coll Cardiol 2006, 47:1418-1426.
46. Beddhu S: The body mass index paradox and an obesity, inflammation, and atherosclerosis syndrome in chronic kidney disease. Seminars in Dialysis 2004, 17:229-232.
47. Ernsberger P, Haskew P: Health implications of obesity: An alternative view. J of Obesity and Weight Regulation 1987, 9:39-40.
48. Ernsberger P, Koletsky RJ: Biomedical rationale for a wellness approach to obesity: An alternative to a focus on weight loss. J Soc Issues 1999, 55:221-260.

49. Lavie CJ, Milani RV, Ventura HO: Obesity, heart disease, and favorable prognosis--truth or paradox? Am J Med 2007, 120:825-826.

50. Gruberg L, Mercado N, Milo S, Boersma E, Disco C, van Es GA, Lemos PA, Ben Tzvi M, Wijns W, Unger F, et al.: Impact of body mass index on the outcome of patients with multivessel disease randomized to either coronary artery bypass grafting or stenting in the ARTS trial: The obesity paradox II? Am J Cardiol 2005, 95:439-444.

51. Lavie CJ, Osman AF, Milani RV, Mehra MR: Body composition and prognosis in chronic systolic heart failure: the obesity paradox. Am J Cardiol 2003, 91:891-894.

52. Schmidt DS, Salahudeen AK: Obesity-survival paradox-still a controversy? Semin Dial 2007, 20:486-492.

53. Kulminski AM, Arbeev KG, Kulminskaya IV, Ukraintseva SV, Land K, Akushevich I, Yashin AI: Body mass index and nine-year mortality in disabled and nondisabled older U.S. individuals. J Am Geriatr Soc 2008, 56:105-110.

54. Olshansky SJ, Passaro DJ, Hershow RC, Layden J, Carnes BA, Brody J, Hayflick L, Butler RN, Allison DB, Ludwig DS: A potential decline in life expectancy in the United States in the 21st century. N Engl J Med 2005, 352:1138-1145.

55. Belluck P: Children's Life Expectancy Being Cut Short by Obesity. New York Times. New York City; 2005.

56. Carmona R: Testimony Before the Subcommittee on Competition, Infrastructure, and Foreign Commerce Committee on Commerce, Science, and Transportation. United States Senate 2004.

57. White House Task Force on Childhood Obesity: Solving the Problem of Childhood Obesity Within a Generation. Report to the White House. 2010.

58. National Center for Health Statistics: Health, United States, 2007. With Chartbook on Trends in the Health of Americans. Hyattsville, MD. 2007.

59. Mathers C, Loncar D: Projections of Global Mortality and Burden of Disease from 2002 to 2030. PLoS Med 2006, 3:2011-2029.

60. Social Security Administration: Periodic Life Table. 2007. (updated 7/9/07)

61. Campos P, Saguy A, Ernsberger P, Oliver E, Gaesser G: The epidemiology of overweight and obesity: public health crisis or moral panic? Int J Epidemiol 2005, 35:55-60.

62. Kruger J, Galuska DA, Serdula MK, Jones DA: Attempting to lose weight: specific practices among U.S. adults. Am J Prev Med 2004, 26:402-406.

63. Strohacker K, McFarlin B: Influence of obesity, physical inactivity, and weight cycling on chronic inflammation. Front Biosci 2010, E2:98-104.

64. Montani JP, Viecelli AK, Prevot A, Dulloo AG: Weight cycling during growth and beyond as a risk factor for later cardiovascular diseases: the 'repeated overshoot' theory. Int J Obes (Lond) 2006, 30(Suppl 4):S58-66.

65. Olson MB, Kelsey SF, Bittner V, Reis SE, Reichek N, Handberg EM, Merz CN: Weight cycling and high-density lipoprotein cholesterol in women: evidence of an adverse effect: a report from the NHLBI-sponsored WISE study. Women's Ischemia Syndrome Evaluation Study Group. J Am Coll Cardiol 2000, 36:1565-1571.

66. French SA, Jeffrey RW, Forster JL, McGovern PG, Kelder SH, Baxter J: Predictors of weight change over two years among a population of working adults: The Healthy Worker Project. Int J Obes 1994, 18:145-154.

67. Guagnano MT, Pace-Palitti V, Carrabs C, Merlitti D, Sensi S: Weight fluctuations could increase blood pressure in android obese women. Clinical Sciences (London) 1999, 96:677-680.

68. Rzehak P, Meisinger C, Woelke G, Brasche S, Strube G, Heinrich J: Weight change, weight cycling and mortality in the ERFORT Male Cohort Study. Eur J Epidemiol 2007, 22:665-673.

69. Lissner L, Odell PM, D'Agostino RB, Stokes J, Kreger BE, Belanger AJ, Brownell KD: Variability of body weight and health outcomes in the Framingham population. N Engl J Med 1991, 324:1839-1844.

70. Diaz VA, Mainous AG, Everett CJ: The association between weight fluctuation and mortality: results from a population-based cohort study. J Community Health 2005, 30:153-165.

71. McDermott R: Ethics, Epidemiology, and the Thrifty Gene: Biological Determinism as a Health Hazard. Soc Sci Med 1998, 47:1189-1195.

72. Brunner E, Marmot M: Social Organization, Stress, and Health. In Social Determinants of Health. 2nd edition. Edited by Marmot M, Wilkinson RG. New York: Oxford University Press; 2006::17-43.

73. Raphael D, Lines E, Bryant T, Daiski I, Pilkington B, Dinca-Panaitescu S, Dinca-Panaitescu M: Type 2 Diabetes: Poverty, Priorities and Policy. The Social Determinants of the Incidence and Management of Type 2 Diabetes. Toronto: York University School of Health Policy and Management and School of Nursing; 2010.

74. Charles MA, Pettitt DJ, Saad MF, Nelson RG, Bennett PH, Knowler WC: Development of impaired glucose tolerance with or without weight gain. Diabetes Care 1993, 16:593-596.

75. Odeleye OE, de Courten M, Pettitt DJ, Ravussin E: Fasting hyperinsulinemia is a predictor of increased body weight gain and obesity in Pima Indian children. Diabetes 1997, 46:1341-1345.

76. Sigal RJ, El-Hashimy M, Martin BC, Soeldner JS, Krolewski AS, Warram JH: Acute postchallenge hyperinsulinemia predicts weight gain: a prospective study. Diabetes 1997, 46:1025-1029.

77. Yost TJ, Jensen DR, Eckel RH: Weight regain following sustained weight reduction is predicted by relative insulin sensitivity. Obes Res 1995, 3:583-587.

78. Halberg N, Henriksen M, Söderhamn N, Stallknecht B, Ploug T, Schjerling P, Dela F: Effect of intermittent fasting and refeeding on insulin action in healthy men. J Appl Physiol 2005, 99:2128-2136.

79. Akram DS, Astrup AV, Atinmo T, Boisson JL, Bray GA, Carroll KK, Chunming C, Chitson P, Dietz WH, Hill JO, et al.: Obesity: Preventing and managing the global epidemic. Report of a WHO consultation on obesity. Geneva, Switzerland: World Health Organization; 1997.

80. Weinsier RL, Norris DJ, Birch R, Bernstein RS, Wang J, Yang MU, Pierson RN Jr, Van Itallie TB: The relative contribution of body fat and fat pattern to blood pressure level. Hypertension 1985, 7:578-585.

81. Ernsberger P, Nelson DO: Effects of fasting and refeeding on blood pressure are determined by nutritional state, not by body weight change. Am J Hypertens 1988, :153S-157S.

82. Schulz M, Liese A, Boeing H, Cunningham J, Moore C, Kroke A: Associations of short-term weight changes and weight cycling with incidence of essential hypertension in the EPIC-Potsdam Study. J Hum Hypertens 2005, 19:61-67.

83. Ernsberger P, Koletsky RJ, Baskin JZ, Collins LA: Consequences of weight cycling in obese spontaneously hypertensive rats. Am J Physiol 1996, 270:R864-R872.

84. Ernsberger P, Koletsky RJ, Baskin JZ, Foley M: Refeeding hypertension in obese spontaneously hypertensive rats. Hypertension 1994, 24:699-705.

85. Chernin K: The Obsession: Reflections on the tyranny of slenderness. New York: Harper & Row; 1981.

86. Cambien F, Chretien J, Ducimetiere L, Guize L, Richard J: Is the relationship between blood pressure and cardiovascular risk dependent on body mass index? Am J Epidemiol 1985, 122:434-442.

87. Weinsier R, James L, Darnell B, Dustan H, Birch R, Hunter G: Body fat: Its relationship to coronary heart disease, blood pressure, lipids, and other risk factors measured in a large male population. Am J Med 1976, 61:815-824.

88. Uretsky S, Messerli FH, Bangalore S, Champion A, Cooper-Dehoff RM, Zhou Q, Pepine CJ: Obesity paradox in patients with hypertension and coronary artery disease. Am J Med 2007, 120:863-870.

89. Messerli FH: Cardiovascular adaptations to obesity and arterial hypertension: detrimental or beneficial? Int J Cardiol 1983, 3:94-97.

90. Gregg EW, Cheng YJ, Cadwell BL, Imperatore G, Williams DE, Flegal KM, Narayan KM, Williamson DF: Secular trends in cardiovascular disease risk factors according to body mass index in US adults. JAMA 2005, 293:1868-1874.

91. Williamson DF, Pamuk E, Thun M, Flanders D, Byers T, Heath C: Prospective study of intentional weight loss and mortality in never-smoking overweight U.S. white women aged 40-64 years. Am J Epidemiol 1995, 141:1128-1141.

92. Williamson DF, Pamuk E, Thun M, Flanders D, Byers T, Heath C: Prospective study of intentional weight loss and mortality in overweight white men aged 40-64 years. Am J Epidemiol 1999, 149:491-503.

93. Andres R, Muller DC, Sorkin JD: Long-term effects of change in body weight on all-cause mortality. A review. Ann Intern Med 1993, 119:737-743.

94. Yaari S, Goldbourt U: Voluntary and involuntary weight loss: associations with long term mortality in 9,228 middle-aged and elderly men. Am J Epidemiol 1998, 148:546-555.

95. Sørensen T, Rissanen A, Korkeila M, Kaprio J: Intention to lose weight, weight changes, and 18-y mortality in overweight individuals without co- morbidities. PLoS Med 2005, 2:E171.

96. Simonsen MK, Hundrup YA, Obel EB, Gronbaek M, Heitmann BL: Intentional weight loss and mortality among initially healthy men and women. Nutr Rev 2008, 66:375-386.

97. Ingram DD, Mussolino ME: Weight loss from maximum body weight and mortality: the Third National Health and Nutrition Examination Survey Linked Mortality File. Int J Obes 2010, 34:1044-1050.

98. Klein S, Fontana L, Young VL, Coggan AR, Kilo C, Patterson BW, Mohammed BS: Absence of an effect of liposuction on insulin action and risk factors for coronary heart disease. N Engl J Med 2004, 350:2549-2557.

99. Manning RM, Jung RT, Leese GP, Newton RW: The comparison of four weight reduction strategies aimed at overweight patients with diabetes mellitus: four-year follow-up. Diabet Med 1998, 15:497-502.

100. Wing RR, Anglin K: Effectiveness of a behavioral weight control program for blacks and whites with NIDDM. Diabetes Care 1996, 19:409-413.

101. Ciliska D, Kelly C, Petrov N, Chalmers J: A review of weight loss interventions for obese people with non-insulin dependent diabetes mellitus. Can J of Diabetes Care 1995, 19:10-15.

102. Howard BV, Manson JE, Stefanick ML, Beresford SA, Frank G, Jones B, Rodabough RJ, Snetselaar L, Thomson C, Tinker L, et al.: Low-fat dietary pattern and weight change over 7 years: the Women's Health Initiative Dietary Modification Trial. JAMA 2006, 295:39-49.

103. Howard BV, Van Horn L, Hsia J, Manson JE, Stefanick ML, Wassertheil-Smoller S, Kuller LH, LaCroix AZ, Langer RD, Lasser NL, et al.: Low-fat dietary pattern and risk of cardiovascular disease: the Women's Health Initiative Randomized Controlled Dietary Modification Trial. JAMA 2006, 295:655-666.

104. Aphramor L: Is A Weight-Centred Health Framework Salutogenic? Some Thoughts on Unhinging Certain Dietary Ideologies. Social Theory and Health 2005, 3:315-340.

105. Aphramor L: Weight management as a cardioprotective intervention raises issues for nutritional scientists regarding clinical ethics. Proc Nut Soc 2009, 67:E401.

106. Sjostrom L, Lindroos AK, Peltonen M, Torgerson J, Bouchard C, Carlsson B, Dahlgren S, Larsson B, Narbro K, Sjostrom CD, et al.: Lifestyle, diabetes, and cardiovascular risk factors 10 years after bariatric surgery. N Engl J Med 2004, 351:2683-2693.

107. Christou NV, Look D, Maclean LD: Weight gain after short- and long-limb gastric bypass in patients followed for longer than 10 years. Ann Surg 2006, 244:734-740.

108. Bacon L, Stern JS, Keim NL, Van Loan MD: Low bone mass in premenopausal chronic dieting obese women. Eur J Clin Nutr 2004, 58:966-971.

109. Van Loan MD, Keim NL: Influence of cognitive eating restraint on total-body measurements of bone mineral density and bone mineral content in premenopausal women 18-45 y: a cross-sectional study. Am J Clin Nutr 2000, 72:837-843.

110. Van Loan MD, Bachrach LK, Wang MC, Crawford PB: Effect of drive for thinness during adolescence on adult bone mass. J Bone Miner Res 2000, 15:S412.

111. Barr SI, Prior JC, Vigna YM: Restrained eating and ovulatory disturbances: Possible implications for bone health. Am J Clin Nutr 1994, 59:92-97.

112. Tomiyama AJ, Mann T, Vinas D, Hunger JM, Dejager J, Taylor SE: Low calorie dieting increases cortisol. Psychosom Med 2010, 72:357-364.

113. Lee DH, Lee IK, Song K, Steffes M, Toscano W, Baker BA, Jacobs DR Jr: A strong dose-response relation between serum concentrations of persistent organic pollutants and diabetes: results from the National Health and Examination Survey 1999-2002. Diabetes Care 2006, 29:1638-1644.

114. Carpenter DO: Environmental contaminants as risk factors for developing diabetes. Rev Environ Health 2008, 23:59-74.

115. Ha MH, Lee DH, Jacobs DR: Association between serum concentrations of persistent organic pollutants and self-reported cardiovascular disease prevalence: results

from the National Health and Nutrition Examination Survey, 1999-2002. Environ Health Perspect 2007, 115:1204-1209.

116. Lee DH, Steffes M, Jacobs DR: Positive associations of serum concentration of polychlorinated biphenyls or organochlorine pesticides with self-reported arthritis, especially rheumatoid type, in women. Environ Health Perspect 2007, 115:883-888.

117. Chevrier J, Dewailly E, Ayotte P, Mauriege P, Despres JP, Tremblay A: Body weight loss increases plasma and adipose tissue concentrations of potentially toxic pollutants in obese individuals. Int J Obes Relat Metab Disord 2000, 24:1272-1278.

118. Lim JS, Son HK, Park SK, Jacobs DR Jr, Lee DH: Inverse associations between long-term weight change and serum concentrations of persistent organic pollutants. Int J Obes (Lond) 2010, in press.

119. Davison KK, Markey CN, Birch LL: A longitudinal examination of patterns in girls' weight concerns and body dissatisfaction from ages 5 to 9 years. Int J Eat Disord 2003, 33:320-332.

120. Holm S: Obesity interventions and ethics. Obes Rev 2007, 8(Suppl 1):207-210.

121. Neumark-Sztainer D, Levine MP, Paxton SJ, Smolak L, Piran N, Wertheim EH: Prevention of body dissatisfaction and disordered eating: What next? Eat Disord 2006, 14:265-285.

122. van den Berg P, Neumark-Sztainer D: Fat 'n happy 5 years later: is it bad for overweight girls to like their bodies? J Adolesc Health 2007, 41:415-417.

123. Stice E, Cameron RP, Killen JD, Hayward C, Taylor CB: Naturalistic weight-reduction efforts prospectively predict growth in relative weight and onset of obesity among female adolescents. J Consult Clin Psychol 1999, 67:967-974.

124. Coakley EH, Rimm EB, Colditz G, Kawachi I, Willett W: Predictors of weight change in men: Results from the Health Professionals Follow-Up Study. Int J Obes Relat Metab Disord 1998, 22:89-96.

125. Bild DE, Sholinsky P, Smith DE, Lewis CE, Hardin JM, Burke GL: Correlates and predictors of weight loss in young adults: The CARDIA study. Int J Obes Relat Metab Disord 1996, 20:47-55.

126. Korkeila M, Rissanen A, Kapriio J, Sorensen TIA, Koskenvuo M: Weight-loss attempts and risk of major weight gain. Am J Clin Nutr 1999, 70:965-973.

127. Neumark-Sztainer D, Wall M, Guo J, Story M, Haines J, Eisenberg M: Obesity, disordered eating, and eating disorders in a longitudinal study of adolescents: how do dieters fare 5 years later? J Am Diet Assoc 2006, 106:559-568.

128. Field AE, Austin SB, Taylor CB, Malspeis S, Rosner B, Rockett HR, Gillman MW, Colditz GA: Relation between dieting and weight change among preadolescents and adolescents. Pediatrics 2003, 112:900-906.

129. Puhl RM, Andreyeva T, Brownell KD: Perceptions of weight discrimination: prevalence and comparison to race and gender discrimination in America. Int J Obes (Lond) 2008, 32:992-1000.

130. Brownell K, Puhl R, Schwartz M, Rudd LE: Weight bias: Nature, consequences, and remedies. New York: Guilford; 2005.

131. Puhl RM, Brownell KD: Confronting and coping with weight stigma: an investigation of overweight and obese adults. Obesity (Silver Spring) 2006, 14:1802-1815.

132. Haines J, Neumark-Sztainer D, Eisenberg ME, Hannan PJ: Weight teasing and disordered eating behaviors in adolescents: longitudinal findings from Project EAT (Eating Among Teens). Pediatrics 2006, 117:e209-215.

133. Neumark-Sztainer D, Falkner N, Story M, Perry C, Hannan PJ, Mulert S: Weight-teasing among adolescents: correlations with weight status and disordered eating behaviors. Int J Obes Relat Metab Disord 2002, 26:123-131.

134. Puhl RM, Moss-Racusin CA, Schwartz MB: Internalization of weight bias: Implications for binge eating and emotional well-being. Obesity (Silver Spring) 2007, 15:19-23.

135. Faith MS, Leone MA, Ayers TS, Heo M, Pietrobelli A: Weight criticism during physical activity, coping skills, and reported physical activity in children. Pediatrics 2002, 110:e23.

136. Storch EA, Milsom VA, Debraganza N, Lewin AB, Geffken GR, Silverstein JH: Peer victimization, psychosocial adjustment, and physical activity in overweight and at-risk-for-overweight youth. J Pediatr Psychol 2007, 32:80-89.

137. Vartanian LR, Shaprow JG: Effects of weight stigma on exercise motivation and behavior: a preliminary investigation among college-aged females. J Health Psychol 2008, 13:131-138.

138. Amy N, Aalborg A, Lyons P, Keranen L: Barriers to routine gynecological cancer screening for White and African-American obese women. Int J Obes Relat Metab Disord 2006, 30:147-155.

139. Puhl R, Brownell K: Bias, discrimination and obesity. Obes Res 2001, 9:788-805.

140. Puhl RM, Heuer CA: The stigma of obesity: a review and update. Obesity (Silver Spring) 2009, 17:941-964.

141. Fagard RH: Physical activity in the prevention and treatment of hypertension in the obese. Med Sci Sports Exerc 1999, 31:S624-630.

142. Appel LJ, Moore TJ, Obarzanek E, Vollmer WM, Svetkey LP, Sacks FM, Bray GA, Vogt TM, Cutler JA, Windhauser MM, et al.: A clinical trial of the effects of dietary patterns on blood pressure. N Engl J Med 1997, 33:1117-1124.

143. Gaesser GA: Exercise for prevention and treatment of cardiovascular disease, type 2 diabetes, and metabolic syndrome. Curr Diab Rep 2007, 7:14-19.

144. Kraus WE, Houmard JA, Duscha BD, Knetzger KJ, Wharton MB, McCartney JS, Bales CW, Henes S, Samsa GP, Otvos JD, et al.: Effects of the amount and intensity of exercise on plasma lipoproteins. N Engl J Med 2002, 347:1483-1492.

145. Lamarche B, Despres JP, Pouliot MC, Moorjani S, Lupien PJ, Theriault G, Tremblay A, Nadeau A, Bouchard C: Is body fat loss a determinant factor in the improvement of carbohydrate and lipid metabolism following aerobic exercise training in obese women? Metabolism 1992, 41:1249-1256.

146. Bjorntorp P, DeJounge K, Sjostrom L, Sullivan L: The effect of physical training on insulin production in obesity. Metabolism 1970, 19:631-638.

147. Finkelstein EA, Trogdon JG, Cohen JW, Dietz W: Annual medical spending attributable to obesity: payer-and service-specific estimates. Health Aff (Millwood) 2009, 28:w822-831.

148. Wildman RP, Muntner P, Reynolds K, McGinn AP, Rajpathak S, Wylie-Rosett J, Sowers MR: The obese without cardiometabolic risk factor clustering and the normal weight with cardiometabolic risk factor clustering: prevalence and correlates of

2 phenotypes among the US population (NHANES 1999-2004). Arch Intern Med 2008, 168:1617-1624.

149. Beaglehole R, Prior IA, Foulkes MA, Eyles EF: Death in the South Pacific. N Z Med J 1980, 91:375-378.

150. Crister G: Fat Land: How Americans Became the Fattest People in the World. New York: Houghton Mifflin; 2004.

151. Heinberg L, Matzon J: Body image dissatisfaction as a motivator for healthy lifestyle change: Is some distress beneficial? In Eating disorders: Innovative directions for research and practice. Edited by Striegel-Moore R, Smolak L. Washington, DC: American Psychological Association; 2001::215-232.

152. Puhl R, Heuer C: Obesity Stigma: Important Considerations for Public Health. Am J Public Health 2010, 100:1019-1028.

153. Leary MR, Tate EB, Adams CE, Allen AB, Hancock J: Self-compassion and reactions to unpleasant self-relevant events: the implications of treating oneself kindly. J Pers Soc Psychol 2007, 92:887-904.

154. Goss K, Allen S: Compassion focused therapy for eating disorders. Int J of Cognitive Therapy 2010, 3:141-158.

155. Aphramor L, Gingras J: That remains to be seen: Disappeared feminist discourses on fat in dietetic theory and practice. In The Fat Studies Reader. Edited by Rothblum E, Solovay S. New York: New York University Press; 2009::97-105.

156. Tribole E, Resch E: Intuitive eating: a revolutionary program that works. 2nd edition. New York: St. Martin's Griffin; 2010.

157. Hirschmann JR, Munter CH: When women stop hating their bodies: freeing yourself from food and weight obsession. 1st edition. New York: Fawcett Columbine; 1995.

158. Matz J, Frankel E: The Diet Survivor's Handbook: 60 Lessons in Eating, Acceptance and Self-care. Naperville, IL: Sourcebooks; 2006.

159. May M: Eat What You Love, Love What You Eat: How to Break Your Eat-Repent-Repeat Cycle. Greenleaf Book Group Press; 2009.

160. Satter E: Secrets of Feeding a Healthy Family: How to Eat, How to Raise Good Eaters and How to Cook. Madison, WI: Kelcy Press; 2008.

161. Cole R, Horacek T: Effectiveness of the "My Body Knows When" intuitive-eating pilot program. Am J Health Behav 2010, 34:286-297.

162. Smith T, Hawks S: Intuitive eating, diet composition and the meaning of food in healthy weight promotion. Am J Health Educ 2006, 37:130-136.

163. Tylka T: Development and psychometric evaluation of a measure of intuitive eating. J Couns Psychol 2006, 53:226-240.

164. Kristeller J, Hallett C: An exploratory study of a meditation-based intervention for binge eating disorder. J Health Psychol 1999, 4:357-363.

165. Smitham L: Evaluating an intuitive eating program for binge eating disorder: A benchmarking study [dissertation]. South Bend, IN: University of Notre Dame; 2008.

166. Hawks S, Madanat H, Hawks J, Harris A: The relationship between intuitive eating and health indicators among college women. Am J Health Educ 2005, 36:331-336.

167. Weigensberg M, Shoar Z, Lane C, Spruijt-Metz D: Intuitive eating (IE) Is associated with decreased adiposity and increased insulin sensitivity (Si) in obese Latina female adolescents. DiabetesPro; 2009.

168. Aphramor L, Gingras J: Helping People Change: Promoting Politicised Practice in the Healthcare Professions. In Debating Obesity: Critical Perspectives. Edited by Rich E, Monaghan L, Aphramor L. U.K.: Palgrave/Macmillan; 2010.

169. Aphramor L, Gingras J: Weight in Practice, Health in Perspective. In Critical Bodies. Edited by Riley S, Burns M, Frith H, Wiggins S, Markula P. Palgrave/Macmillan; 2007::155-117.

170. Bacon L: Reflections on Fat Acceptance: Lessons Learned from Privilege. [http://www.lindabacon.org/Bacon_ThinPrivilege080109.pdf] Keynote Speech, National Association to Advance Fat Acceptance conference; Washington, DC 2009.

171. Marmot MG: Status syndrome: a challenge to medicine. JAMA 2006, 295:1304-1307.

172. Clarke P, O'Malley PM, Johnston LD, Schulenberg JE: Social disparities in BMI trajectories across adulthood by gender, race/ethnicity and lifetime socio-economic position: 1986-2004. Int J Epidemiol 2009, 38:499-509.

173. Chandola T, Brunner E, Marmot M: Chronic stress at work and the metabolic syndrome: prospective study. BMJ 2006, 332:521-525.

174. Vitaliano PP, Scanlan JM, Zhang J, Savage MV, Hirsch IB, Siegler IC: A path model of chronic stress, the metabolic syndrome, and coronary heart disease. Psychosom Med 2002, 64:418-435.

175. Raikkonen K, Matthews KA, Kuller LH: The relationship between psychological risk attributes and the metabolic syndrome in healthy women: antecedent or consequence? Metabolism 2002, 51:1573-1577.

176. Aphramor L: Disability and the Anti-Obesity Offensive. Disability & Society 2009, 24:897-909.

177. Lebesco K: Fat Panic and the New Morality. In Against Health: How Health Became the New Morality. Edited by Metzl J, Kirkland A. New York: New York University Press; 2010::72-82.

178. Klein R: What is Health and How Do You Get It? In Against Health: How Health Became the New Morality. Edited by Metzl J, Kirkland A. New York: New York University Press; 2010::15-25.

This chapter was originally published under the Creative Commons Attribution License. Bacon, L., and Aphramor, L. Weight Science: Evaluating the Evidence for a Paradigm Shift. Nutrition Journal 2011: 10(9). doi:10.1186/1475-2891-10-9.

CHAPTER 18

GAUGING FOOD AND NUTRITIONAL CARE QUALITY IN HOSPITALS

ROSA WANDA DIEZ-GARCIA, ANETE ARAÚJO DE SOUSA,
ROSSANA PACHECO DA COSTA PROENÇA,
VANIA APARECIDA LEANDRO-MERHI,
and EDSON ZANGIACOMI MARTINEZ

18.1 BACKGROUND

Changes in population age distribution and lifestyle require that these institutions undergo modifications, in order to meet the current demands of society such as increased life expectancy and new disease profiles [1-4]. As part of the national health systems, these changes had an impact on the hospitals. The emergence of novel technologies, the constant need for recycling of knowledge and abilities due to reformulations of scientific paradigms, and the hospital costs implied in this recycling justify the need for assessment of quality and efficacy in this health segment [5].

Nutritional status in hospital inpatient has been the object of many studies [6-11], but there are only a few literature works on quality indicators concerning hospital food and nutrition services (HFNSs) as well as food and nutritional care actions conducted by dietitians in health institutions [12-15]. Hospital expectations often place the food and nutrition service as an undervalued support service [16], even though changes and improvements in hospital diets and nutritional care can prevent nutritional aggravations [7,8,12,17] that have a negative impact on the length of hospital stay and hospitalization costs [10,11,18-20]. Moreover, such amelioration can also impact patient's perception of the hospitalization experience positively [21,22].

European research on food and nutritional care in hospital has recognized that it is necessary to define responsibilities, promote staff qualification, enable patients' participation in nutritional decisions, and integrate the health care team into nutritional care [14]. A comparative study on nutritional care management involving two hospital institutions, namely a French hospital and a Brazilian hospital, has detected fragmentation of dietitians' actions due to existence of different interlocutors and to the unpredictability inherent to food preparation procedures [23].

Food and nutritional care actions regarding both patient assistance and food quality must be well delineated and become an effective practice in health institutions. Different management sectors, namely the clinical and administrative areas, should be involved in the process, and actions should be recognized and evaluated by regulating agencies concerned with hospital quality control.

Standardization of nutritional care practice in the United States was implemented by the American Dietetic Association (ADA) in 1987. In 1993, the Clinical Nutrition Management executive committee selected professionals who later developed and assessed the standard nutritional practices that should be employed for management of the clinical nutritional area, which gave rise to a standard reference for this field [24]. Knowledge about the actual state of food and nutritional care is a crucial stage for delivery of good quality hospital assistance. This kind of diagnosis enables future comparisons and allows for evaluation of implemented changes, which is essential for action planning [25].

This study aimed to detect and compare actions relative to food and nutritional care quality in hospital in public and private hospitals.

18.2 METHODS

Thirty-seven hospitals were investigated. Twenty-seven hospitals were located in municipalities of the state of São Paulo, more specifically

Campinas and Ribeirão Preto, whereas ten hospitals were located in the city of Florianópolis, capital of the state of Santa Catarina. Both Campinas and Ribeirão Preto are important scientific-technological health centers with various services of nationwide recognition. The cities included in the present work are home to various public (federal and state) and private universities. Campinas, Ribeirão Preto, and Florianópolis have an estimated population of 1,039,297; 547,417; and 396,723 inhabitants, respectively.

In the states of São Paulo and Santa Catarina there are 2.29 (0.58 public and 1.71 private) and 2.66 (0.67 public and 1.99 private) hospital beds/1,000 inhabitants, respectively. The metropolitan region of Florianópolis holds a larger concentration (72.7%) of public beds (2.61 of the 3.59 hospital beds/1,000 inhabitants are public), while the metropolitan region of Campinas has a larger proportion (74.6%) of private beds (1.47 of the 1.97 hospital beds/1,000 inhabitants are private) [26].

The following inclusion criteria were considered: hospitals located in the studied municipalities, regardless of the type—general, specialized, public, private, small (up to 50 beds), medium-sized (between 51 and 150 beds), or large (more than 150 beds)—that agreed to take part in the research. Psychiatric hospitals, day hospitals, nursing homes, and shelters were not included. Hospitals that did not have a dietitian responsible for the Hospital Food and Nutrition Service (HFNS) were excluded because this is compulsory according to the Brazilian law and hospitals that refused to participate in the study were not included, either. Although the healthcare team is responsible for nutritional screening and other actions, the piece of this investigation was to evaluate the dietitians actions of the hospitals food and nutritional services. An informed consent for the participation in the research was obtained from both the interviewee and a representative of the participating institution. The project was approved by the Research Ethics Committee of Faculdade de Medicina de Ribeirão Preto, University of São Paulo.

Data was collected by means of a structured interview, using a questionnaire designated Instrument for Evaluation of Food and Nutritional Care in Hospital—IEFNCH [27]. This questionnaire contained open and closed questions that helped diagnose hospital activities supporting food and nutritional care. The questions were directed to the hospital nutrition service coordinators during two visits that had been pre-arranged with the institution. The present IEFNCH was based on instruments published in similar works [13-15,24,28-30]. After the application of IEFNCH, a data bank containing information about various aspects of the institutions under study was built. We organized these data as criteria, according to these references used to qualify this instrument [27]. The size of the HFNS was measured by the number of hospital beds per dietitian, the number of HFNS staff members (kitchen staff) per dietitian, the number of produced meals per HFNS staff member, and the number of produced meals per dietitian. In these cases all dietitians that worked in these hospitals were considered, which include, clinical dietitian, dietitian who works in the management of meal production and the dietitian coordinator, if there was one.

Activities carried out by the HFNS were divided into two corpora of criteria, one relative to nutritional care quality (NCQ) and another concerning quality of the actions related to hospital food service (FSQ). Descriptive statistics was accomplished for the NCQ and FSQ criteria in terms of the legal nature and location of the institution. Differences in the criteria between public and private hospitals were considered substantial, moderate, and small when they were equal to 30%, less than 30 to 15%, and less than 15%, respectively (Table 1).

The criteria were subdivided into 8 groups of actions, designated NCQ and FSQ indicators (4 groups of actions for each corpus). These indicators, consisting of between 3 and 6 criteria, were measured as a percentage of existence of that group of actions in a certain institution. Each indicator thus corresponded to 25% of the total NCQ and FSQ value. Food and Nutritional Care Quality in Hospital (FNCQH) was determined as the mean percentage that each institution complied with the NCQ and FSQ indicators, and comparisons in terms of the legal nature, type (general or specialized), size, and location of the hospital as well as the presence of a clinical dietitian were made. It was considered "clinical dietitian" the professional who works in the infirmary with the patient's nutritional care. The existence of actions was assessed; however, the extent of their coverage was not evaluated.

Descriptive statistical data analysis was also performed, and ANOVA models were employed for comparison of NCQ and FSQ among the studied institutions. Such model assumes that the residues obtained from the

TABLE 1: Criteria comprising the nutritional care quality (NCQ) and food service quality (FSQ) indicators

Ncq indicators (100%)	Employed Criteria
Inpatient dietary coverage actions (a) (25%)	A1.Duty shift system in the area of clinical nutrition
	A2.Supervision of meal distribution in the ward
	A3.Routine visits to patients
Evaluation and monitoring of nutritional status actions (b) (25%)	B1.Nutritional status evaluation (complete)
	B2.Nutritional status monitoring
	B3.Entry of nutritional care information in the medical record
	B4.Filling in forms about nutritional care
	B5.Nutritional guidance at discharge
	B6.Assistance protocols
Actions on integration of nutritional assistance activities within the team (c) (25%)	C1. Diet prescription in the medical records
	C2. Interconsultations on nutritional care
	C3. Team visits to patients
	C4. Participation in activities outside the HFNS
	C5. Nutritional support team
Actions supporting diet therapy (d) (25%)	D1.Diet manual
	D2.Information about energy supply
	D3.Selection of nutritional supplements
	D4.Mechanisms for patients to require changes to the diet
Fsq indicators (100%)	Employed criteria
Mediation actions with users and other hospital sectors (a) (25%)	A1. Duty shift in the area of meal production
	A2. Formal evaluation of the HFNS regarding user satisfaction
	A3. Planning and goal-setting for the HFNS
	A4. HFNS participation in other hospital sectors
Autonomy and management control actions (b) (25%)	B1. HFNS responsibility for purchases
	B2. Budget autonomy
	B3. Control of cost/meal or cost/daily produced food
	B4. Statistical control by the HFNS
	B5. Statistical control of the produced diets

TABLE 1: *Cont.*

Meal production qualification actions (c) (25%)	C1. Standard prescription form
	C2. Dietetic kitchen
	C3. Routine tasting of diets
	C4. Good practice manual
	C5. Diet manual (*)
	C6. Production of nutritional supplements
Staff qualification actions (d) (25%)	D1. Staff evaluation
	D2. Instrument for staff evaluation
	D3. Periodic training program

(*) This criteria was considered important in both NCQ and FSQ.

difference between values predicted by the model and the observed values have normal distribution with average 0 and constant variance. In situations in which this assumption was not confirmed, transformed-response variables were utilized [31]. Models were adjusted with the aid of the software SAS version 9.

18.3 RESULTS

Sixty-seven point six percent of the sample consisted of private hospitals, including philanthropic institutions (10 hospitals), whilst 32.4% were public hospitals, 18.9% of which were university hospitals and 13,5% were government institutions. In Florianópolis the majority of the sample was comprised of public hospitals (70,0%), whereas the cities of the state of São Paulo had a larger number of private institutions (81.5%) (Table 2). However, in terms of the public beds, Florianópolis had 79%; Ribeirão Preto had 67% and Campinas had 51%. Considering beds in specialized hospitals, we had 13,0% in Campinas (90,0% public beds), 7,3% in Ribeirão Preto (38,5% public beds) and 19,4% in Florianópolis (88,4% public beds). The investigated hospitals corresponded to 82.4% of the hospital beds available in the referred municipalities (Campinas 82.5%; Ribeirão Preto 87.5%; Florianópolis 76.0%), which represented a coverage of 5,566 beds [26]. There were 2 hospitals in Florianópolis, 2 in Ribeirão Preto and 2 in Campinas that did not accept to participate. There were 2 more hospitals in Florianópolis that were not included because one was being renovated and the other did not have a dietitian at that moment; and one in Campinas did not have a dietitian when we were collecting the data of the investigation.

As for HFNS human resources ratio, the average number of hospital beds per HFNS staff member and per dietitian was 3.81 (SD 1.98) and 68.04 (SD 43.26), respectively. Both indicators had a large coefficient of variation (Cv) (52.01% and 63.58%, respectively). Concerning meal production per staff member and per dietitian, the average number of produced meals was 20.55 (SD 14.61 and Cv 71.08%) and 320.65 (SD 173.67 and Cv 54.16%), respectively. There were a significant statistical difference between public and private hospitals to the number of hospital beds per HFNS staff member ($p = 0.02$) and per dietitian ($p < 0.01$) (Table 3). These variables were also significantly different for the hospitals located in Florianópolis, as compared to institutions situated in Campinas ($p < 0.01$) and Ribeirão Preto ($p = 0.04$).

TABLE 2: Characteristics of the hospitals

Hospital Characteristics	Campinas	Ribeirão Preto	Florianópolis	Total	
	(n=17)	(n=10)	(n=10)	(n=37)	%
Legal nature					
Public (n=12)	3	2	7	12	32.4
Private (n=25)	14	8	3	25	67.6
Total	17	10	10	37	100.0
Type					
Specialized	3*	2**	2***	7	18.9
General	14	8	8	30	81.1
Total	17	10	10	37	100.0
Size					
Small	2	1	3	6	16.2
Medium	11	6	4	20	54.1
Large	4	3	3	10	27.0
Total	17	10	10	37	100.0

*Maternity, oftalmologic and women hospital; ** maternities; ***maternity and infections and contagious disease hospital.*

TABLE 3: HFNS human resource indicators*

Hospitals	n.b/HFNS sm	n.b/dt	n. HFNS sm /dt	n.meals/ HFNS sm	n.meals/ dt
Legal nature					
Public hospitals (=12)					
Mean (sd)	3.26±(2.72)	36.32±(13.56)	14.01±(6.87)	25.4±(20.5)	297.67±(159.42)
Median	2.11	32.50	13.25	20.35	262.00
Coefficient of Variation	83.41	37.34	49.04	80.7	53.55
Minimum	1.72	16.54	3.20	11.4	98.00
Maximum	11.51	66.67	32.30	85.70	637.00
Private hospitals privados (=25)					
Mean (sd)	4.07±(1.51)	83.27±(44.48)	22.16±(13.28)	18.2±(10.5)	331,68±(182.22)
Median	4.02	70.00	21.00	15.83	308,00
Coefficient of Variation	37.07	53.42	59.94	57.8	54,94
Minimum	1.88	16.00	6.00	2.30	80,00
Maximum	9.33	169.00	60.00	50.0	780,00
Institution type					
Municipalities					
Campinas					
Mean (sd)	4.48±(2.47)	77.28±(46.62)	20.98±15.01	19.28±(18.48)	281.82±(180.32)
Median	3.89	56.00	15.00	13.71	220.0
Coefficient of Variation	55.07	60.32	71.53	95.87	63.98
Minimum	2.25	30.00	3.20	2.33	80.0

Hospitals	n.b/HFNS sm	n.b/dt	n. HFNS sm /dt sm	n.meals/ HFNS sm	n.meals/ dt
Maximum	11.51	169.00	60.00	85.71	780.0
Ribeirão Preto					
Mean (sd)	3.82±(1.17)	84.29±(41.29)	22.18±(9.76)	18.21±(8.68)	363.5±(164.85)
Median	3.57	75.00	19.00	20.50	348.0
Coefficient of Variation	30.64	49.67	44.01	47.65	45.35
Minimum	2.11	25.00	11.90	6.25	115.0
Maximum	5.58	145.00	40.00	31.07	665.0
Florianópolis					
Mean (sd)	2.67±(1.11)	36.09±(16.76)	14.36±(7.13)	25.06±(11.81)	343.8±(173.74)
Median	2.08	32.50	14.00	22.39	332.00
Coefficient of Variation	41.75	46.44	49.64	47.11	50.53
Minimum	1.72	16.00	8.00	11.72	98.00
Maximum	4.63	66.67	32.30	50.00	637.00

* n.b HFNS sm = number of beds per HFNS staff member; n.b/dt = number of beds per dietitian; n. HFNS sm /dt = number HFNS staff members per dietitian; n.meals/ HFNS sm = number of produced meals per HFNS staff member; n.meals/dt = number produced meals per dietitian.

TABLE 4: NCQ criteria in hospitals

NCQ criteria	Private Hospitals (n=25)		Public Hospitals (n=12)		Difference*	Campinas (n=17)		Ribeirão Preto (n=10)		Flori-anópolis (n=10)	
	n	%	n	%	n	n	%	n	%	n	%
A - Inpatient dietary coverage actions											
A1. Duty shift system in the area of clinical nutrition	4	16.0	3	25.0	9.0	2	11.8	3	30.0	1	10.0
A2. Supervision of meal distribution in the ward	7	28.0	4	33.3	5.3	6	35.3	2	20.0	3	30.0
A3. Routine visits to patients	16	64.0	12	100.0	36.0	12	70.6	6	60.0	10	100.0
B – Evaluation and monitoring of nutritional status actions											
B1. Nutritional assessment (complete)**	4	16.0	8	66.7	50.7	7	41.2	1	10.0	4	40.0

TABLE 4: *Cont.*

NCQ criteria	Private Hospitals (n=25)		Public Hospitals (n=12)		Difference*	Campinas (n=17)		Ribeirão Preto (n=10)		Florianópolis (n=10)	
B2. Nutritional status monitoring	8	32.0	6	50.0	18.0	7	41.2	4	40.0	3	30.0
B3. Entry of nutritional care information in the medical record	9	36.0	7	58.3	22.3	7	41.2	2	20.0	7	70.0
B4. Filling in forms about nutritional care	7	28.0	4	33.3	5.3	5	29.4	1	10.0	5	50.0
B5. Nutritional guidance at discharge	24	96.0	12	100.0	4.0	16	94.1	10	100.0	10	100.0
B6. Assistance protocols	9	36.0	6	50.0	14.0	10	58.8	3	30.0	2	20.0
C - Actions on integration of nutritional assistance activities within the team											
C1. Diet prescription in the medical records	15	60.0	7	58.3	1.7	12	70.6	4	40.0	6	60.0
C2. Interconsultations on nutritional care	7	28.0	5	41.7	13.7	5	29.4	3	30.0	4	40.0

TABLE 4: *Cont.*

NCQ criteria	Private Hospitals (n=25)		Public Hospitals (n=12)		Difference*	Campinas (n=17)		Ribeirão Preto (n=10)		Florianópolis (n=10)	
C3. Team visits to patients	9	36.0	7	58.3	22.3	9	52.9	3	30.0	4	40.0
C4. Participation in activities outside the HFNS	18	72.0	9	75.0	3.0	11	64.7	9	90.0	7	70.0
C5. Nutritional support team	7	28.0	3	25.0	3.0	5	29.4	4	40.0	2	20.0
D – HFNS actions supporting diet therapy											
D1. Diet manual ***	16	64.0	4	33.3	30.7	14	82.4	3	30.0	3	30.0
D2. Information about energy supply	14	56.0	6	50.0	6.0	13	76.5	3	30.0	4	40.0
D3. Selection of nutritional supplements	7	28.0	4	33.3	5.3	5	29.4	4	40.0	2	20.0
D4. Mechanisms for patients to require changes to the diet	12	48.0	11	91.7	43.7	11	64.7	3	30.0	9	90.0

* Difference (in %) between Private and Public Hospitals; ** Nutritional assessment (complete) include patient's history and anthropometric and biochemical data; *** This criteria was considered important in both NCQ and FSQ.

Evaluation of the presence of actions related to criteria of the NCQ corpus revealed that the difference between public and private hospitals varied between 1.7% and 50.7%, and that the average of this difference were 17.4% (SD 14.9%). The actions with the most differences ($\geq$30%) between public and private institutions were presence of routine visits to patients, evaluation of nutritional status, and existence of mechanisms for patients to require changes to the diet (Table 4), all of which predominated in the former type of health institution.

In all the studied cities, actions related to inpatient dietary coverage were rarely present in public and private hospitals (between 12% and 35% of the institutions developed these actions). A slightly better situation was found in terms of actions concerning assessment and nutritional status monitoring, which existed in 33.3% to 66.7% of the public hospitals. Nutritional guidance at discharge was one of the actions that were most present in both public and private institutions. As for the remaining actions, they occurred in approximately a third of the private hospitals.

When it comes to municipalities, hospitals in Florianópolis stood out particularly for entry of nutritional care information in the medical record and existence of a printed form specially designed for nutritional care.

As for actions related to integration of the health care team into nutritional care activities, over 70% of the HFNS of public and private hospitals participated in events held outside the institution, evidencing engagement of the service with nutritional issues. On the other hand, actions related to insertion of the dietitian into the health care team were more frequent in public hospitals; for instance, routine visits to inpatients and requirement for nutritional care interconsultation with the HFNS took place in public institutions more often.

Information about the diet energy supply, present in approximately half of the hospitals, and the choice of nutritional supplement offered by the HFNS, which occurred in approximately one third of the institutions, indicated that HFNS actions supporting dietotherapy must be implemented and valued, since they are essential for efficient delivery of inpatient nutritional care.

Evaluation of the criteria of the FSQ corpus revealed that the difference between public and private hospitals in terms of the presence of actions related to meal production was 17.3% (SD 13.5%) on average, varying between 1.0% and 39.3%. A higher number of private hospitals had a good practice manual, a diet manual, an instrument for staff evaluation, and a periodic training programme (Table 5).

TABLE 5: FSQ criteria in hospitals

HMPQ criteria	Private Hospitals (n=25)		Public Hospitals (n=12)		Difference*	Campinas (n=17)		Ribeirão Preto (n=10)		Florianópolis (n=10)	
	n	%	n	%		n	%	n	%	n	%
A - HFNS mediation actions with users and other hospital sectors											
A1. Duty shift in the area of meal production	7	28.0	3	25.0	3.0	5	29.4	5	50.0	0	0.0
A2. Formal evaluation of the HFNS regarding user satisfaction	7	28.0	3	25.0	3.0	6	35.3	3	30.0	1	10.0
A3. Planning and goal-setting for the HFNS	11	44.0	7	58.3	14.3	9	52.9	6	60.0	3	30.0
A4. HFNS participation in other hospital sectors	19	76.0	9	75.0	1.0	11	64.7	10	100.0	7	70.0
B - Autonomy and management control actions											
B1. HFNS responsibility for purchases	14	56.0	2	16.7	39.3	8	47.1	7	70.0	1	10.0
B2. Budget autonomy	5	20.0	1	8.3	11.7	4	23.5	2	20.0	0	0.0
B3. Control of cost/meal or cost/daily produced food	19	76.0	9	75.0	1.0	13	76.5	8	80.0	7	70.0
B4. Statistical control by the HFNS	21	84.0	12	100.0	16.0	14	82.4	9	90.0	10	100.0

TABLE 5: *Cont.*

HMPQ criteria	Private Hospitals (n=25)		Public Hospitals (n=12)		Difference*	Campinas (n=17)		Ribeirão Preto (n=10)		Florianópolis (n=10)	
B5. Statistical control of the produced diets	17	68.0	11	91.7	23.7	13	76.5	8	80.0	7	70.0
C - Meal production qualification actions											
C1. Standard prescription form	10	40.0	4	33.3	6.7	7	41.2	4	40.0	3	30.0
C2. Dietetic kitchen	13	52.0	8	66.7	14.7	8	47.1	8	80.0	5	50.0
C3. Routine tasting of diets	15	60.0	4	33.3	26.7	12	70.6	5	50.0	2	20.0
C4. Good practice manual	21	84.0	6	50.0	34.0	14	82.4	6	60.0	7	70.0
C5. Diet manual **	16	64.0	4	33.3	30.7	14	82.4	3	30.0	3	30.0
C6. Production of nutritional supplements	7	28.0	5	41.7	13.7	6	35.3	4	40.0	2	20.0
D – Staff qualification actions											
D1. Staff evaluation	13	52.0	2	16.7	35.3	5	29.4	5	50.0	4	40.0
D2. Instrument for staff evaluation	8	32.0	4	33.3	1.3	1	5.9	4	40.0	7	70.0
D3. Periodic training program	15	60.0	3	25.0	35.0	6	35.3	5	50.0	5	50.0

* *Difference (in %) between Private and Pubic Hospitals; ** This criteria was considered important in both NCQ and FSQ.*

Management control actions were strongly influenced by the legal nature of the institution, many of which reflected in the differences found between public and private hospitals. Among the actions that were detected in most of the institutions, HFNS participation in other hospital administrave spheres and cost control can be mentioned. In contrast, less than a third of the hospitals conducted evaluation regarding user satisfaction. It is noteworthy that less than half of the institutions had a standard diet prescription form (nutritional contents of food preparations furnished by the Service). There was a larger difference between public and private hospitals with respect to the meal production qualification actions. In the same way, it is important to note that few public institutions carried out staff qualification actions.

The mean percentage of compliance with the NCQ criteria in private and public hospitals was 41.6% (SD 19.8) and 51.8% (SD 16.1), respectively, and the median was 39.2% and 53.0%, respectively. As for FSQ criteria, compliance values were 49.1% (SD 20.7), median of 46.7% and 42.4% (SD 16.6), median of 42.7%, respectively.

Among the variables analyzed in Table 6, NCQ was positively influenced by hospital type (general) and presence of clinical dietitian. FSQ was affected by hospital size: medium-sized and large institutions were significantly better than small hospitals.

18.4 DISCUSSION

HFNS human resources, measured in terms of number of hospital beds and produced meals, are heterogeneous and characterized by a wide coefficient of variation, thus suggesting that there are no preset parameters for human resources ratio in this area.

The relation number of staff members per hospital bed, an indicator of hospital human resources in Brazil, varies between 1.0 and 7.2, while in public institutions this indicator varies from 4.0 to 9.0 [32]. Using this same relation for the number of HFNS staff members per hospital bed, an average of 0.27 (SD 0.09) and median of 0.25 is obtained. Differences found between human resources ratio in public and private hospitals with respect to the number of hospital beds per dietitian and the number of HFNS staff members per dietitian evidences a more favorable situation in public institutions in terms of graduated professionals. The difference among the investigated cities is probably a consequence of the larger concentration of public hospitals in Florianópolis. In a study on eight hospitals of four different Brazilian states [33] was observed a relation varying from 50 up to 150 patients per dietitian, associated with a situation of very precarious in same action analised about nutritional care.

Viabilization of nutritional care through evaluation of nutritional status and establishment of actions that suit their clinical and nutritional status along the duration of hospital stay depend on the relation number of hospital beds per dietitian [34]. Even if screening criteria are created and nutritional care levels are defined [35], values of 30 and 15 hospital beds per dietitian are recommended for general hospitals and more complex units, respectively [30]. The study that evaluated how nutritional risk is assessed and managed in European hospitals with twenty one thousand patients, found a range between 21% and 73% of the units from different regions that reported nutritional screening routine. The presence of dietitian, nutrition team and the screening nutrition routine increased the probability of to identifing nutritional risk [36].

More heterogeneous conditions were detected for the productivity indicator (number of produced meals per staff member). The number of meals produced for other segments such as hospital staff members and visitors may distort the aims of the HFNS and redirect human resources from the nutritional care sector to meal production. An increase in administrative demands may also deteriorate inpatient nutritional care actions [16,33].

Comparison between public and private health institutions in terms of NCQ criteria reveals that there are more actions related to nutritional care in public hospitals (routine visits to patients, evaluation of nutritional status, mechanisms for patients to require changes to the diet, entry of nutritional care information in the medical record, among others). Such actions may avoid or detect nutritional problems that can be handled during the hospital stay, thereby preventing nutritional aggravations [37]. This difference can be attributed to the presence of a larger number of clinical dietitian in public hospitals and to the fact that there are more university hospitals of public legal nature. The lack of nutritional assessment, diet prescription, and entry of nutritional information in medical records has also been detected in another work on Brazilian and Italian hospitals [16,33,38].

TABLE 6: Food and Nutritional Care Quality in Hospital measured as percentage of NCQ and FSQ

Variables	INCQ (%)						HMPQ (%)					
Hospitals	Mean (SD)	Median	Coef Var	Minimum	Maximum	p	Mean (SD)	Median	Coef Var	Minimum	Maximum	p
Legal Nature												
Public (n=12)	51.82 (16.07)	52.95	31.01	23.80	80.40	0.11	42.38 (16.55)	42.70	39.05	14.20	78.30	0.37
Private (n=25)	41.62 (19.84)	39.20	47.68	9.20	85.40		49.14 (20.69)	46.70	42.10	12.50	100.00	
Type												
General (n=30)	48.47 (17.79)	47.49	36.70	21.70	47.90	0.01	49.84 (19.78)	49.80	39.69	14.20	100.00	0.06
Specialized (n=7)	29.73 (18.09)	22.50	60.85	9.20	58.80		34.54 (12.78)	33.80	37.00	12.50	50.40	
Clinical dietitian												
yes (n=22)	39.11 (17.91)	37.70	45.80	9.20	85.40	0.02	50.15 (21.95)	48.55	43.78	12.50	100.00	0.32
no (n=15)	53.46 (18.05)	55.40	33.77	21.70	83.30		42.25 (14.59)	42.10	34.53	23.30	78.30	
Size												
Small (n=6)	31.82 (16.54)	30.85	51.97	9.20	52.90	a	29.4 (14.44)	29.80	49.10	12.50	46.30	b

TABLE 6: *Cont.*

Medium (n=21)	46.63 (18.65)	48.30	39.99	21.70	85.40	49.57 (18.57)	50.40	37.47	18.30	100.00
Large (n=10)	49.21 (19.83)	51.05	40.29	21.70	80.40	51.96 (19.64)	49.80	37.80	30.00	91.70
Municipality										
Campinas (n=17)	51.49 (20.06)	51.30	38.95	20.80	85.40 c	46.94 (19.15)	50.40	40.80	12.50	78.30 d
Ribeirão Preto (n=10)	36.05 (18.20)	31.05	50.50	9.20	62.90	57.01 (22.25)	48.55	39.03	31.70	100.00
Florianópolis (n=10)	42.64 (15.43)	45.85	36.19	21.70	65.80	36.89 (12.05)	35.85	32.67	14.20	56.70

a – no significant difference; b – significant difference between small and medium-sized hospitals (p=0.01) and between small and large hospitals (p=0.01) and no significant difference between medium-sized and large hospitals; c – significant difference between institutions in Campinas and Ribeirão Preto (p=0.04), no difference for the others; d – significant difference between Ribeirão Preto and Florianópolis (p=0.03), no difference for the others.

Some actions are lacking in both public and private institutions, with a difference smaller than 15% between them. Such lack of NCQ actions denotes little technical qualification for very important actions. Only half of the hospitals provide information about energy supply, whereas only a third has appropriate forms for registration of nutritional care, participation of the dietitian in meal distribution, and production of nutritional supplements by the HFNS. The legally prescribed nutritional support team [39] exists in a quarter of the hospitals only. These data reinforce the need for professional qualification and nutritional care action descriptors for the hospital segment [38].

Differences in FSQ criteria demonstrate that there is greater concern about staff evaluation and standardized procedures such as good practice and diet manuals in private institutions. Slight differences emerge when most of the NCQ and FSQ criteria are compared between public and private hospitals and among municipalities, which highlights the need for establishing general quality standards for an HFNS.

Among the FSQ actions, up to a third of the hospitals have duty shift in the area of meal production, carry out staff evaluation, and conduct formal evaluation of the HFNS regarding user satisfaction. There are actions that call for closer attention, since they take place in less than a third of the hospitals. For instance, despite being present in most of the public hospitals and in half of the private institutions, supervision of patient nutrition in the ward would very much facilitate establishment of mechanisms for patients to require changes to the diet if patient food ingestion was directly observed. Unfortunately, this contact between the dietitian and the patient has been overlooked [33,40]. As for differences concerning the responsibility of the HFNS for purchases, they are due to regulations regarding this procedure in public hospitals.

Request of nutritional care by physicians and other professionals by means of interconsultations demonstrates recognition of this type of action by the multiprofessional team. Nevertheless, this takes place in less than a third of private institutions. In public hospitals, the situation is slightly better, though below the desired frequency. Similar results indicating that food and nutritional care is still incipient in health institutions have also been reported by De Seta et al. [33].

Herein, the legal nature of the institution did not influence the food and nutritional care quality, in spite of the larger number of dietitian present in public hospitals. Evaluation of HFNS human resources ratio did not necessarily imply in better quality, since it also depends on professional qualifications and skills. Nevertheless, hospitals with clinical dietitians had substantially better NCQ, and 80% of the 15 institutions that hired a dietitian were public. The presence of a specialized professional in this area may make all the difference in terms of nutritional care quality not only because of qualification, but also because of the existence of institutional policies valuing these actions. However, it is noteworthy that an array of conditions should also exist, so that this type of care can be improved [37,41]. Professional qualification, institutional policies for the sector, nutritional care quality programmes such as accreditation and institutional evaluation [42], and sufficient number of professionals [34] can better qualify food and nutritional care in hospitals.

The more complex structure of general hospitals favors NCQ. A higher demand due to the diverse nutritional problems that may arise in general institutions may contribute to this result. Although there are no significant differences in relation to FSQ, data for general (49.8%) and specialized (34.5%) hospitals suggest that more complex units are more qualified in this area. Results concerning hospital size can be analyzed in the same light. Larger hospitals have higher FSQ. Additionally, size does not significantly influence NCQ, but scores rise with increasing hospital size. Furthermore, university hospitals may influence hospital nutritional care positively, once they are placed among general institutions. It should be borne in mind that five of the seven university hospitals included in this work are large.

The significant difference between the NCQ scores of hospitals located in two cities of the same state (both cities proportionally having the same number of university hospitals) and the lack of any difference as compared to institutions located in Florianópolis, where public hospitals are the majority, suggest that other factors operate when service qualification is being analyzed. Even if no differences among these municipalities exist in terms of staff qualification, differences regarding professional skills may be present.

18.5 CONCLUSION

Food and nutritional care quality in hospital must be evaluated and qualified for improved efficacy of health institutions. The legal nature and size of hospitals may interfere in the examined segments, human resources score, NCQ, and FSQ. However, results from the present analysis lead to the conclusion that nutritional care is still incipient, and that actions concerning patient care and food service take place on an irregular basis in hospitals. This study allowed for attainment of a qualitative panorama of these actions and human resources indicators concerning hospital food and nutrition services.

The fact that coverage of the assessed actions was not verified is a limitation of the present work, which might have generated biased data. For instance, it is possible that some hospital units have excellent nutritional care teams while the care delivered to inpatients of some wards is deficient. The other limitation of the study was the frequency that these actions were developed. Both are important aspects that can influence in the quality of care. Some criteria influenced by the legal nature of the hospital may have given rise to some distortions.

Put together, our results show the performance of the actions developed by the HFNS. Although we cannot measure the coverage and the frequency of the actions, this study made a profile of the food and nutritional care in hospitals, an important step in guidelines for nutritional care in hospitals.

REFERENCES

1.   Allison S: w?>Clinical nutrition: the view from Europe. Nutrition 1996, 12(4):287-288.
2.   Succi MJ, Alexander JA, Lee SYD: Change in the population of health systems: From 1985 to 1998. J Healthc Manag 2001, 46(6):381-393.
3.   Lee SYD, Alexander JA: Managing hospitals in turbulent times: Do organizational changes improve hospital survival? Health Serv Res 1999, 34(4):923-946.
4.   Gerkens S, Merkur S: Belgium: health system review. Health Syst Transit 2010, 12(5):1-266.

5. Mckee M, Healy J: Hospital in a Changing Europe (European Observatory on Health Care System). First edition. World Health Organization, Buckingham Philadelphia; 2002::59-80.

6. Leistra E, Neelemaat F, Evers AM, van Zandvoort MH, Weijs PJ, van der van Bokhorst-de Schueren MA, et al.: Prevalence of undernutrition in Dutch hospital outpatients. Eur J Intern Med 2009, 20(5):509-513.

7. Leandro-Merhi VA, Diez Garcia RW, Mônaco DV, de Oliveira MR M: Comparación del estado nutricional, consumo alimenticio y tiempo de hospitalización de pacientes de dos hospitales, uno público y otro privado. Nutr Hosp 2006, 21(1):32-37.

8. Hickson M, O'Flynn J, Peake H, Foster D, Frost G: The prevalence of malnutrition in hospitals can be reduced: Results from three consecutive cross-sectional studies. Clin Nutr 2005, 24(6):1078-1088.

9. Penie JB, Malnut CGSH: State of malnutrition in Cuban hospitals. Nutrition 2005, 21(4):487-497.

10. Correia MI, Waitzberg DL: The impact of malnutrition on morbidity, mortality, length of hospital stay and costs evaluated through a multivariate model analysis. Clin Nutr 2003, 22(3):235-239.

11. Chima CS, Barco K, Dewitt ML, Maeda M, Teran JC, Mullen KD: Relationship of nutritional status to length of stay, hospital costs, and discharge status of patients hospitalized in the medicine service. J Am Diet Assoc 1997, 97(9):975-978.

12. Donini LM, Castellaneta E, De Guglielmi S, De Felice MR, Savina C, Coletti C, et al.: Improvement in the quality of the catering service of a rehabilitation hospital. Clin Nutr 2008, 27(1):105-114.

13. Flanel DF, Fairchild MM: Continuous quality improvement in inpatient clinical nutrition services. J Am Diet Assoc 1995, 95(1):65-74.

14. Ovesen L, Beck AM, Balknas UN, Furst P, Hasunen K, Jones L, et al.: Food and nutritional care in hospitals: how to prevent undernutrition-report and guidelines from the Council of Europe. Clin Nutr 2001, 20(5):455-460.

15. Beck AM, Balknas UN, Camilo ME, Furst P, Gentile MG, Hasunen K, et al.: Practices in relation to nutritional care and support-report from the Council of Europe. Clin Nutr 2002, 21(4):351-354.

16. Garcia R: Hospital diet from the perspective of those involved in its production and planning. Rev Nutr 2006, 19(2):129-144.

17. Kondrup J, Bak L, Hansen BS, Ipsen B, Ronneby H: Outcome from nutritional support using hospital food. Nutrition 1998, 14(3):319-321.

18. Leandro-Merhi VA, de Aquino JL, Sales Chagas JF: Nutrition status and risk factors associated with length of hospital stay for surgical patients. J Parenter Enteral Nutr 2011, 35((2):241-248.

19. Pichard C, Thibault R, Chikhi M, Clerc A, Darmon P, Chopard P, et al.: Assessment of food intake in hospitalised patients: A 10-year comparative study of a prospective hospital survey. Clin Nutr 2011, 30(3):289-296.

20. Amaral TF, Matos LC, Tavares MM, Subtil A, Martins R, Nazare M, et al.: The economic impact of disease-related malnutrition at hospital admission. Clin Nutr 2007, 26(6):778-784.

21. Belanger MC, Dube L: The emotional experience of hospitalization: its moderators and its role in patient satisfaction with foodservices. J Am Diet Assoc 1996, 96(4):354-360.
22. Stanga Z, Zurfluh Y, Roselli M, Sterchi AB, Tanner B, Knecht G: Hospital food: a survey of patients' perceptions. Clin Nutr 2003, 22(3):241-246.
23. Sousa AA, Pacheco RPC: Technology of management of nutritional care: recommendations to qualifying the attendance in hospital food and nutrition services. Rev Nutr 2004, 17(4):425-436.
24. Witte SS, EscottStump S, Fairchild MM, Papp J: Standards of practice criteria for clinical nutrition managers. J Am Diet Assoc 1997, 97(6):673-678.
25. Øvretveit J: What are the best strategies for ensuring quality in hospitals?. WHO Regional Office for Europe, Copenhagen; http://www.euro.who.int/document/e82995. pdf. November 2003)
26. Ministério da Saude / DATASUS: Datasus. Departamento de Informática do SUS; 2008.
27. Diez-Garcia RW, Sousa AA, Proença RPC: Qualifying instrument for evaluation of food and nutritional care in hospital. Nutr Hosp 2012, 27(4):1154-1161.
28. Vogelzang JL, Roth-Yousey LL: Standards of professional practice: Measuring the beliefs and realities of consultant dietitians in health care facilities. J Am Diet Assoc 2001, 101(4):473-480.
29. Ministério da Saúde: Manual Brasileiro de Acreditação Hospitalar. Secretaria de Assistência à Saúde. 3a, Edição Brasília; 2002.
30. Conselho Federal de Nutricionistas: Regulamenta a profissão de nutricionista e determina outras providências. Lei N 8.234, 17 de setembro de 1991 (DOU 18/09/1991). 1991.
31. Montgomery DC: Design and Analysis of Experiments. John Wiley & Sons I, New York; 2000.
32. Zuchhi PB: OJNV Funcionários por leito: estudo em alguns hospitais públicos e privados. Rev Adm Saude 2002, 4(14):1-7.
33. De Seta Mod G, Henriques P, Sales GLP: Nutritional care in public hospitals of four Brazilian states: contributions of health evaluation to health surveillance services. Cien Saude Colet 2010, 15(Supl. 3):3413-3422.
34. Byham-Gray L: Managing Human Resources, Nutrition Dimension. 2010. www.NutritionDimension.com
35. Duchini L, Brito TA, Jordao AA, Diez-Garcia RW: Assessment and monitoring of the nutritional status of hospitalized patients: a proposal based on the opinion of the scientific community. Rev Nutr 2010, 23(4):513-522.
36. Schindler K, Pernicka E, Laviano A, Howard P, Schütz T, Bauer P, Grecu I, Jonkers C, Kondrup J, Ljungqvist O, Mouhieddine M, Pichard C, Singer P, Schneider S, Schuh C, Hiesmayr M, Nutrition Day Audit Team: How nutritional risk is assessed and managed in European hospitals: a survey of 21,007 patients findings from the 2007–2008 cross-sectional nutritionDay survey. Clin Nutr 2010, 29(5):552-559.
37. Council of Europe Committee of Ministers: Resolution ResAP (2003) 3 on Food and Nutritional Care in Hospital. 2003.
38. Donini LM, Riti M, Castellaneta E, Ceccarelli P, Civale C, Passaretti S, et al.: A survey on diet manuals in Italian hospitals. Ann Ig 2009, 21(6):575-585.

39. Ministério da Saúde (Brasil): Regulamento Técnico para fixar os requisitos mínimos exigidos para terapia de nutrição enteral. Resolução - RDC n 63, de 6 de julho de 2000. Diário Oficial da União da República Federativa do Brasil, Brasília; 2000.
40. Diez-Garcia RW, Padilha M, Sanches M: Hospital food: proposals for qualification of the Food and Nutrition Service, evaluated by the scientific community. Cien Saude Colet 2012, 17(2):473-480.
41. Kondrup J: Proper hospital nutrition as a human right. Clin Nutr 2004, 23(2):135-137.
42. Vecina-Neto G, Malik AM: Trends in hospital care. Cien Saude Colet 2007, 12(4):825-839.

This chapter was originally published under the Creative Commons Attribution License. Diez-Garcia, R. W., de Sousa, A. A., Pacheco da Costa Proença, R., Leandro-Merhi, V. A., and Zangiacomi Martinez, E. Gauging Food and Nutritional Care Quality in Hospitals. Nutrition Journal 2012: 11(66). doi:10.1186/1475-2891-11-66.

AUTHOR NOTES

CHAPTER 1

Competing interests
None of the authors have any conflict of interest to declare.

Authors' contributions
As conceived of the original idea and aided with the experimental design, writing the final manuscript, and data interpretation. MR and SD carried out the all of the subject interviews, collection of data, data interpretation, and writing of the manuscript. FH, FS and MV carried out the study design, recruitment of patients, review of the original data and their compilation. AH and MG carried out data analysis, manuscript revision, critical revision of the manuscript for important scientific content. All authors read and approved the final manuscript.

Acknowledgments
We thank Ghazaleh Shimi, Saeedeh Nasiri, and Majid Goharinejad for specimen processing, anthropometric, and dietary data collection. Dr. Mehdi Hedayati and colleagues are acknowledged for biochemical analyses. We acknowledge Ms. Nilufar Shiva for language editing of the manuscript. This clinical trial was supported by grants from Tehran University of Medical Sciences (grant no. 852) and the Research Institute for Endocrine Sciences, Shahid Beheshti University of Medical Sciences (grant no. 293).

CHAPTER 2

Competing interests
The authors declare that they have no competing interests.

Authors' contribution

UT conducted research, wrote the manuscript and performed statistical analysis; UT and MK analysed data; UT and GJ designed research and had primary responsibility for final content. All authors read and approved the final manuscript.

Acknowledgments

We thank VCI (Verband der Chemischen Industrie e.V.) for financial support and for supplying the supplement. The study sponsor was not involved either in data interpretation or in authoring the manuscript. Technical assistance from Ute Helms is greatly appreciated. We thank Nasim Kroegel for language editing.

CHAPTER 3

Competing interests

The authors declare that they have no competing interests.

Authors' contributions

All authors participated in the preparation of the manuscript and approved the final manuscript.

CHAPTER 6

Conflict of Interests

The authors declare that they have no conflict of interests.

CHAPTER 7

Competing interests

The author(s) declare that they have no competing interests.

Authors' contributions

WFM conducted literature search, prepared the manuscript and assisted in presentation of final draft, LEA and NRR conceived the idea, organized contents and participated in preparation of final manuscript.

CHAPTER 8

Acknowledgment

The authors are supported by FIS PS09/00447, PI10/00072, EUS2008/03565, Fundacion Lilly, cvREMOD, ISCIII-RETIC REDin-REN/RD06/0016, Comunidad de Madrid/CIFRA/S-BIO0283/2006, S2010/BMD-2378, Sociedad Española de Nefrología, ERA-EDTA, Rio Hortega FIS and, Programa Intensificación Actividad Investigadora (ISCIII/Agencia Laín-Entralgo/CM) to A. Ortiz.

CHAPTER 9

Competing interests

The authors declare that they have no competing interests.

Authors' contributions

GC conceived of the study. GC and AF participated in the design of the study, performed the statistical analysis and have been involved in drafting the manuscript and revising it critically for important intellectual content. AC and PDL carried out the acquisition, the analysis and interpretation of data. All authors read and approved the final manuscript.

Clinical relevancy statement

Dieters of 21st century want instant weight loss and do not want to lose "only" a few pounds each week. Finding a fast and safe weight loss treatment could be the crucial battle to win in the war on obesity. Ketogenic Enteral Nutrition is a modified approach that allows a fast weight loss. It was tested on thousands of patients and it turned out to be safe and inexpensive, we can say to our patients that the treatment will cost about the same amount as eating their normal diet for 10 days.

CHAPTER 10

Competing interests

The author has no competing interests.

Authors' contributions

NW carried out the literature search, reviewed the papers and prepared the manuscript.

Acknowledgments

The author kindly acknowledges the assistance of Mr ADN Scott and Dr David Gerrett in reviewing and commenting on the manuscript.

CHAPTER 11

Competing interest

All authors declare no competing interest; they are all independent from funders. SCB and ADM are part of the Competence network of obesity, which is largely funded by a research grant of the Federal Ministry of Education and Research, Germany; within this network, the research group of SCB is funded in part by Nestlé HealthCare Nutrition GmbH, Munich, Germany. The sponsors had no influence in study design, analysis, and interpretation of data, as well as in the writing of the manuscript. No other relationships or activities exist that could appear to have influenced the submitted work.

Authors' contributions

The study was designed by ADM and SCB. ADM and GW carried out the study, collected, and analyzed the data. ADM drafted the manuscript. SCB reviewed the manuscript. All authors read and approved the final manuscript.

Acknowledgment

This work was supported by the "Competence Network of Obesity", research group "Obesity and the GI tract,"funded by the Federal Ministry of Education and Research, Germany (No. FKZ 01GI0843 to SCB), and by Nestlé HealthCare Nutrition GmbH, Munich, Germany, who is part of the "Competence Network of Obesity"

CHAPTER 12

Acknowledgments

We thank Science & Medicine for editorial support and Abbott Nutrition for funding to develop this manuscript.

An abstract of this work was presented at the 71st Annual Meeting of the American Diabetes Association, June 24–28, 2011, San Diego, California. Additionally, abstracts related to certain methodologic aspects of this work were submitted to and/or accepted by the Asia Pacific Congress of Diabetes Education, the Asian Congress of Nutrition, the European Association for the Study of Diabetes, the European Society for Clinical Nutrition and Metabolism, and the Canadian Diabetes Association. These submitted and/or accepted abstracts focus on different aspects of the diabetes-specific nutrition algorithm presented in this work. The abstract submitted to the Asian Pacific Congress of Diabetes Education focuses on the application of the algorithm in culturally diverse populations, whereas the abstract submitted to the Asian Congress of Nutrition focuses on the applicability of the algorithm in Asian societies. The European Association for the Study of Diabetes and the European Society for Clinical Nutrition and Metabolism abstract submissions focus on the patient algorithm for nutrition therapy (PATH), which combines nutrition recommendations from major diabetes organizations and geographic and ethnocultural factors to optimize diabetes care. The abstract submitted to the Canadian Diabetes Association focuses on the transcultural diabetes nutrition algorithm, which is intended to supplement CPGs and provide evidence-based information on lifestyle modifications, including physical activity and nutrition interventions for patients with diabetes.

Disclosure

Conflicts of interest: The development of this article was funded by Abbott Nutrition. The content was created and enriched solely by task force members through a process of ongoing literature searches, independent contributions and reviews, and group interactions for consensus. Other support may have been provided to task force members as indicated in the following statements. Caroline Apovian has received financial support from Amylin, Merck, Johnson & Johnson, Arena, and Sanofi-Aventis;

and research funding from Eli Lilly, Pfizer, Orexigen, Amylin, and Meta-Proteomics. Alexander Koglin Benchimol has served as a board member for Abbott, MSD, and Novo Nordisk; served as a consultant for Abbott, MSD, and Novo Nordisk; served as a speaker and developed educational presentations for Abbott, MSD, Novo Nordisk, Libbs, Sanofi-Aventis, and Torrent; and received funding for travel and accommodations from Abbott, MSD, Novo Nordisk, Libbs, Sanofi-Aventis, and Torrent. Peter H. Bisschop has received financial support for consultancy and research from Abbott Nutrition; also received funding for travel from Abbott Nutrition. Alexis Bolio-Galvis has nothing to disclose. Osama Hamdy has served as a consultant for Abbott Nutrition and a speaker for Amylin/Eli Lilly. Refaat A. Hegazi is employed by Abbott Nutrition; the material presented in this article is based on the best-known clinical evidence and is not affected by this financial relationship. David Jenkins has served as a consultant for Solae, Unilever, and Haine Celestial; served as an advisory board member for Herbalife International, Nutritional Fundamentals for Health, Pacific Health Laboratories, Metagenics/MetaProteomics, Bayer Consumer Care, and Orafti; received research funding from Solae, Unilever, Haine Celestial and Orafti; and received honorarium from Unilever. Miguel Leon Sanz has nothing to disclose. Albert E. Marchetti has received financial support for research and the development of educational materials from Eli Lilly, Takeda, GlaxoSmithKline, Bristol-Myers Squibb, and Abbott Nutrition International. Jeffrey Mechanick has received financial support for the development of educational presentations from Abbott Nutrition. He has received financial support for consultancy and for writing and reviewing the manuscript from Abbott Nutrition. He has received fees for participation in review activities such as data monitoring boards, statistical analysis, and end point committees from Abbott Nutrition International. He has received funding for travel and accommodations from Abbott Nutrition. Enrique Mendoza has received financial support for consultancy from Abbott Nutrition; He has received funding for travel and accommodations from Abbott Nutrition. Wayne Huey-Herng Sheu has received financial support for consultancy from Abbott Nutrition, Pfizer, GSK and Bayer. Patrizio Tatti received financial support for participation in review activities for Abbott Nutrition. He has received funding for travel from Abbott Nutrition. Man-Wo Tsang has nothing to disclose.

CHAPTER 13

Competing interests
The authors declare that they have no competing interests.

Authors' contributions
All authors were involved in the development of the study protocol. ASC performed subject recruitment, data collection and was responsible for the day-to-day running of the study. ASC and SG performed statistical analysis and drafted the final version of the manuscript. All authors approved and read the final manuscript.

CHAPTER 14

Competing interests
The authors declare that they have no competing interests.

Authors' contributions
RJK drafted the manuscript, UK drafted figures and parts of the manuscript, both authors finalized the manuscript. All authors have read and approved the final manuscript.

Acknowledgments
We are grateful to the two anonymous referees for their suggestions that helped to improve this paper. We also would like to thank Bill Lemke and Sebastian Baier for fruitful discussions and comments on a previous version of this paper. UK appreciates a research grant from the "Deutsche Gesellschaft für Ernährungsmedizin (DGEM)". This publication was funded by the German Research Foundation (DFG) and the University of Würzburg in the funding program Open Access Publishing

CHAPTER 15

Conflict of Interest
The authors have no potential conflict of interest to disclose.

CHAPTER 16

Competing interests
The authors declare that they have no competing interests.

Authors' contributions
SNK, DGG, AP and DPN designed research; IS, HB, FP and VH conducted research; IS analysed the vitamin D forms; AP analyzed the data; SNK, DGG, AP and DPN wrote the paper; DPN and BCT had primary responsibility for final content. All authors read and approved the final manuscript.

Acknowledgments
Supported by grants from Kingston University Research Development funds and Hellenic Society for the Study of Bone Metabolism (EEMMO).

CHAPTER 17

Appendix
[1]Critics challenge the value of using BMI terminology, suggesting that BMI is a poor determinant of health and the categories medicalize and pathologize having a certain body. We accept this argument; we have used "overweight" and "obese" throughout this paper when necessary to report research where these categories were used. We recognize, however, that "normal" does not reflect a normative or optimal value; that "overweight" falsely implies a weight over which one is unhealthy; and that the etymology of the word "obese" mistakenly implies that a large appetite is the cause.
[2] Health at Every Size/HAES is a pending trademark of the Association for Size Diversity and Health.

Conflict of interests Disclosure
Linda Bacon and Lucy Aphramor are HAES practitioners. Both also speak and write on the topic of Health at Every Size and sometimes receive financial remuneration for this work.

Authors' contributions
LB initiated the collaboration. Both authors contributed to conceptualizing and drafting the review. LB was lead researcher and undertook the system-

atic review and designed and completed the tables. Both authors approved the final manuscript.

Acknowledgments
Deb Burgard conceptualized the obesity cost analysis. The authors thank Deb Burgard, Sigrún Daníelsdóttir, Paul Ernsberger, Janell Mensinger, Elise Paradis, Jon Robison, Camerin Ross, Abigail Saguy, and Evelyn Tribole for their contributions and critical review. Lucy Aphramor thanks the WM NMAHP Research Training Awards for financial support.

CHAPTER 18

Competing interests
The authors declare that they have no competing interests.

Authors' contributions
RWDG was the mentor of the work, was involved in the protocol and study design, data collecting and analysis, carried out the statistical analysis and wrote the manuscript. AS and RPCP participated in the planning of work, discussion and data collection in Florianópolis. VALM participated in the planning of work, discussion and data collection in Campinas. EZM made the statistical analysis and corrected the manuscript. All authors read and approved the final manuscript.

Acknowledgments
This study was supported by FAPESP (Fundação de Amparo à Pesquisa do Estado de São Paulo) and FAEPA HCFMRP-USP.

INDEX

α-tocopherol 66, 202–203
ß-carotene xxvii, 200, 202–203

A

acute pancreatitis (AP) xxiv, 103, 105, 107, 109, 111, 113, 115, 117–119, 159, 170, 288, 329, 361
adolescent 15–16, 34, 37, 44, 46–48, 50, 205, 252, 353, 360–362
albumin 61–62, 71, 79, 89, 92, 106, 110–111, 116
Alzheimer's disease 282
American Diabetes Association (ADA) 212–213, 215, 220, 234, 237–239, 252, 366, 395
American Society for Enteral and Parenteral Nutrition (ASPEN) xxx, 297
ammonia 61, 75, 81–82, 92, 95–96, 401
analysis of covariance (ANCOVA) 11, 191
analysis of variance (ANOVA) xxii–xxiii, 40, 368
anemia 301
antioxidant xxiv, 43–44, 49–50, 56–57, 74–75, 89, 100, 151, 171, 180, 202–203, 206, 242, 253, 308
appetite xxiii, 2, 16, 58, 61, 139, 172, 253, 349, 354
areas under the curves (AUC) xxii, 26–27, 29
ascites xxiv, 78–80, 94
asthenia xxvi, 165, 168

B

bariatric surgery xiv, 172, 187, 204, 217, 234, 238, 359
basal metabolic rate (BMR) 105–106, 115
behavior modification 353
bilirubin 92, 158
Bioelectrical Impedance Analysis 5, 10, 79, 171, 188
body mass index (BMI) xxvi, xxi, 5, 8–11, 25, 60, 67, 79–80, 160, 162, 165, 188, 192, 204–205, 212–215, 217, 230, 234, 245, 325, 340, 345–347, 355–356, 358, 363
bone xviii, 16, 28–31, 98, 142, 148–150, 308–310, 330, 359
brain function 80
branched-chain amino acids (BCAAs) xxiii, 61, 70–71, 74–75, 88–89, 99–100
Brenner Hypothesis 127
buccal mucosa cells (BMCs) xxvii–xxviii, 187–189, 196, 198–203, 206, 235, 289

C

calcitonin 29, 31
calcium xxii, xxxi, 2, 7–11, 15–16, 19, 21, 23–31, 91, 123, 139–140, 150, 152, 163, 187–188, 195–196, 200–201, 218, 296, 303, 308, 325, 330
    calcium phosphate vii, 19, 21, 23, 25, 27, 29–31

cancer xxix–xxx, 30, 69, 71, 168,
171, 179, 182–183, 206, 242, 252,
255, 257, 259–261, 263, 265–267,
269, 271–273, 275–291, 361
carbohydrate (CHO) xxiii–xxx, 8, 11,
25, 53–54, 56, 62, 70, 74–75, 122,
134–135, 138–139, 148, 163–165,
171–172, 200, 215, 218–220, 229,
237–238, 252, 255, 257, 259, 261,
263, 265, 267, 269, 271–273, 275,
277–283, 285, 287–291, 361, 401
cardiac arrhythmias 159–160
children xxii–xxiii, 14–15, 33–35,
37–38, 40–42, 44, 46–50, 79, 94,
143, 235, 252, 305, 307–310, 329,
339, 352, 356–357, 361
    Children's Depression Inventory
    (CDI) xxiii, 35, 37, 49–42, 48–49
cholesterol xxiii, 30–31, 53, 55, 59,
65–66, 134, 149, 215, 218, 232, 235,
237–239, 342, 351, 356
chronic hepatitis C (CHC) xxiii,
53–54, 57–59 66–69, 100
chronic kidney disease (CKD) xxv,
28, 30–31, 121–124, 126–127, 129,
135–136, 141, 143–153, 338, 355
cirrhosis xxiii, 54, 62, 66, 68–72,
74–76, 79–80, 85, 89, 91–101
Clinical Global Impressions (CGI)
xxiii, 34–35, 37–42, 49
clinical practice guidelines (CPGs)
xxviii, 137, 210–211, 220–221,
229–230, 233–235, 395
constipation xxvi, 148, 165, 168
cytokines 61, 86, 94, 96, 98, 100,
119, 202, 287

D

dehydration 129
depression xxii–xxiii, 33–35, 37–38,
40–50, 335–336

diabetes-specific nutrition algorithm (tDNA) xxviii, 209, 211, 213,
215, 217–219, 221–223, 225, 227,
229–231, 233, 235, 237, 239, 395
diet
    Dietary Approaches to Stop
    Hypertension (DASH) 213, 218,
    234, 238
    dietary energy intake 56–57, 60
    dietary record xxvii, 187–188,
    191–192, 200, 203
    dietary reference intake (DRI)
    xxvii–xxviii, 122, 134, 150,
    186–187, 194–195, 197, 199, 201,
    205, 330
discrimination xxxii, 334, 344,
351–352, 360–361
disease management 230
DNA 188–189, 402
dopamine 44, 96
Dual X-Ray Absorptiometry (DXA) 10
dysplasia 300, 302, 308

E

enteral nutrition therapy 168
ethics xxxii, 3, 48, 188, 350,
352–353, 357, 359–360, 367
European Society for Clinical Nutrition and Metabolism (ESPEN) 69,
94, 98, 104, 117–118, 395

F

fasting 22, 134, 157–158, 170–171,
183, 213, 218, 251, 278–279, 281,
283, 285–286, 288, 357
fat mass (FM) xxi–xxii, xxvi, 1–3,
5, 7–13, 15–17, 136–137, 158, 162,
164–165, 169, 238, 340, 361
Fibroblast Growth Factor 23 (FGF23)
xxv, 142, 144, 151–152

fluoxetine xxii–xxiii, 33–35, 40–42, 45, 47
folate 187–188, 194, 196, 200, 205
free radical 43–44, 151, 300
fruit viii, xxix, 148, 241–247, 249–253

G

gender 30, 40, 123, 136, 186, 191–193, 211, 245, 344, 346, 360, 363
 female xxi–xxii, xxix, 1–2, 7, 9, 14, 16, 30–31, 105, 126, 130–132, 134, 136, 139–140, 143, 160, 162, 165, 172, 192, 194, 200, 204, 206, 212, 214, 217, 245, 249–250, 253, 283, 286, 290, 314, 323, 329, 335–336, 340, 346, 353–363, 371
 male xix, xxii, xxix, 5, 14, 28, 31, 105, 123, 130, 132, 134–135, 138–139, 160, 162, 165, 172, 192, 194, 200, 204–205, 209, 212, 214, 217, 239, 283, 286, 353, 357–358, 360
genomics 211, 403
glomerular xxv, 133, 141, 170
 glomerular filtration rate (GFR) 122, 125–128
 glomerulosclerosis 139
glucose xxx, 15, 28–29, 62–63, 70–71, 75, 94, 106, 115, 134, 139, 158, 163, 165, 171, 213, 218, 220, 231–232, 235, 237, 242, 249, 251–252, 257, 260–261, 263, 265, 267, 270, 272–273, 277, 280, 284, 286–287, 304, 357, 403
 glucose availability xxx, 263, 265
 glucose intolerance 62–63
glutamine xxvii, 96, 180, 183
glycemic

glycemic control xxviii–xxix, 134, 138, 214–215, 237, 241–243, 245, 247, 249–251, 253, 280, 342
glycemic index (GI) 71,117, 215, 219–220, 229, 234, 237, 249, 279–280, 282–283
glycogen 61, 74–75, 86, 158, 281, 287
glycolysis 260–262, 280, 284, 286

H

"Health at Every Size" (HAES) xxxii, 334–336, 347–350, 352–353
hepatic encephalopathy (HE) xxiii–xxiv, 14, 62–63, 71, 73–75, 85–86, 89, 91–92, 96, 98–99, 101, 135–137, 158, 164, 167, 171, 206, 286
hepatocellular carcinoma (HC) xxiii, 69–70, 91, 100, 172, 236
high protein (HP) xxiv–xxv, 122–123, 128–133, 137–139, 143, 158, 170, 183, 289–290
homeostasis 31, 128, 150, 180, 202
hospital xiii–xx, xxiv, xxvii, xxxii–xxxiii, 22, 34, 48, 105–107, 116, 179–181, 188, 259, 330, 365–369, 371, 378, 380–382, 384–389
hospital food and nutrition service (HFNS) 365, 367–369, 371–373, 376–378, 380–381, 384–386, 388
hyperammonemia 82, 95
hypercatabolic 116
hypercholesterolemia 66, 239
hyperglucagonemia
hyperinsulinemia 71, 134, 287, 357
hyperparathyroidism 10, 14
hyperphosphatemia 28, 145, 149, 151–152
hypertension 123, 135–136, 163, 165, 172, 213, 218, 232, 236, 238, 338–341, 346, 351, 355, 357–358, 361, 403

hyponatremia xxiv, 79, 94
hypothalamus 2, 61

I

infants, xxx–xxxi, 295, 297–298,
300–305, 307–310, 327, 330
insulin xxiv, xxx, 15–16, 53, 57–58,
61, 65–68, 71, 74–75, 78, 99, 139,
143, 158, 172, 193, 205, 231–232,
235–238, 249, 252, 260–261, 273,
276, 278, 280, 283, 285–290,
304–305, 309–310, 339–340, 342,
344, 351, 357–359, 361–362
    insulin receptor (IR) 16, 260–261,
    276, 280
    insulin resistance xxiv, xxx, 15,
    53, 57–58, 65–68, 71, 74–75, 78,
    139, 143, 287–288, 339–340, 351
interferon xxiii, 67–69, 100
International Physical Activity Questionnaires 5
intestine
    intestinal dysbacteriosis xxv, 148
    intestinal motility 162
intuitive eating 348–349, 353–354, 362
iron xxiii, xxvii–xxviii, 43, 54, 59,
66–69, 187–188, 195–196, 200–202,
206

K

Ketogenic Enteral Nutrition (KEN)
xxvi, 157, 159–165, 167–169, 171,
173
ketone bodies (KB) xxx, 158,
268, 270, 272–273, 279, 281, 286,
288–289
kidney xxv, 28, 30–31, 121–124,
127–133, 135–141, 143, 145, 147,
149–153, 170, 217, 219, 234, 338,
355, 402

kidney viii, xxv, 28, 30–31,
121–122, 127, 130, 133, 135–136,
141, 143, 145, 147, 149–153, 338,
355, 402
kidney stone 121, 132–133, 140

L

L-carnitine 74, 84
lean body mass (LBM) xxv, 7, 75,
134, 158, 160
lipids xxiii, xxxii, 15, 44, 49, 56,
65–66, 119, 134, 143, 168, 173, 238,
284, 288, 290–291, 299, 302, 308,
334, 337, 344–345, 358, 361
liver xxiii–xxiv, 31, 53–57, 59, 61,
63, 65–75, 77, 79–81, 83, 85–87, 89,
91–101, 170, 202, 281, 285, 310
    liver cirrhosis (LC) xxiii, xxxi, 54,
    60–64, 69–72, 74–75, 89, 93–97,
    99–101, 170, 289, 326–327, 330,
    387
    liver disease xxiii–xxiv, 53,
    65–66, 69, 74–75, 79, 91, 93–98,
    100–101
    liver failure vii, xxiii–xxiv, 73–75,
    77, 79–81, 83, 85–87, 89, 91,
    93–95, 97, 99–101
    liver transplantation 85–86,
    97–98, 101
    liver X receptor 65
lung disease 302

M

macronutrient 5, 122, 134, 136, 253,
282
major depressive disorder (MDD) vii,
xxii–xxiii, 33–35, 37, 39, 41, 43–47,
49
malnutrition xxiii–xxv, 59–62,
74–77, 79–80, 82, 86, 93–95, 98,

103, 116, 145–146, 148, 152, 181,
204–205, 387
manganese 83, 96–97, 204
medical nutrition therapy (MNT)
xxix, 137, 213, 219, 236–237, 251
metabolic equivalent task (MET) 5,
8, 302
micronutrients xxvii–xxviii, xxx,
xxxv, 5, 48, 123, 185–201, 203–205,
207, 216
mitochondria 279
Modification of Diet in Renal Disease (MDRD) 127–128, 135, 138,
150
mortality xxiv–xxvi, xxxii, 14, 28,
30, 71, 79, 104, 107, 110, 112–113,
116–117, 119, 143, 145–146, 150–
151, 171, 232, 275, 282–283, 285,
297, 309–310, 338, 340, 355–358,
387
multivitamin (MVI) xxx, 75, 91,
296–297, 302–303, 307
muscle
    muscle catabolism 158–159
    muscle tissue 158, 281

nutrition therapy xxiii, xxviii–
xxix, 53–55, 57–61, 63–65,
67, 69, 71, 137, 168, 213, 219,
229–230, 235–237, 251, 395, 403
enteral nutrition viii, xxiv, xxvi,
62, 69–70, 94, 98, 100, 103–104,
116–119, 157, 159–161, 163, 165,
167–169, 171, 173, 177–179,
182–183, 297, 403
immunonutrition 180
parenteral nutrition (PN) xxiv,
xxvi–xxvii, xxx, 103–107, 109,
111, 113, 115–119, 137, 159,
178–180, 182–183, 288–289,
295, 297–303, 305, 307–309,
311, 401
Total Parenteral Nutrition (TPN)
xxvi, 118–119, 179, 182–183,
296–297, 307–308
nutritional care quality (NCQ)
xxxii–xxxiii, 365–371, 373–377,
379–385, 387, 389
nutritional depletion xxvi–xxvii,
176, 180–182
nutritional therapy 86, 103, 107,
219

N

N-acetylcysteine (NAC) 90, 100, 308
nasogastric tube xxvi, 159, 164, 167
National Health and Nutrition Examination Survey (NHANES) 135, 309,
340, 358, 360, 362
nausea 166, 168
necrosis 57, 70, 94, 117, 287, 290
neutropenia 158, 170, 301
nonalcoholic fatty liver disease
(NAFLD) xxiii, 53–57, 65–66
nonalcoholic steatohepatitis (NASH)
53–54, 56, 60, 65, 100
nutrition

O

obesity xiii, xvi, xxi, xxiii, xxv, 2,
9, 14–16, 53, 58, 62, 64–65, 69,
71, 123, 134–135, 155, 157–161,
163, 165, 167–173, 188, 198, 202,
204–206, 212, 214–215, 217–218,
229, 234–238, 285, 338–341, 345,
347, 351–358, 360–363
    obesity paradox 338, 355–356,
    358
oral antidiabetic drugs (OADs) 245,
247, 251
osteoclasts 29

P

pancreatitis xxiv, 103, 105, 107, 109, 111, 113, 115–119, 159, 401
parathyroid hormone (PTH) xxv, xxxi, 7–8, 10–11, 14, 16, 30, 141–142, 149, 319, 325
persistent organic pollutants (POPs) 359–360
phlebotomy 67, 69
phosphatonin 142
phosphorus xxv, xxxi, 8, 11, 25–26, 28–31, 93, 141–147, 149–153, 163, 308, 325, 330
    phosphorus binders xxv, 143, 146–147, 149, 151
physical activity 5, 8, 11, 14–15, 136, 172, 214–215, 234–235, 237, 244–245, 248, 250–252, 334, 340, 344, 353, 361, 395, 405
pneumonia 104, 118, 181
positron emission tomography (PET) 259–260, 284
pregnancy xxxi, 3, 126, 134, 138, 143, 160, 284, 301–302, 309–310, 314, 323, 325–327, 330
probiotics xxiii–xxiv, 30, 71, 74–75, 91–92, 101
prostate 272–273, 276–277, 283, 287, 289–290
protein xxiii–xxv, xxviii, xxx, 2, 8, 11, 15, 25, 60–62, 66, 70–71, 74–77, 87, 89, 93–94, 98–101, 103, 107, 115–116, 121–140, 142–146, 148, 150–151, 158–160, 162, 168–173, 181, 188, 200–201, 215, 218, 238, 261, 272–273, 277, 280, 282, 284–286, 289–290, 304, 308, 405
    protein synthesis 74, 89
    proteinuria xxv, 124, 135, 143

R

randomized controlled trial (RCT) xxix, 47, 71, 119, 151, 216, 221, 237–238, 253, 334, 337
renal disease xxv, 121–124, 126–128, 131, 133, 135–136, 138, 149–151, 407
renal function xxiv–xxv, 30, 100, 121–131, 133, 135–139, 142
resting energy expenditure 58, 61, 67
Resting Metabolic Rate 10, 118

S

selective serotonin reuptake inhibitor (SSRI) 34
selenium xxvii, xxx, 59, 83, 96, 187–188, 196, 200–201, 204, 296–297, 300–301, 303, 308–309
self-esteem xxxii, 334–337, 348, 352
sepsis 119, 171, 179, 182
serum albumin 61–62, 89, 106, 110–111, 116
side effects xxii, 35, 56, 67, 92, 139, 249, 334
small-for-gestational age (SGA) 80
socioeconomic status 145, 151
sodium 151, 163, 194, 218, 238, 296
soft drinks 54, 144–145
starvation xxvi, 28, 49, 158, 168, 170–171
Subjective Global Assessment 80, 95
substance abuse 33
suicide 33, 44, 47, 49–50

T

technology xvi, 354, 388
thrifty genotype hypothesis

trace elements 95–96, 100, 296, 300–301, 308

transculturalization 221–222, 231, 235

tumor xxix–xxx, 57, 70, 257, 260, 262, 267, 272–273, 275–277, 280–281, 284–287, 289–290

tumorigenesis xxx, 260, 280, 284, 290

Tumour Necrosis Factor 94, 287

type 2 diabetes (T2DM) xxviii–xxix, 134, 139, 155, 213, 217, 231–232, 234–238, 241–242, 249–253, 285, 290–291, 338, 340, 342, 357, 361

U

ultraviolet B (UVB) xxxi, 317, 319, 325

undernourishment xxiii

urea 129, 136, 138, 159

V

vegetables xxv, 74, 88, 98–99, 144, 148, 200, 219, 249, 252–253, 275, 280

visceral adipose tissue 9, 15

vitamin B1(thiamine) xxx, 85, 97, 100, 194, 297, 303, 307

vitamin B12 187–188, 194, 196, 205

vitamin C (ascorbic acid) vii, xxii–xxiii, xxvii–xxviii, 33–35, 37, 39–45, 47–50, 59, 100, 187–188, 190, 194, 196, 198–203, 205–206, 251, 296, 303

vitamin C deficiency 34–35, 45, 48

vitamin D xxi, xxxi–xxxii, 2–3, 5, 7–11, 14–16, 35, 59, 68, 91, 101, 142, 149–150, 187, 194, 200, 206,

303–305, 309–310, 313–315, 317, 319–321, 323, 325–327, 329–331

vitamin D deficiency 2, 7, 14, 309, 323, 326, 329

vitamin D receptor 2, 15, 304, 310

vitamin D3 xxi–xxii, 1–3, 5, 7–11, 13, 15–17, 59

vitamin E 49, 56, 59, 100, 187–188, 194, 196, 200–201, 302–303, 309–310

W

Warburg effect 258, 260, 280

weight

weight cycling 186, 339–340, 356–358

weight loss xxiv, xxvi, xxix, xxxii, 9–10, 16, 58, 66–67, 122, 134–135, 137–138, 157–159, 164, 167–169, 172, 181–182, 186, 188, 191–192, 201–202, 205–206, 215, 217, 236, 250, 253, 272, 275, 281–282, 285, 287–288, 290, 334, 336–337, 341–344, 347, 349, 351, 353–355, 358–360

Wernicke's Encephalopathy

World Health Organization (WHO) xxxi, 5, 8, 15, 25, 35, 44–45, 68, 91–92, 104, 138, 159–160, 165, 168, 176, 199, 205, 214, 216–217, 230, 234, 300, 305, 334, 339–340, 342, 344–346, 357, 366, 368, 388

Z

zinc xxiii, xxviii, xxx, 59, 71, 74, 82, 95–96, 187–188, 195–196, 201, 296, 301, 303

zonulin 280, 291